Allergy Free Eating

Allergy Free Eating

Key to the Future

Liz Reno, M.A.

and

Joanna Devrais, M.A.

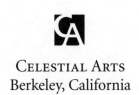

CELESTIAL ARTS
Berkeley, California

Cover design by
Text design and composition by FORM FOLLOWS FUNCTION

Originally published by Vision Books International 1992

First Printing Celestial Arts printing 1995

Library of Congress Cataloging-in-Publication Data

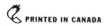

PRINTED IN CANADA

1   2   3   4   5 — 99   98   97   96   95

Dedication

THIS BOOK IS DEDICATED to all our clients whose need, love, and support has helped to make this possible. It is also dedicated to everyone in recovery from allergies, immune disorders, substance abuse, and eating disorders. To everyone seeking health and wellness and the means to achieve that goal, this book is dedicated to you.

❦ Acknowledgments

LIZ RENO WOULD LIKE TO THANK the following:

My clients for their persistence, patience, and encouragement; Joanna Devrais, my friend and collaborator on this work, for her gentle support, sweet spirit, wisdom and inspiration, research, and delicious recipes; my children, for their understanding, patience, and sacrifice of time; my husband Mike, for his support, love, patience, and the many hours in helping to do the preliminary editing; Dr. Jeffrey Bland, Dr. Robert A. Buist, Marshall Mandell, M.D., Russel Jaffe, M.D., Dr. Stephen Levine, Joseph Beasley, M.D., James Braly, M.D., for their friendship, encouragement, and support; and I wish to thank the Lord for His inspiration and for providing the means to accomplish this work.

To all of you, much love and thanks!

JOANNA DEVRAIS WOULD LIKE TO THANK the following:

Paul for bringing Liz and I together for this collaboration; the clients of Heart Cuisine who inspired me to create some of the recipes; Liz Reno for her extensive knowledge and the opportunity to work with her; my many friends, especially Selma and Howard Aslin and Marge Moench, who supported me through this time and provided a place to stay while writing; my family members, in particular Barbara and Ron Surz and my son, Matthew, for his understanding; and my friend Stephen for his guidance. This book was created with love for all who choose joy and healthy lifestyles, and who look to the future and hold harmony for our world.

The authors would both like to recognize the research, knowledge, and experience of such notable professionals as: Theron Randolph, M.D., Marshall Mandell, M.D., Orian Truss, M.D., William Crook, M.D., William Philpott, M.D., Dean Ornish, M.D., Gabriel Cousens, M.D.,

Michael Rosenbaum, M.D., Jeffrey Anderson, M.D., Carl Pfieffer, M.D., Russell Jaffe, M.D., Robert Buist, Ph.D., Stephen Levine, Ph.D., Parris Kidd, Ph.D., Jeffrey Bland, Ph.D., Alexander Schauss, Ph.D., and Charles Rudy, Ph.D.

❧ Table of Contents

Part III: Food and Recipes

Appendices

🦋 Foreword

by James Braly, M.D.

GOOD MEDICINE CANNOT BE practiced without a solid grasp of food allergy. Many patients haven't healed, and may never heal, I'm sorry to say, until their food allergies are properly diagnosed and treated. With over 50 medical conditions and literally hundreds of common medical symptoms identified in the scientific literature as caused or provoked by food allergy, it follows that no single subspecialty in medicine is more fundamentally important to the proper diagnosis and treatment of human disease that food allergy (or for that matter, no area of medical research is more appealing: research into food allergy's role in insulin-dependent diabetes, sudden infant death syndrome, duodenal ulcers, rheumatoid arthritis, epilepsy, and asthma).

Paradoxically, no subspecialty of medicine is submerged in more controversy and misinformation than food allergy; the unbending belief system that food allergy is rare in adults, for example, has been the official mantra of too many American physicians for too long, to the serious detriment of tens of thousands of food allergic patients.

Particularly today, with all the new research involving food allergy and its attending controversy and misinformation, there's an urgent need for a comprehensive, yet clear-headed book allergy free eating, a book based not only on solid theory, but hands-on, "in the trenches" clinical experience, a book both for the health professional and his food allergic patients.

Liz Reno and Joanna Devrais' *Allergy Free Eating* is exactly that book.

Recommending and complying with an allergy free diet is a formidable challenge, until now more an art form than a science. Through much of the 1980s my patients and I too often struggled with following "the program"–the allergic patients' all-too-human eating habits that badly needed an overhaul, their basic lack of knowledge about good nutrition (a well balanced diet of allergic foods is *not* good nutrition), their physical addiction to allergic foods (with consequent withdrawal-like symptoms when they gave up those foods), their predictable complaints when asked to give favorite, but allergic foods. "How can you expect me to live without my favorite foods!" remains an all-too-familiar chant of the food allergy sufferer; that chant becomes a shriek if giving up a favorite food is unaccompanied by an easy to prepare, tasty, alternative nonallergenic food–available right now! Oh, if only Reno and Devrais' book had been there early on to guide us!

Liz Reno understands her subject well. Her thoughtful and compassionate discussion of the *psychology of eating and changing of habits was especially prized*–no single human act is more difficult than changing a habit (particular if that habit is a favorite food), and Liz makes it appear easy. Her grasp of the underlying causes of food allergy, especially the "leaky gut syndrome," and what the allergy sufferer can do to reverse and "clear" from food allergy may well be worth the price of the book alone. You'll also appreciate the near encyclopedic list of alternative foods and recipes, the "shopping and eating out" hints, and her excellent treatment of the rotation diet.

If you are a food allergy sufferer (and the probability is high that you are), *Allergy Free Eating* is a book you need to read and keep nearby in your personal library. If you're a health professional who sees food allergic patients in your practice (this includes most health care professionals whether they recognize the patients or not) *Allergy Free Eating* becomes the prefect gift for yourself, your staff, and your patients.

James Braly, M.D.
Medical Director and Editor
Immuno Labs, Inc.
Fort Lauderdale, Florida

❦ Authors' Introduction

ALLERGIES AFFECT APPROXIMATELY 50 million Americans, with annual health costs of $5 billion. Another $40 billion is spent on the weight loss business. Health concerns are increasingly at the forefront of our attention. Good health cannot be replaced or bought and it seems to be alluding the average person. Perhaps you have picked up this book because you have health concerns and want information to make the needed changes surrounding food and health, or you have read about and been told by a health practitioner that you have a specific ailment which you suspect may be related to a poor diet. If you have been told to eat whole grains–where do you buy them and how do you cook them? Perhaps you have never even been to a health food store. Now what?

Individuals with severe Candida, allergies, addictions, immune deficiency disorders, or in the early stages of recovery can be overwhelmed. It is sometimes difficult to find the food and information they need to survive. If you suffer from an allergy to MSG, how do you know which products are safe? If dairy and dairy products are an issue where they are hidden in food, how are they replaced? If you give up your favorites, are foods going to be bland, boring, tasteless, or strange? The purpose for this book comes from the above questions and the needs of my own clients. The purpose and inspiration of this work is to provide complete and clear allergen free information without extremes or gimmicks and represents fifteen years of research and experience in the clinical nutrition field. We are indebted to the research, knowledge, and experience of such notable professionals as Theron Randolph, M.D., Marshall Mandell, M.D., Orian Truss, M.D., William Crook, M.D., William Philpott, M.D., Dean Ornish, M.D., John McDougall, M.D., Gabriel Cousens, M.D., Michael Rosenbaum, M.D., Jeffrey Anderson, M.D.,

Carl Pfieffer, M.D., Russell Jaffe, M.D., Robert Buist, Ph.D., Stephen Levine, Ph.D., Parris Kidd, Ph.D., Jeffrey Bland, Ph.D., Alexander Schauss, Ph.D., and Charles Rudy, Ph.D.

The compilation of material holds keys to provide support and to help motivate people, or clients/patients, to make the necessary changes in their lifestyle. This book creates a bridge to change for the individuals seeking a healthy lifestyle and for the health care professional (physicians, chiropractors, clinical ecologists, acupuncturists, nutritionists, eating disorders counselors, and chemical dependency therapists) to provide a tool for their clients/patients to use.

Change is difficult and this book will explore the nature of change in Part One: Food Addiction and Changing Your Ways. In Part Two: The Healthy Diet and Tools for Change, we will present important guidelines for implementing change. The questions surrounding what to substitute, how to rotate, and the new foods and how to prepare them will be answered. The recipes in Part Three will provide you with interesting and fun foods while addressing the problems of allergies, addictions, and healthy food choices. The recipes are traditional foods made from non-allergenic fresh wholesome ingredients. Simplify and substitute are major keys to recipe creations. Although we both believe in a basically vegetarian diet, meat and fish recipes have been included. These recipes support the theories of Dean Ornish, M.D.

This work is not an attempt to present a new theory or gimmick. Important material is organized so everything you need is in this one volume. Each person is biochemically unique, and no one diet program works for everybody. The principles offered can be applied individually whether you are in recovery, suffering from allergies, Candida, other immune dysfunctions, or simply desire a healthy lifestyle. One delightful side effect of applying these principles is weight loss.

The creation of these recipes has been a joyful experience. During the process of co-creating this work, we joined to share our knowledge, skills, love of beauty, and our love of cooking. Our memories of sun-filled days laughing over the joyful process of creating names for the recipes or the foggy winter days we spent making and eating dozens of muffins made from different grains and various fruits, nuts, eggs, egg replacers, and sweeteners will always remain with us. We often wished that you, the reader, could have shared in the joy of the experience. Even though the information is heavy, we hope that you will also see the lightness, humor, and love with which it is presented.

NOTE: Based on their experiences with clients, the authors refer to specific situations in the first person, particularly in chapters one through seven, which were written by Liz Reno.

PART I

Food Addictions
and Changing Your Ways

Knowledge is power and a motivating force for change. The following information regarding allergies, immune disorders, eating disorders, and alcohol/drug addiction provides important keys to understanding how your diet and lifestyle affects you and the uses of the rotation diet.

CHAPTER 1

The Nature of Change

The greatest discovery in my generation is that by changing your attitude you can change your circumstances.

—William James, philosopher and teacher

T HE PROSPECT OF CHANGE can be frightening. The uncertainty that accompanies change can create anxiety and fear. Change is difficult! It could be starting school, moving to a new location, switching careers, getting married, going through a divorce, or even the death of a loved one. For most of these situations, we exercise our ability to choose. For some, like the death of a loved one, we have no control or choice. In the areas where we can make a conscious decision, information is gathered and sorted, alternatives are weighed, then our attitude regarding it is altered, and an action is decided upon. We survive the change.

Some people put off making any changes and remain stuck in an unpleasant job, an unhappy marriage, or with bad habits. They believe they cannot behave in a different way. They seek the familiar and want to remain in their comfort zone. No matter how unpleasant, the pain is familiar and it can be handled. The rules are known and there are no real surprises. This behavior is unproductive and there is no growth from the experience.

For others, attempts to change are made in one way or another. Maybe a new exercise program is begun, only to stop after a couple of weeks. Or a new diet is tried with the familiar diet yo-yo — lose a few pounds, gain a lot. The end result of these efforts is a loss of some self-respect and self-esteem, and may add more self-defeating behaviors. Change is not a matter of simply exercising will power.

A diagnosis from your health professional, or your own inner knowledge that you are not feeling right, has led you to consider dietary changes. You could be looking for a healthier lifestyle. This will require major changes in the way you perceive food and eating. Change takes time and old habits will yield slowly. To change without shocking your system or alienating your family, you cannot throw out everything and begin a totally new life instantaneously, or can you?

Most diets promise control from an exterior set of rules and conditions. For instance, if you follow a certain diet plan, you will lose weight. You make no decision, other than to put your life and health into someone else's hands, and have little or no choice. Eventually frustration, boredom, or resentment sets in. If you succeed in losing the weight, but have made no real or permanent change in your regular diet, you gain back the weight. Our purpose is to teach you correct principles, give you a richer set of choices, and encourage you to govern yourself. The secret to change lies within yourself. Knowledge is power and applying it will empower you.

In order to obtain self-control and make those changes, there are certain principles that must be understood. A conscious, informed decision is the first step in making or effecting change. There are three main ideas that must be understood emotionally, as well as mentally, in order for it to be a fully conscious decision. Change, in order to be effective and lasting, has to be mental as well as emotional. Understanding becomes knowledge as it makes that two-foot drop in the gut. You not only "see" it, but you "feel" it. Now you know it! Unless it makes that two foot drop, it will not stay. It will not motivate permanent change.

It will be far easier for you to understand mentally—you will probably quickly agree and say, "Hey, that's right!" It will be harder still for you to get your rebellious and illogical emotions under control. The following three main ideas will help you achieve that first step:

Understanding the nature of the problem
Understanding the nature of change
Understanding how to change

🦋 The Nature of the Problem

Understanding the nature of the problem provides a foundation of information that you can absorb. There are two parts to the nature of the problem: the physical, and the mental/emotional. The physical provides facts, usually minus an emotional hook. The mental/emotional deals with your belief systems and how you view yourself and the world, and often carries with it a big emotional hook.

Unfounded fear is a disease state completely within the imagination which arises mainly out of a lack of knowledge. Remember that knowledge is power, and so it is important to arm yourself with the facts. It is important to understand how Candida or allergies are acting or reacting within the body, how they affect the immune or adrenal systems, and what causes the allergic reactions. Are there cause and effects because of what you eat or the supplements you take? What does Candida do in the body and can it be controlled? How do the physical effects of eating disorders or alcohol/drug addiction affect recovery? Due to time factors, my clients can only receive a limited amount of information during an office visit. When I encourage them to go to one of my lectures, receive more information, facts, and a better understanding of what exactly is going on inside themselves. They go home inspired and motivated to fully implement the program they have been given. They are empowered with knowledge, and the best way to dispel unfounded fears regarding change in lifestyle is with knowledge, a knowledge that breeds confidence, a confidence that formulates beliefs, and beliefs that result in positive actions. The first few chapters of this book will provide a foundation of information, hopefully supplementing what you already have.

Your mental/emotional attitudes are governed by your belief systems. Actions come from your belief system and behavior is created because of an internalized, external belief system. Your reality around food originates from social concepts and perceptions towards supermarkets, fast food chains, and the four food groups, and family, regional, and ethnic traditions. Up to fifty percent of beliefs, values, and attitudes are formed by the age of four. Another thirty percent are added between ages of four and eight, fifteen percent between ages eight and eighteen, and only five percent from age eighteen and onward. With that foundation formed in the early years, you can see why there is a tremendous emotional attachment to food, associating it with comfort or nurturing. Often when feeling helpless, powerless, or victimized, people lose touch with the physical realities of the body, and continue to eat, drink, or do those things which are harmful. The mental physical link is disconnected; there is no longer a choice and the person is being acted upon.

Those from dysfunctional homes were deprived from the beginning. With inadequate rules and distorted belief systems, you attempt to solve the problems of life, the distresses of the body, and the anxieties of the mind with food, use of alcohol or drugs, or engage in other addictive behaviors. There is a great fear surrounding not eating, and because of the headaches, weakness, or distress associated with an attempt to fast or to skip meals, you become convinced that food or drugs are the answer to your problems, or unconsciously use food to exert control over your own body and/or other people. When the issue of taking something away from you occurs in the form of a major diet change, you reject it, and are overwhelmed, angry, and sad.

Social concepts mold belief systems from infancy. The modern diet and sedentary lifestyle is a sad testament to these concepts. How many people will fight to find a parking place right in front of a store rather than walk? The foods today have changed considerably from fifty years ago. Sometimes the structure of the food has been destroyed and the nutritional value lost. The convenience of fast foods has altered the type of foods consumed, or even desired to eat. An American child watching television on a Saturday morning will see many food commercials but few will promote a reasonably nutritious product. Take the same child into a supermarket or on a drive through the local fast food strip and the exposure to nonfood is reinforced. At school, the child is taught the basic four food groups, only one of which is really healthy. This same child lives in a home with parents that have been victims of the same process and add their family traditions, or ethnic or regional customs to the education of the child. What has the child learned? What is their perception of food, of self-responsibility for health?

Not only do fast foods help to create addictions, but they are also full of common allergens (corn, wheat, sugar, yeast, dairy, salt, peanut, and soy). These foods are a major contributing factor to current medical and physical problems. Over the past twenty years, a growing body of legitimate scientific research has linked diet to such health problems as obesity, heart disease, diabetes, immune dysfunction, and cancer. The United States is quickly becoming the only nation of overweight and malnourished people on the earth.

The emotional attachment to food can be very powerful. On a subconscious level there is a belief that eating can satisfy emotional hungers, like the need for love. Eating is used to fill the emptiness inside and reduce other psychological tensions, such as loneliness, depression, boredom, or unhappiness. It provides comfort, nurturing, and can numb you out. These problems often have their roots in subconscious programs learned in childhood. In the conscious mind, you may be aware that eating food cannot satisfy emotional hungers; at a subconscious level, there is the belief that when starved for love, eating will make you feel better. An irrational desire to eat when tense or unhappy is referred to as pseudo-hunger, the use of food to reward, comfort, and offer solace in an unhappy or troubled existence. This desire is unproductive, solves nothing, and is self-defeating and self-destructive.

Another belief system is a misguided sense of one's own will power, and the belief that will power alone will motivate change. If self-defeating patterns continue, there is a loss of valuable self-esteem, and instead of having power, are rendered powerless. The disappointment is not with the program or anticipated change, but with yourself. Because of a lack of superhuman will power, and not knowing what else to do, self-respect is lost. This is tragic, because genuine self-esteem is one of a person's most valuable assets. Everyone needs all they can get. Repeating this process several times reinforces self-defeating attitudes.

🦋 The Nature of Change

In any conflict between the rational will to change and an irrational compulsion (like overeating), the irrational compulsion wins almost every time. In other words, the body wins every time. Instead of mind over matter, it really is matter over mind. Will power by itself is not enough.

In order for a program to succeed, change is necessary. It's easier to change clothes styles or hair styles than it is to change eating habits. This is due in part because we are surrounded by food every day and must eat to live. The food system you are involved with usually does not support or make easy the healthy choices you need to make. Healthy choices are hard. Your spouse may not eat the same way and sometimes even sabotage your efforts. The office offers donuts, candy, coffee, and the inevitable birthday cakes. Fast food restaurants, delicatessens, and junk food confront you at every turn. To be successful in your new program, change your attitudes toward food and yourself and fight the inertia that prevents you from getting started.

During the launching of the lunar voyages of Apollo, more energy was spent in the first few minutes of lift-off from the earth than in the rest of the journey. The gravity pull before the spacecraft could break through the earth's atmosphere was tremendous. The internal thrust had to be greater than both the pull of gravity and the resistance of atmosphere. Now look at yourself and your habits. Your problems do not stem so much from ignorance as they do from not applying what you know to be right. The problem not only lies in your ignorance but also in your habits. When you do not finish what you start, it is easy to lose faith in your ability to keep the promises you make to yourself, and you lose self-esteem. You are dealing with your basic character structure. You need to desire to overcome the gravitational pull of habits like procrastination, laziness, and stubbornness.

Change has to come from a place of choice within, a place where you have no more desire to continue negative behavior. Change requires effort and it will be difficult at first until new habits are formed and the desire for the old ways has changed. If you overcome the pull and the inertia, you will have won. You will have kept your resolve. You can then move to other things. By small things, great things are accomplished. These concepts that will help you understand more about yourself and your behavior.

Change demands effort and an alteration in attitude, a new way of looking at things, viewing it with a different eye, and expanding your choices. Change can be rewarding, bring growth, and can even be fun.

🦋 How to Change: Honesty, Open-Mindedness, and Willingness

Knowing that change requires effort and that old belief systems keep you blocked are important pieces of information. Both the physical and the mental/emotional come into play for any change to take place. The mental/emotional is concerned with the means of change and the altering of attitudes by fighting an idea with an idea. The physical part applies the principles of simplifying your basic eating habits, substituting one food for another food, and making these changes slowly so that you do not create expectations which cause you to abandon your attempts to make changes. The most important words for your new diet are: simplify, substitute, slowly.

First, be totally honest with yourself and admit you do have an illness or allergy. Accept that concept. Next, recognize whatever your weaknesses may be: procrastination, laziness, self-willed, or denial about yourself and your problems. Look at any resentments, anger, or fears. Get honest about what really happened in the past, including childhood. Search your current belief systems to see if they are still valid. Be honest with yourself and others about your feelings. Learn not to "people please" and give in to the desire to be accepted or approved by others, and do not seek that approval regardless of whether or not it is good for you. Do not try to rationalize and justify your actions—I eat or drink because of circumstances, my wife, the boss, or the kids. Realize that you seek to hide from the pain involved in difficulties. You are running from the fear and pain of really knowing yourself. Honesty is the foundation of change.

Open-mindedness means to be willing to expand your view and perceptions of things. Be open to new concepts and ideas without pre-judgments or criticism. Let new ideas flow in and study, compare, sort, and ponder the new material.

Desire motivates willingness and willingness is the catalyst for change. You become willing by admitting you do not have all the answers, that you are not perfect, that you have a problem, and that you need to change. Surrender to the problem by acceptance. Acceptance can do what will power can never accomplish. Surrender and acceptance release the energy needed for healing. Your energy is no longer being used to fight the problem, the disease, or the concept. Willingness frees your perception to accept new ideas and information and expands your vision. It opens your attitudes and beliefs to transformation.

Attitude is the transformer of reality. Let's fight an idea with an idea. What is your attitude about yourself? Each person is an individual with unique talents and abilities; each person is of worth. When you daydream or think of yourself, how do you imagine yourself? Healthy, at an ideal weight, and looking attractive? You deserve to be the very best that you can be. It is beliefs and attitudes, not you, that hold you back. You are of great worth and have within the potential to make great changes.

You eat to live, not live to eat. When you live to eat, food has control and power over you and your life. Food can become a powerful drug and, with the enticements from the food and marketing industry, you lose control and the ability to choose. If you eat to live, then you have control over your life and what happens to you. If you eat to live, you act as an agent for yourself, rather than being acted upon; participate instead of looking on; become actively involved, as opposed to passively listening; create rather than respond to pressures, expectations, or stimuli from others.

🦋 Love Needs

As you move toward implementing dietary changes, what are your limitations regarding food? What is your relationship to food? Do you feel deprived or overwhelmed? What kind of feelings emerge? Let's fight an idea with an idea and examine basic love needs. One reason we cling to food is that it represents mother to us—love, comfort, and nurturing. Learn to nurture yourself by understanding your love needs and breaking old, self-defeating patterns.

Each of us has one major and one minor love need. Knowing these needs, what they are, and how to get them, gives powerful self-knowledge. You can then use them to comfort and nurture yourself instead of eating your fears and problems away. The basic love needs are:

To be listened to and understood
To be touched, tenderly, nonsexually
To deeply communicate with an adult
To be praised and encouraged
To be given personal space

Self-knowledge is the key to the power and mastery of yourself. If you know, then you can master, and finally give of yourself. There are three main ways in which we react to our environment.

Physical response (the five senses)
Visual (color, design, beauty, order)
Audio (music, conversation, sounds)

Think about what your basic love needs are and learn how to use that knowledge. Do not be afraid to ask for what you need. Be clear, honest, and try not to be demanding or manipulate others. Learn to nurture yourself. One special method is to think of a time when you needed comforting and did not receive what you needed. Go back to that time in your mind and recreate the scene. This time nurture and comfort yourself by words, a touch, or whatever feels right for you. Make a nurturing list that has no relationship to food. It might contain a hot bath, a fire in the fireplace, a walk in the woods, reading a book, watching a film, or a massage. When you are in recovery, don't label yourself "bad" when you do not keep your commitment and goals around food and diet changes. This is a learning experience and disapproval does not improve your self-worth. When the urge to eat something unhealthy surfaces, choose a nurturing activity and do it. Deciding to do something, then doing it, empowers you. Immediately you will sense a surge of freedom. It will create the desire for more freedom. In this moment, you can choose to act, and any act will free you.

Twelve step programs are supportive and self-help groups have much to offer all people. Whichever twelve step program applies to your particular situation can be a tremendous help in achieving change. The cost is a small donation or they are free. There are also a lot of good books focused around the twelve step programs. Private therapy is also another alternative which can assist you in opening the way for change.

Still the question remains: how do I make these changes? Change comes by repetition and by learning to simplify, substitute, slowly, making small changes in small steps. How do you eat an elephant? One bite at a time!

Simplify

In this complicated age, nothing is simple, including our foods. Ice cream is not entirely real. A McDonald's shake can be tolerated by someone with a milk allergy, because it is not made from milk. Labels have to be constantly read, because products may contain chemicals, additives, or hidden sugars. The container may say no sugar added and when you find the fine print, it lists sucrose as the first ingredient. Sucrose is regular, processed white sugar.

Contemporary cooking and eating habits favor fancier and more complicated meals: sauces, gravies, seven-course meals, and fancy desserts. Either we carefully prepared the meals ourselves, or, to make matters worse, purchase a processed, prepackaged product loaded with chemicals and heated in a microwave oven. Hours are spent in the pursuit of food: thinking about it, shopping for it, preparing it, eating it, and cleaning up after it. Wouldn't it be nice to be free from this cycle and improve our health in the bargain? When addictive foods are eliminated from the diet, food no longer has control over you. Cravings and hungers disappear. You eat to live. You are drawn to lighter and simpler foods, and your mind is freed to pursue other interests.

You will simplify your life and basic eating habits as you learn to substitute slowly and apply the changes in your diet. You will simplify both the product and the process. You will eat more raw and basic foods, prepared in a simpler manner. The most wholesome and nutritious foods are raw foods, such as fruits, vegetables, and nuts and seeds, which require little preparation.

Substitute

In the process of simplifying your diet, substitute sometimes slowly and cautiously, and at other times immediately, one item for another. For instance, you cannot suddenly throw out everyone's soda pop without some type of substitute. What do you do? Pure fruit juice can be substituted for the sweetened variety right away, and is about the same price. For a while, diet sodas can replace the sugared ones as you explore other choices. Sparkling seltzer water and fruit juice make a wonderful soda, and seltzer water by itself is very refreshing. Another area of extremely poor nutrition is Jell-O. If your family loves Jell-O fruit salads, don't panic. Explore Salads on page 247 for delightful and delicious surprises.

Slowly

The secret will be to proceed slowly. People are basically resistant to change, preferring to remain in a comfort zone and do that which is familiar. Change is possible, but can be difficult. Therefore, so you will not alienate your family, be labeled a food fanatic, or harm your digestive system, proceed slowly. In regard to some of the changes, your family will say, Why didn't you do this sooner? Other changes will require a step-by-step method.

If you have Candida, food allergies or addictions, are in recovery, or have other immune dysfunction that demand changes be accomplished quickly, proceed as fast as you can. Remember to nurture yourself, be kind to yourself, and do not beat yourself up if you cannot do it all at once. Moving slowly and thoroughly will produce a permanent change.

Substitution is the most important aspect of a transition in foods. Be honest with yourself, open your mind, and be willing to explore the variety and rich set of choices that await you. Be adventurous! The material in the following chapters will deal with the problem of what to substitute and how to accomplish this. The secret will be to do this slowly. As you substitute you will find that you have simplified your life, and improved your health and the health of your family.

CHAPTER 2

Allergies and Addictions

Allergy may occur without addiction but generally addiction is always accompanied by allergy.

—Stephen Levine, Ph.D.

According to the cover story in the June 22, 1992 issue of *Time Magazine*, "Allergies Nothing to Sneeze At," allergies and asthma affect as many as 50 million people in the United States, costing up to $5 billion annually and accounting for one of every nine visits to the doctor, including one of every five trips to a pediatrician for children. The word "allergies" presents someone having a definite reaction to a food or substance. It could be a reaction to bee stings, pollen, dust, molds, medicines, or from a food. The correlation is usually clear: hay fever reaction from pollen, hives from allergic reactions, or asthma from a food. On the other hand, the word "addiction" means the cigarette smoker or drug addict who cannot quit. Though these may be the common definitions to these words, new concepts and information have been presented in the last twenty to forty years. With all the knowledge available, it is amazing to me when I present a lecture, the number of people who only know these limited definitions.

The type of allergy described above is a "fixed" or conventional allergy, also known as a Type I response, IgE (immunoglobulin E). It is strictly immune in nature and is easy to detect with established testing procedures. A Type I response is associated with inhalant and airborne allergies, or food allergies in which symptoms may appear less than one hour or two after eating. Only between one to five percent of the people with food-related problems actually have "fixed" allergies. The person will always be allergic to the substance. Generally, there is a predictable response like hives, asthma, rash, or eczema. If the substance is not eaten for many years, a reaction will still occur whenever the substance is ingested. Sometimes the body will adapt for a time and change the symptoms, but the allergy remains constant. This adaptation, which seems to decrease with time, later manifests itself with different symptoms and may include allergies to other foods or substances.

Most allergies are what is called food intolerances or sensitivities— Type II, III, or IV responses, frequently involving IgG (immunoglobulin G) antibodies. Food intolerance is a state of sensitivity to a specific substance that would be harmless to most people, like cucumbers. Because of certain conditions, the body becomes sensitive to these foods. Studies have found that as many as two thirds of adults are forced to avoid one or more specific foods.[1] Food intolerance and sensitivity are manifestations of inflammatory damage and an impaired immune system resulting from free radical damage. Unfortunately, it can escalate with food intolerances increasing, even leading to chemical sensitivities, or vice versa (see table on page 17).

According to the *Journal of Allergy and Applied Immunology*, allergic reactions are probably the most frequently unrecognized cause of illness in the United States. Sadly, some "experts" have dismissed food allergies, especially adult allergies, and are not taken seriously unless they are a Type I response. Even among children, the "experts" claim that it is rare and quickly outgrown. However, extensive research, numerous international symposiums on food allergy, and personal experience sheds a new light on the truth about food allergy.

What are the Facts?

1. Food allergy is not rare. It clearly affects the majority of the American people.

2. The effects of food allergy are not limited to just the air passages, the skin, and the digestive tract.

3. Most food allergies are delayed reactions, taking anywhere from two hours to three days to show themselves, and are therefore much harder to detect.

Immediate Onset Versus Delayed Onset Food Allergy

Immediate "Fixed"	Delayed Intolerance
1 (or 2) foods are involved in eliciting allergic symptoms	3 to 10 food allergens clinically involved (20 to 30 foods in some rarer cases have been reported)
As a rule, allergic symptoms appear 2 hours or less after the consumption of the offending food	Allergic symptoms appear from 2 to 72 hours (or longer) after consumption
Common in children, rare in adults	Very common in children and adults
Primarily digestive tract, skin, and airways affected	Virtually any system, organ, or tissue of the human body can be affected (over 70 medical conditions are thought to be associated with delayed onset food allergies)
Except for young children is commonly self-diagnosed	Rarely self-diagnosed in any age group
Involves rarely eaten foods	Involves frequently eaten foods
Rarely involves addictive cravings or withdrawal symptoms	Commonly involves addictive cravings and withdrawal symptoms (25 to 35 percent of patients)
Small amounts of food trigger intense allergic reactions	Larger amounts of foods commonly are needed to cause allergic reactions
Often a permanent, fixed allergy to a food	Allergic reactions commonly clear following 3 to 6 months of avoidance and is reversible
Frequently skin test and/or IgE ELISA/RAST blood test positive	Frequently skin test and IgE ELISA/RAST blood test negative; IgG ELISA/RAST blood test positive
IgE antibody-mediated (Type I) allergic reaction	IgG (Type II), IgG-immune complex (Type III), and/or immune cell-mediated (Type IV) allergic reactions

(Condensed from *Dr. Braly's Food Allergy and Nutrition Revolution* by James Braly, M.D., New Caanan, CT: Keats Publishing, 1992.)

4. Delayed food allergy appears to be simply the inability of your digestive tract to prevent large quantities of partially digested and undigested food from entering the bloodstream.

5. When allergic sensitivities begin to develop-for whatever reasons-they have far-reaching, unsuspected effects.

6. Most of the causes of allergy are under our control and can therefore be minimized, corrected, or eliminated.

(Condensed from *Dr. Braly's Food Allergy and Nutrition Revolution* by James Braly, M.D., New Caanan, CT: Keats Publishing, 1992.)

When allergens are present, the body rejects the food much in the same way that the body tries to reject an organ transplant, creating an allergen/antigen reaction. Reasons for the development of food intolerances are: repeated exposure to the same food; exposure to chemicals in food; water, air, and physical environment; a compromised immune system; severe stress; Candida albicans and other immune disorders; eating disorders; alcoholism/drugs; impaired digestion (leaky gut syndrome); or poor nutritional status. The presence of these other conditions, with their various symptoms, often mask the related symptoms caused by the food intolerances. Sometimes the symptoms will not appear for several days or hours after ingesting the offending substance, causing what are known as hidden food allergies. This creates confusing messages for the individual and his or her health care practitioner.

The leaky gut syndrome is a by-product of many common causes and conditions. Small openings, or channels, occur in the small intestine. Because of these small openings in the small intestine, macromolecules (large molecules of undigested or partly undigested food) enter the bloodstream. In a healthy, well-functioning body this occurs on a small scale, but is easily handled. When it occurs more pervasively, the immune system has to labor to clear the bloodstream of the offending matter. The signal to the immune system is that this is an allergen which leads to the formation of IgG antibodies to these foods. Symptoms occur anywhere the blood can go, which is throughout the body. This syndrome explains what happens when you have figured out the offending food(s) and have removed it from your diet and within three to two eight weeks the symptoms are back. Because of the leaky gut, you have only switched "allergens." This also explains why there can be so many multiple allergies.

Common Causes of the Leaky Gut

1. Premature birth

2. Bottle feeding or whole food exposure before 6 months of age (except near-complete hydrolyzed baby formulas such as Nutraminagen)

3. Infections (bacteria, viruses), infestations (parasites) of the digestive tract (Candidiasis, amebic dysentery)

4. Inflammatory bowel diseases (Crohn's disease, ulcerative colitis, Celiac disease [gluten gastroenteropathy])

5. Cancer radiation therapy of abdomen (colon, uterus)

6. All alcoholic beverages

7. All non-steroidal anti-inflammatory drugs (Motrin, Advil)

8. Corticosteroids (prednisone, decadron)

9. Secretory IgA insufficiency

10. Zinc and/or vitamin A insufficiency

11. Amino acid insufficiency (glutamine, arginine, taurine, BCAA's)

12. Conditional bioflavonoid insufficiency (Quercetin)

13. Excessive stress (distress such as found in endurance exercise, injuries, surgery, psychological distress)

14. Poor digestion (underproduction/release of hydrochloric acid in stomach [hypochlorhydria]), underproduction/release of bile acids [gall bladder disease, liver disease], underproduction/release of pancreatic digestive enzymes [alcoholic pancreatitis], too rapid transport of foods through intestines [diarrhea], insufficient chewing/too rapid swallowing of foods.

15. Consumption of allergic foods with non-allergic foods may create new allergic foods.

16. Lack of variety and rotation in the diet (Too frequent consumption of the same foods in too large amounts—80 percent or more of the total daily calories consumed by the average American come from the same foods and is not compatible with our genetic heritage.)

17. Famine, starvation (leads to poor digestion, leakiness of intestinal lining [mucosa], diarrhea, malnutrition)

18. Antibiotic therapy/excessive simple sugars in diet (leads to over-growth of unfriendly microorganism [fungus, bacteria])

19. Acquired Immune Deficiency Syndrome (AIDS)

(Compiled by James Braly, M.D.)

Hope

There is hope. Hidden food allergies are not a permanent situation. Type IV responses are not fixed allergies. When the immune and adrenal systems are supported, the allergens are removed from the diet for about two months and the rest of the foods are rotated, the food intolerance often disappears. A few foods may surface as a fixed allergy, some may remain a problem because of their addictive and psychological natures, and the rest can be reintroduced into the diet in moderation.

Allergy or allergic-like sensitivities nearly always accompany addiction. As Stephen A. Levine, Ph.D. states in his *More About Allergy and Addiction,* allergy may occur without addiction but generally addiction is always accompanied by allergy. Food sensitivities may cause allergic people to crave foods to which they are allergic. It may not be clinical in the sense of withdrawal symptoms and cravings. The food-sensitive individual is usually physically and psychologically addicted to their food of choice, with many food allergies and food intolerances.

Psychologically, addictive foods are used to physiologically block discomfort. Food can be used to make a person feel high, nurtured, comforted, loved, rewarded, or revengeful. It may release anger or numb a person and suppress real feelings.[2] Endorphins and neurotransmitters (brain chemicals) provide further clues to understanding addiction. Dr. Michael Rosenbaum of the Allergy Research Group believes that food sensitivity exerts its most profound effect on the limbic portion of the brain. This section of the brain houses the control centers of emotions, as well as memory and vegetative functions including body temperature, sexuality, blood pressure, sleep, hunger, and thirst. Food allergies affect most of these vital functions.[3]

This neurophysiological analysis is shared by author William Philpott, M.D., a clinical ecologist, who has written extensively on the subject. Dr. Philpott speculates that frequent contact with allergenic foods trigger a rise in the brain opioid enkephalin. Enkephalin is a narcotic produced by the body that is as addictive as externally supplied narcotics.[4]

If one accidentally or deliberately picks up an addictive substance, several reactions may occur:

Nothing, and the person assumes the substance is safe and continues to indulge, then after several days symptoms reoccur, and they find themselves addicted again.

Immediate cravings and bingeing.

Adverse physical reactions such as headache, nausea, bloating, palpitations, fatigue, drowsiness, and depression—even suicide.

It is necessary to discern all the addictions.[5] The understanding of these principles provides a foundation for the client to make intelligent and knowing choices.

According to food allergy specialists Barbara Solomon, M.D., Marshall Mandell, M.D., and Stephen Levine, Ph.D., it takes four days for the offending food to be eliminated from the system. The fifth day acts as a buffer zone. I usually recommend an extended rotation plan for foods that are questionable, anywhere from seven to fourteen days. Questionable foods are those that have a mild reaction indicated on an allergy test, but not a full allergic response. Foods in the questionable category can produce a bingeing response or physical symptoms, and the client must eliminate them if either of these responses occur. The extension of the time between eating the same food lessens the chance of a negative reaction. The rotation plan (see page 65) allows clients to experience a wider variety of foods, lessening feelings of restriction and deprivation.

Physiologically, when a person (often a child) first has contact with an offending food, there is an unfavorable response in the form of headache, nausea, vomiting, gas, discomfort, asthma, congestion, rash, or irritability. As the person continues to eat the food, the symptoms reduce and finally disappear. The allergy is considered to be outgrown, along with the stuffy nose, ear infections, or upset stomach. In actuality, the food has now become habit and the symptoms are masked or delayed. The body has adapted to the offending substance and the body learns to live with it. Later on in life, depending upon the body's integrity, the allergies reappear with a new set of symptoms such as irritable bowel syndrome, sinus infections, bronchial asthma, ulcers, or migraine.

Medical Conditions Provoked or Caused by Food Allergy

Acute gastroenteritis
Allergic enteritis
Allergic rhinitis (non-seasonal)
Anaphylaxis
Angioedema
Angioneurotic edema
Anxiety, acute or chronic
Aphthous ulcers
Arthralgia
Arthritis
Asthma
Attention deficit
Atopic dermatitis
Baker's asthma
Bedwetting
Bronchial asthma
Bronchitis
Celiac disease
Chronic diarrhea
Chronic fatigue syndrome
Chronic urticaria
Colic
Colitis
Croup
Eczema
Enuresis
Enterocolitis
Eosinophilic gastroenteritis
Exercise-induced anaphylaxis
Diabetes mellitus, type I insulin
    dependent
Depression
Dermatitis herpetiformis
Diarrhea
Failure to thrive
Food-induced
    gastroenteropathies
Hay fever
Headaches (migraine and
    non-migraine)

Heiner's syndrome
Hyperactivity/hyperkinesis
Inflammatory bowel disease
Insomnia
Iron deficiency anemia (secondary to gi blood loss)
Laryngeal edema
Learning disorders
Malabsorbtion syndrome
Movement disorders
Myalgia
Nephritis
Occupational-induced rhinitis
Post-infectious enteritis
Primary pulmonary hemosiderosis
Protein-losing enteropathy syndrome (also known as "eosinophilic gastroenteritis")
Rhinitis
Sleep disorders
Tension-fatigue syndrome
Urticaria
Vasculitis

Additional Food Allergy Conditions

Acne vulgaris
Allergic sore throat
Ankylosing spondylitis
Bulimia
Candidiasis
Chronic constipation
Crohn's disease
Conjunctivitis
Delusions
Dyslexia, transient
Edema (weight fluctuations of 3 to 10 pounds)
Epilepsy (in association with migraine headaches)
Fever (up to 104 degrees fahrenheit)
Gastric and duodenal ulcerations
Hallucinations
Hashimoto's thyroiditis/ hypothyroidism
Hoarseness (or complete loss of voice)
Hypochlorhydria
Irritable bowel syndrome
Juvenile rheumatoid arthritis
Loss of voice
Malnutrition, food allergy-induced
Memory loss
Ménière's disease
Mental incapacitation
Multiple sclerosis
Obesity/overweight
Otitis media (middle ear infections and inflammations)
Premenstrual syndrome
Psoriasis
Rheumatoid arthritis
Sore throat, alleric
Tinnitus
Vertigo

(Lists compiled from lectures, citations, and abstracts presented at the Eighth International Food Allergy Symposium on July, 1993, sponsored by the American College of Allergy and Immunology.)

🦋 The Adaptation Process

As the adaptation process continues, it produces stress on the system. In a confused effort to deal with the problem, the body mistakes the offending substance for a nontoxic substance, and actually becomes used to and dependent on the food. It is during this adaptation or masking phase that addiction takes place. The physiological compensation for allergy takes its toll in chronic stress. The adaptation is so strong that the person becomes dependent on the food, eating it at regular intervals to avoid withdrawal symptoms. When the food is not consumed for a period of time, or the person tries to quit, their body craves the substance, causing the allergy-addiction syndrome.

During the final stages of stress, the body fails to maintain adaptation and experiences allergic and addiction symptoms simultaneously. During this stage, the chronic symptoms of disease emerge. Scientists call this stage exhaustion. During exhaustion, the allergy and/or new allergies re-surface full force.

The first organ of failure during stress is the pancreas. The pancreas is responsible for blood sugar regulation and insulin response, and digestive enzymes. The allergic reaction itself can result in a drastic reduction in blood sugar with the accompanying symptoms of weakness, hunger, and irritability. Author of several books on nutrition, Carlton Fredericks, considers erratic blood sugar levels to be a cause of behavior disorders. Allergens, hormones (especially those released during stress), sugar, processed grains and foods, and birth control pills, aspirin, and other drugs all raise blood sugar levels. Insulin is one of the two hormones which will lower blood sugar, the other being insulin-like growth factor 1 (IGF-1). Falling blood sugar levels, with accompanying hypoglycemic symptoms, are a result of hyperinsulinism, or too much insulin. Testing clients with their favorite allergic-addictive foods would result in a more accurate test for hypoglycemia. Hypoglycemic reactions can even occur from protein foods, the very foods suggested for a hypoglycemic diet.

Without the digestive enzymes from the pancreas and adequate hydrochloric acid, food is improperly assimilated. Without proper assimilation, the nutrients needed for metabolism cannot be extracted. In addition to the internal damage on deep cellular levels, the everyday symptoms can be extremely uncomfortable. Symptoms may vary from bloating and flatulence to esophageal hernia (gastroesophageal sphincter) and spastic colon.[6]

The adrenal and immune systems are interconnected by their effect on one another. Prolonged stress will weaken the immune system, and a weakened immune system will produce stress in the body. Common nutrient needs are required for the metabolic functioning of both systems: B5 (pantothenic acid), vitamin C, and potassium. Adequate levels of vitamin A, zinc, iodine, and other B complex vitamins should also be present. Sufficient levels of the other antioxidant nutrients vitamin E and selenium are required to prevent free radical damage. Supplements should always be taken in their proper balance (especially minerals) and individual nutrient deficiencies corrected. It may be necessary for a relatively short time to take pancreatic enzymes or hydrochloric acid to support the pancreas and ensure proper digestion. It is also important to correct the flora in the gut to assist in healing and restore normal growth of protective microorganisms (such as lactobacillus acidophilus).

Many physical conditions are complicated by the presence of food intolerances. Allergies can be manifested by a wide variety of symptoms, depending upon which target organ or system has been affected. They can be cerebral (mental/emotional, memory loss, irritability, foggy thinking, headaches), respiratory (ear infections, sinus problems, bronchitis, asthma, colds, hay fever), digestive disorders (colitis, irritable bowel, gas, cramps, constipation, diarrhea), or seemingly unrelated (arthritis, PMS, alcoholism, drug addiction, Candida albicans, dermatitis, eczema, hypoglycemia, hyperactivity in children, Ménière's disease, thrombophlebitis, eating disorders, chronic fatigue syndrome, environmental illness [EI], AIDS, Epstein-Barr, and other inflammatory or autoimmune disorders).

In my practice, I have substantiated that if a person has tested allergic to rye grass in the field, walnut trees, or wool, they will also be allergic to rye, walnuts, and lamb. If cow's milk is a problem, then beef will also be an allergen. It is interesting to watch the ironic addictive nature of allergies emerge. When dairy is mentioned, client responses include

I don't drink milk or eat cheese, or even I hate milk. When asked what their favorite desserts are, the answers will be I love frozen yogurt, cheese cake, or ice cream. Once I had a client who said she was very allergic to mustard grass. Upon questioning, she admitted that her favorite condiment was mustard. In working with allergies, it is important to find and eliminate all hidden sources of addictions. When the internal allergy source (like rye) is removed, the external reaction to rye grass, or the hay fever response, lessens or even disappears.

New research collaborates this information. Recently it was discovered that an albumin molecule in egg yolk, alpha livetin, is also found in the feathers and droppings of chicken. Other interesting developments are the antigenic connection between isolated protein molecules that are the same in ragweed and watermelon. These two foods are not even in the same food family. This new information may help to explain why people react differently to varieties within the same food family. I have clients who can have a Granny Smith apple but are allergic to a gala apple, or can have a russet potato but not a red potato.

Fixed allergies, and even some food sensitivities can be hereditary. Dr. Stephen Wasserman, chairman of the medicine department at the University of California at San Diego, said "Probably there is a genetic predisposition to respond with IgE (immunoglobulin E antibody), and if you're unlucky enough to have both the exposure and the predilection, then you're more likely to have allergies." A recessive gene has been discovered that may be responsible for allergies.[7] If both parents have allergies, then 70 percent or more of their offspring will also. Other recent research has identified a gene inherited from the mother that may make offspring susceptible to asthma and hay fever attacks. The people with the particular variant of the gene were unusually likely to have high blood levels of IgE.

The increase in food and chemical sensitivity reflects the modern day changes to food production and processing. During the past sixty years, the chemical stress load on people has increased at an alarming rate and our immune (or anti-oxidant) system has not been equipped handle this strain. This also reflects the constant exposure to common allergens in daily food. Dairy, wheat, eggs, soy, corn, sugar, and yeast are found in most processed foods and foods that should be clean. Dextrose (corn sugar) can be found in whipping cream, sugar can be found in salt, whey (dairy) can be found in hot dogs and lunch meats. The list goes on.

Young children are of particular concern. Parents feel that kids should have fun and frequently feed them fun or junk food. Children are targeted by television and other advertising, and pressured because all their friends eat these nonfood foods. If parents start very young, from the womb, many of the problems with irritable, moody, sick, or hyperactive children can be avoided. Mothers should avoid eating known allergens when pregnant. Known allergens should also be avoided when nursing as the allergens will come through the breast milk. A baby can be sensitive to a food that the mother is not. If there is a genetic predisposition to Type I insulin-dependent diabetes mellitus, the mother should avoid all dairy, beef, and food products with dairy in them. "Research over the last decade forcefully argues that prevention of insulin-dependent diabetes may now be possible through careful immunological monitoring, exclusive breast feeding and strict elimination of cow's milk from the diet of the newborn during the first months of life." (From an article by James Braly, M.D. in *The Immuno Review,* Volume 1, Number 2, Fall 1993.) Mothers should watch for symptoms like colic and rotate the foods consumed to reduce the child's exposure to potential allergens. Introduce new foods slowly to children. Provide enough time between new foods to see if there is a reaction and present a wide variety of food choices. As the child becomes older, explain to them why they cannot have certain foods. If they are not addicted, they will cooperate. "Fun food" can be saved for very special occasions, or not at all (see the recipe section of this book for delicious alternatives). If the parents are eating healthy, the children will follow.

No More Trips to the Emergency Room

Allergies, whether they are internal (food intolerances) or external (hay fever), are miserable to live with. They elicit many trips to the doctor or corner drugstore for some kind of cure. Researchers are unraveling the complex process that can provoke the immune system into an irrational IgE response. Dr. Stephen Wasserman has stated, "What has changed dramatically over the past decade is an appreciation of how the inflammatory response is orchestrated. We are beginning to understand the fundamental regulators of the entire process."

With allergies, the immune system perceives the food protein or pollen protein as a threat. Antibodies (IgE, or immunoglobulin E) which are positioned on mast cells, are released. If the exposure continues, then histamines and other chemicals are released. Antihistamines are prescribed to counteract the symptoms, which are all too familiar to the hay fever sufferer, caused by histamine. Some foods, like tuna or wine, will naturally release histamine even if there is no allergy to them.

Credit for the growing interest in allergies within the scientific community goes mainly to the holistic health revolution. As an increasing number of physicians and allergists accept and implement the growing body of knowledge about all forms of allergies (fixed or sensitivities), support, help, and healing will be available for the millions of sufferers. Much important information and substantiated research already exists on this subject and more comes forth almost daily. When the immune and adrenal systems are supported, there is adequate allergy testing, known allergens are removed, and dietary variety is provided through use of a rotation diet when necessary, relief is possible. Through this process, one of my clients reduced his use of asthma inhalers and medication by eighty percent and no longer required any trips to the emergency room.

🦋 Types of Allergy Testing

Avoid and Challenge

This testing method is often recommended and is frequently used in clinical ecology units in a clinic or hospital. It is best used under medical supervision. Severe reactions to foods or substances can occur upon testing (challenging). If there are multiple allergies or severe reactions of any kind, do not use this method. In a hospital setting, the patient is put on a spring or distilled water fast for a number of days to detox the system and alleviate symptoms. The patient is then challenged with suspected foods and the results recorded. If a reaction occurs, the medical staff is there to assist the patient. In the home, if one or two foods are suspect, eliminate it from the diet for one to two weeks, then challenge yourself with a good-sized helping. If symptoms reoccur, then the problem has been located. If it is a hidden food allergy, the suspect food has to eaten two or three more times before symptoms reoccur. The time lapse may often confuse the results. Unfortunately, the chances of it being only one food are very slim.

Applied Kinesiology

Applied kinesiology is a part of a system called Touch For Health, developed by John F. Thie, D.C. It is based upon the biomechanical (muscles—kinesiology) and electromagnetic energy (meridians) in the body. The energy pathways, or meridians (the same in acupuncture) are used for the testing. The deltoid muscle in the upper arm and shoulder governing the stomach meridian is the one applied for the test. Other muscles can also be used. The test is administered in two ways. One method has the client eat a small amount of the food, the muscle is tested, and then the client thoroughly rinses his or her mouth with distilled water. The other method has the client hold the suspect food in one hand and the opposite arm is tested (the skin is a very porous organ and absorbs quickly). Administered by a well-trained person, the test can be very accurate. Applied kinesiology is noninvasive. Everything can be tested, and the price is reasonable. Recently, a machine has been developed that eliminates the need for a person to administer the test. It is not a medical test and its validity is questioned in the medical community. However, I have found its results substantiated by comparable tests like RAST or ELISA.

Intradermal, Scratch, Sublingual

These are the old standbys still in use today by medical allergists. With intradermal and scratch tests, a small amount of the suspected allergen is injected under the skin on the back or upper arm. If the area swells, reddens, or itches, then an allergy exists or it could also be a reaction to being irritated by the procedure. With sublingual testing a small amount of a suspected allergen, usually of a chemical origin, is placed under the tongue. Again, if the patient responds with symptoms, a possible allergen is found. Drugs and/or neutralizing doses are the treatment associated with this type of testing. Neutralizing doses are a minute amount of the offending substance administered by injection or drops. The purpose is to immunize the patient against the allergen.

RAST (radioallergosorbent)
The RAST test measures the amount of antibodies (or IgE or IgG) present in the blood. It labels the antigen—antibody reaction with a radioactive substance. The intensity of the reaction is then measured by a Geiger-counter-like device. The RAST test is more accurate than the intradermal, scratch, or sublingual form of testing. However, the radioactive waste from the RAST test is becoming an environmental concern.

ELISA (enzyme-linked immunosorbent assay)
The ELISA test is widely used in immunology (environmental medicine or clinical ecology) for the detection of IgG antibodies against food antigens. With the leaky gut syndrome, the incompletely digested food molecules act as antigens. The immune system responds by forming IgG antibodies to these foods. The test depends upon the characteristic that an antigen or antibody links to an enzyme while it retains both immunological and enzymic activity in the person. Since most reactions are not fixed allergy (Type I) responses, the ELISA test is excellent for uncovering hidden food allergies, intolerances, or hypersensitivities (Type IV). It is performed by a blood draw and approximately 100 foods are tested at one time.

Miscellaneous Tests
The cytotoxic (or leukocytotoxic) test is performed by a blood draw. Approximately 150 items can be tested. The results depend upon the laboratory that is used. It is not very accurate. Other possible tests are: FAST (fluoroallergos orbent), MAST (autoradiographic), IP (immunoperoxidase), and PRIST (the sophisticated paper radioimmunosorbent test).

Most food allergy/hypersensitivity reactions, especially in adults, are not due to immediate-onset skin test positive, IgE-mediated reactions. The signs and symptoms of food allergy are more often delayed for many hours or up to three days after the multiple food allergens are eaten. This can make the laboratory and clinical diagnosis of allergic, offending foods very difficult. A handful of the more innovative American laboratories have now modified and improved the ELISA to better detect these more pervasive delayed-onset, IgG (Immunoglobulin G) blood test positive food allergies.

As a consequence of the leaky gut syndrome, partially digested, larger-than-normal food molecules enter into the bloodstream. These perceived-as-harmful foreign invaders regularly provoke a defensive immune system response, leading to formation IgG antibodies to these foods. The stronger the protective immune response to each of these foods the higher the IgG blood level to each food. The IgG ELISA is based on the detection of these food-specific IgG antibodies in the bloodstream of food allergic individuals.

The IgG ELISA, measuring only delayed onset reactions, becomes an excellent tool for the laboratory detection of this more common form of food allergy. The ELISA test has been made simple, requiring a single blood draw. The blood serum is then immediately picked up and delivered to an allergy specialty laboratory where 100 or more foods are quickly and efficiently tested all at one time. The IgG ELISA is as sensitive and specific as the RAST method, but because it is capable of more computerization and automation than the RAST, it is much faster, less predisposed to human error, and less expensive. For the environmentally concerned, the ELISA is totally free of the radioactive contamination and waste disposal problems seen with the RAST.

Immuno Laboratories in Fort Lauderdale, Florida is a state and federal licensed clinical laboratory, servicing thousands of physicians and other health care professionals throughout the United States and Europe. Immuno Labs uses a highly computerized, state-of-the-art modification of the IgG ELISA blood test for delayed onset (hidden) food allergies. Immuno Labs also tests for immediate food and airborne allergies utilizing the IgE CAP. In addition, it can provide yeast levels (Candida albicans), and an Epstein-Barr virus antibody profile. I personally endorse this company, the integrity and efficiency of their lab services, the follow-up doctor-patient support and education they offer, and the high degree of professionalism of their staff. For more detailed information phone Immuno Laboratories at (800) 231-9197. Sidney MacDonald Baker, M.D. of the Princeton Bio-Center in Skillman, New Jersey said, "I have used the IgG food allergy testing (Immuno Lab's immuno I bloodprint) for several years. The results of the immuno I bloodprint get me an exact reading often enough to make the test worth doing in any patient in whom food sensitivity is a consideration. And it is hard to find a patient with complex chronic illness in whom food sensitivity is not a possibility."

The issue of food sensitivities and intolerances is recognized by allergists from the mainstream, conventional, and clinical ecology field. Even C. Everett Koop, M.D., the Surgeon General of the United States during the Reagan Administration, said, "Qualified health professionals should advise persons with food allergies and intolerances on the diagnosis of these conditions and on diets that exclude foods and food substances that induce symptoms." The main difference of opinion surrounds the validity of the various forms of allergy testing. Education and information are the keys.

Food sensitivities can change with time and circumstances, so retesting within one year is probably necessary. Adherence to a program— taking supplements to replace deficiencies and build the immune and adrenal systems, avoiding offending foods, and rotating the remaining foods—will bring relief to allergy sufferers. One very pleasant side effect of all this effort, besides the reduction or cessation of symptoms, is weight loss. Cravings disappear. Control and choice become a part of your life.

Notes

1. Stephen A. Levine, Ph.D. and Parris M. Kidd, Ph.D. "Biochemical Pathologies Initiated by Free Radical Oxidant Compounds in the Etiology of Food Hypersensitivity," *International Clinical Nutrition Review,* Volume 5, Number 1, January 1985.
2. "Elliot Blass, a psychologist at John Hopkins University, finds that eating sweets may stimulate endorphin production. Adam Drewnowski, a psychologist and biochemist at the University of Michigan notes that stress also affects endorphins. 'The more stress a person is under, the higher the endorphin level in the blood,' he says." Paul Raeburn, "The Pistachio Ice Cream Neurotransmitter." *American Health,* December 1987.

3. Stephen A. Levine, Ph.D. *Food Addiction, Food Allergy, and Overweight* (San Leandro, CA: DBA Research Group, 1982)

4. "Sarah Leibowitz of the Rockefeller University, New York says, 'The focus of this activity appears to be in the hypothalamus, a region near the base of the brain. Experiments with rats have shown hunger-stimulating substances administered directly to the hypothalamus can cause regularly fed rats to binge.'" Paul Raeburn, "The Pistachio Ice Cream Neurotransmitter." *American Health,* December 1987.

5. Theron Randolph, M.D. *An Alternative Approach to Allergies* (New York: Bantam Books, 1981)

6. "If the stomach contents have not been sufficiently acidified, reflex secretions from the duodenum and by the pancreas (i.e., the flow of bicarbonate and pancreatin) are diminished. A reduction in quantity of activated pancreatic enzymes (i.e. activated by pancreatic bicarbonate excretion into the duodenum) can lead to incomplete digestion of protein based antigens and other large macromolecules which can subsequently gain entry to the body through the intestinal wall.

    "Any diminution of the digestive processes may facilitate the passage of large antigenic molecules through the intestinal cells to gain systemic entry causing production of reagins (IgE), precipitins, cellular immune responses and non-specific release of histamines. These events result in possible interference with nutrient uptake, alimentary allergy, and adverse reactions to food additives, yeasts, bacteria, and chronic immune deficiency." Robert Buist, Ph.D. "Food Intolerance—A Growing Phenomenon. Current Concepts in Development, Manifestation and Treatment." *International Clinical Nutrition Review,* January 1986.

7. Leon Jaroff. "Allergies—Nothing To Sneeze At." *Time Magazine,* June 22, 1992.

CHAPTER 3

Immune Disorders

HE FIRST HALF OF this century witnessed the curtailing of common contagious diseases like typhoid, cholera, and smallpox. Vaccines also became available for polio, measles, mumps, and whooping cough. The human life span was extended by improved trauma care and intricate surgeries. However, when life spans seemed to be extending, degenerative diseases began to rise in the second half of this century. Heart disease, arthritis, diabetes, and cancer either shorten life or limit its quality. In the final phase of the twentieth century, general health continues to deteriorate with the appearance of immune disorders. Diseases thought to be declining, like malaria and tuberculosis, are reappearing with a more virulent strain of microbe. New retroviruses such as AIDS, and spirochetes such as Lyme disease, complicate the picture. These retroviruses destroy the immune system, and there is no known medical cure.

Despite advanced technology, the proliferation of information, and new discoveries, the quality of health continues to decline. Wellness remains elusive except for those who are directly seeking health, health education, and who are applying those principles. Profit is the motivating factor behind the food industry, causing chemicals in the form of fertilizers and pesticides to permeate the food chain. Antibiotics and hormones can be found in almost all dairy and meat products. Sugar, salt, and fats are consumed at levels never even thought of a hundred years ago. The perfection of the refining process of grains has become a marketing art. Common allergens, such as dairy, corn, wheat, yeast, soy, sugar, and MSG, are distributed freely and hidden in many products as a filler or flavor enhancer. These allergen foods, especially in the refined forms, can be highly addictive. Repeated consumption of them either exacerbates already existing allergies or creates new ones, weakening our adrenal and immune systems. Water and air supplies are polluted; the latest research indicates that dioxin (a component used in many manufacturing processes and in Agent Orange, a defoliant) at common levels of exposure through the natural food chain may cause reproductive and developmental problems and suppress human immune systems. Even the destruction of the ozone layer has been linked with the weakening of our immune systems.[1] Americans no longer have to chop wood, carry water, walk, or do much physical labor. Occupations are more sedentary and autos provide transportation for even the shortest distances.

Despite this gloomy picture, much new knowledge and information has come from the alternative health care field. This information continues to be substantiated by solid clinical and medical research. Understanding has emerged regarding vitamins, minerals, and good nutrition in health.[2] Prevention has become a key word, wellness and health a possibility. We have learned that if we exercise, eat correctly, and take needed vitamin and mineral supplements, we can prevent or correct problems such as heart disease, adult onset diabetes, and osteoporosis. In addition, clinical application of sophisticated tests, products, and information have advanced the treatment of allergies, Candida, and other immune disorders to the point where recovery, or at least arresting the disease, is possible.

Immune disorders range from only a disorder to the actual destruction of the immune system. Babies are being born without an immune system, and other people's immune systems are actually self destructing. Immune disorders are another manifestation of degenerative diseases. When the same destructive elements enter two different people, one may develop heart disease and the other environmental illness (EI). Many factors, including hereditary genetic predisposition (like weak lungs and respiratory problems), lifestyle (foods, stress, exercise, smoking, drugs, alcohol), psychological and emotional experiences (victimization, abuse, incest), and environmental toxins (exposure to pollutants, chemicals, molds, radon), determine how the immune system will respond and how the disease process will manifest.

❧ Causes

Stress
Whether it is mental, physical, or emotional, stress weakens the adrenal system and compromises the immune system. Key nutrients are required for adequate adrenal support which are depleted during stressful periods. The modern lifestyle, with overwork, insufficient rest, and limited exercise, creates a tremendous load of stress. The fight-or-flight response to burn off toxins is not utilized; instead of fighting or running, the anger, frustration, and fear is repressed. Toxins that would be eliminated while physically fighting or running away remain in the system.

Processed Food
The contemporary food supply is comprised mainly of processed and refined products devoid of nutrients and fiber, and loaded with chemicals, pesticides, preservatives, additives, and artificial colors. People knowingly and unknowingly consume allergens and frequently eat the same foods day after day creating food intolerances and sensitivities, weakening both the adrenal and immune systems. Awareness is increasing, but the average diet is high in fat, salt, sugar, and protein.

Pollution
Every day people are exposed to many sources of pollution in the air and water, and chemicals, molds, exhaust fumes, formaldehyde, detergents, cosmetics, and other pollutants which exist in the modern world.

Drugs
The use of drugs is common. Drugs can be recreational (alcohol, caffeine, tobacco, or illegal street drugs) or medical (including over-the-counter or prescription). Many of the drugs can be immunosuppressant, such as antibiotics or chemotherapy.

There are many more sources for the continued contamination of the immune system, the rise of degenerative disease, and decline in the overall quality of health. By examining how the immune system functions, it can be better understood why it is failing and how to support it.

❦ The Immune System

The immune system is an extensive, protective barrier against disease, germs, and free radicals (allergens, pollutants, and stressors). There are many layers and organisms involved in this system: bone marrow, spleen, liver, lymph nodes, thymus, thyroid, adrenal glands, mucus membranes, enzymes in connective tissue between the skin and bone, and beneficial bacteria in the intestines. The entire immune system is divided into the nonspecific immune system and the specific immune system.

The nonspecific immune system, or the reticuloendothelial system, is the body's emergency system. It is an extremely important front defense against any foreign invader (virus, bacteria, or chemical substance) and is not specific against just one type of particle. The reticulum cells are a group of cells from bone marrow (hemocytoblasts, and myeloblasts), lymph nodes (lymphocytes), and tissue (tissue histiocytes), which wander through the body and perform the function of phagocytosis. Reticulum cells are also found in abundance in the spleen and liver. Phagocytosis is the ingestion of foreign organisms or foreign material. In addition, the body will produce antibacterial and immune-stimulating substances called cytokines and interferons. They increase the number of phagocytes and help to regulate the immune system.

The specific immune system, or antibody formation, provides a solid rear defense. It is comprised of the body's natural immunity and the formation of a trained group of cells, called antibodies, that have developed a memory of specific foreign invaders. These cells arise in the spleen, the lymphatic system, and bone marrow and are stimulated by the thymic hormone. Lymphocytes circulate freely in the body, are mainly present in the lymph system, and the main line of defense in the specific immune system. The lymphocytes are also present in the thymus gland, spleen, and bone marrow. The lymphatic system is the foundation for an adequate specific immune system. It is important that the lymph system be kept clean of mucus and toxins. If it becomes overloaded with debris, the toxins will back up into other body systems.

The functions of lymphocytes are extremely complex. They need to be able to recognize a substance and decide whether it is friend or foe, self or nonself. The substance (an antigen) may be a bacteria, a virus, an environmental toxin, a fungus or parasite, or even a common food. Tissue and organ transplants also can act as antigens because the body may label the tissue as foreign, and naturally reject the unfamiliar tissue. Once the decision has been made that an enemy is present, then the lymphocytes respond to the problem by organizing an attack with the assistance of the nonspecific immune system. When the battle is over, the immunological memory remembers the enemy and provides immunity should the same enemy strike again.

In autoimmune disease, immunity is developed against the body's own tissue proteins. It may be a condition that has existed since birth. It may develop because of the similarity of the body's own proteins to foreign antigens or it may occur following exposure of the body to certain haptens. Common haptens are usually drugs, chemical components of dust, various industrial chemicals, and breakdown products of dandruff and skin from animals. Haptens combine with some of the body's natural proteins. In turn, the body forms immunity against both the hapten and its conjugated protein. Thereafter the immune system attacks the body's own proteins. AIDS, Epstein-Barr, lupus, chronic fatigue syndrome, Candida, environmental illness, and allergies are all forms of autoimmune disease.

Four major metabolic systems are involved in the proper functioning of the immune system: the thyroid gland, the adrenal glands, the lymph system, and the process of digestion and elimination. The thyroid is responsible for the body's basic metabolic rate and metabolism of proteins, carbohydrates, and fats by the release of the thyroid hormone thyroxin from its principal cells. The principal cells, T3 (triiodothyronine) and T4 (tetraiodothyronine), manufacture the thyroid hormones. Thyroxin is synthesized from iodine and an amino acid called tyrosine.

Whether the thyroid is overactive (hyperthyroid) or underactive (hypothyroid), it has a profound effect on metabolism and general health and energy. Thyroxin increases the reactivity of the nervous system, which causes an increase in heart rate and motility of the gastrointestinal tract. If insufficient carbohydrates and fats are available for energy, thyroxin causes rapid degradation of proteins to be used for energy through either gluconeogenesis or ketogenesis. A vitamin deficiency can occur when excess thyroxin is secreted. Key vitamins are B_1 (thiamine), B_{12}, other B complex vitamins and vitamin C. A small amount of thyroxin is also necessary for the conversion of carotenes into vitamin A in the liver. Iodine is often low in the average diet; one milligram of iodine per week is required to provide adequate iodine for proper thyroid functioning. Although it is easily absorbed from the gastrointestinal tract, iodine does not remain very long in the system and within the first three days, two thirds of the ingested iodine is excreted in the urine. The remaining one third is removed from the blood stream and utilized by the thyroid. Stress upon the body, whether from an internal or external source, profoundly affects the thyroid and basic metabolism. Prolonged stress will deplete iodine and thyroxin.

Located superior to each kidney are the adrenal glands, which are responsible for our fight-or-flight response to stress. The adrenals are divided into two sections: the cortex and the medulla. The cortex oversees three main functions: electrolyte homeostasis through the mineralocorticoids and the release of aldosterone; the release of the glucocorticoids (mainly hydrocortisone) hormones to maintain normal metabolism and to assist the body in resisting stress; and the gonadocorticoids, which secrete a small amount of both male and female hormones. The medulla consists mainly of hormone-producing cells releasing epinephrine and norepinephrine, which also help the body resist stress.

Aldosterone regulates mineral metabolism, especially concentrations of sodium and potassium. It acts upon the kidneys causing them to retain sodium and decrease the reabsorption of potassium. As a result of stress, large amounts of potassium can be lost in the urine. Sodium and potassium are balanced with calcium and magnesium. If the sodium/potassium balance is altered, then the calcium/magnesium balance will be affected. All four minerals are responsible for electrolyte homeostasis, and healthy nerves, muscles, and bones.

The first hormone secreted in women during stress is estrogen. Estrogen release elevates blood sugar levels and affects the nervous system. This creates more stress resulting in the release of epinephrine. Epinephrine increases blood pressure, accelerates the rate of respiration, decreases the rate of digestion, increases the efficiency of muscular contractions, increases blood sugar levels, and stimulates cellular metabolism. The process of stress requires many nutrients and depletes them quickly. Potassium, B_5 (pantothenic acid), other B complex vitamins, and vitamin C are key nutrients for stress support. The release of aldosterone during stressful periods will aid in the excretion of potassium through the kidneys. The B vitamins and vitamin C are water soluble and the B vitamins are crucial to the body's basic energy cycle (Krebs cycle). The stress response will metabolize the B and C vitamins, and the increased urine output will eliminate any excess from the system. Interestingly, vitamins C, B_5, B_1, B_6, and potassium also play a major role in immune support.

The lymphatic system is not well understood by the general public. It is an extremely important component for the immune system. Two major functions of the lymphatic system are to produce lymphocytes and to develop immunities. The lymphatic system is comprised of lymph, lymph vessels, lymph nodes, and three body organs (tonsils, thymus, and spleen). The lymph nodes and vessels are found mainly in the center of the body, along the spine, in the groin, the armpit, the neck and head. They are a part of the blood circulatory system. Their major function is to drain from tissue spaces protein-containing fluids and accumulated toxins that escape from the blood capillaries. These fluids are deposited into the veins for reabsorption or elimination. Because of the abundance of toxins we are exposed to in the air, water, and food supplies, it should not be surprising that lymph systems frequently are clogged with debris. This accumulation of toxins, which will block the proper functioning of this portion of the immune system, contributes to chronic disease. Luc Chaltin, M.D., states in *SIMILIA Newsletter* (Volume 1, Number 2, January-February 1992), "The first observation is that all chronic diseases start with an abnormal accumulation of toxins." A healthy, well-functioning lymphatic system is vital to good health. Proper muscle contraction and healthy respiratory and circulatory systems provide support for the lymphatic system.

The fourth major component for a healthy immune system is proper digestion and elimination. The pancreas, which is responsible for blood sugar regulation and digestive enzymes, is the first organ of failure in stress. If food cannot be completely digested and the nutrients absorbed, metabolism will break down and non-end product metabolites and oxidants will result. Eventually, a disease state will be manifested. Digestion begins in the stomach with the release of hydrochloric acid (HCL) from the partial cells. Most of the absorption of nutrients occurs in the small intestine and some in the colon. A healthy intestine consists of adequate muscle contraction (peristalsis), adequate fiber and fluids in the diet, and a balanced microflora in the stomach. Candida, alcohol/drug abuse, allergies, environmental illness, and other immune disorders are prime results of compromised digestion, elimination, and an imbalance in the microflora.

🦋 Immune Disorders

Candida, Epstein-Barr, chronic fatigue syndrome, environmental illness, and AIDS all profoundly affect the mental/emotional and physical state of the individual. Feeling overwhelmed, fearful, and unable to cope with everyday life are common manifestations. Key nutrient deficiencies, impaired adrenal and immune systems, poor digestion and elimination, allergies, and food intolerances are all similar. The disease state can be arrested (provided that the disease state is not too far advanced, the body has integrity, and the immune system has not been destroyed) and life can once more have meaning. The process requires commitment and persistence, diligence and study, and a change of attitude and lifestyle.

Candida albicans
Vaginal yeast infections, some bladder infections, athlete's foot, thrush, and fungus infections of the skin or nails are usually outward manifestations of Candida albicans, the yeast organism responsible for the problem. The symptoms associated with Candida are poly-symptomatic and can affect the entire organism. Symptoms vary from indigestion, bloat-

ing, anal itching, acne, bronchitis, sinus and ear infections, and asthma, to hormonal imbalances affecting thyroid malfunction, adrenal failure, blood sugar regulation, and ovarian and uterine failure. The hardest and vaguest symptoms to trace can affect the central nervous system and the psychological response with headaches, withdrawal, depression, confusion, fog, nervousness, PMS, loss of memory, and irritability.

Those most susceptible to Candida are infants (contracted in the birth canal), women, and postoperative patients; people who have used antibiotics, birth control pills, and cortisone; alcoholics, people with a history of drug abuse or eating disorders, and those with HIV and AIDS infection; people taking immunosuppressive drugs or undergoing chemotherapy, patients with recent bacterial infection of the colon, known allergic people, and those with other immune disorders.

Candida is a yeast (fungus) found in the mouth, throat, and intestinal tract of normal people, and can be cultured from the mouth, vagina, or feces. When those who are susceptible to Candida use antibiotics and other drugs, and/or other conditions are present which upset the natural flora in the intestinal tract, the friendly, healthy bacteria (acidophilus and lactobacillus) are destroyed. Candida, being very tenacious, survives. Diets high in sugar, refined carbohydrates, and even junk food are highly favored by the Candida organism. If not enough food is available, the yeast will change into a fungal form and migrate throughout the body in search of food. The fungal form will also establish colonies in other sections of the body, such as the brain or respiratory system. In Candida's search for food, macromolecules of partly digested food are released into the blood stream, creating stress on the immune and adrenal systems. The macromolecules are treated as an allergen by the immune system, creating intolerances and allergies where previously no allergy occurred. This creates further stress upon the metabolism. The body demands the offending substance, and an addiction is created to the foods causing the problems. The downward spiral has begun. The person becomes increasingly sensitive to their environment, with chemical sensitivities complicating any progress.

The increased stress load and demand upon the immune system depletes major nutrients: B complex vitamins, B$_5$, vitamin C, iodine, potassium, vitamin A, zinc, magnesium, and amino acids. In addition, the metabolism of Candida produces acetaldehyde, the same by-product of alcohol metabolism. Acetaldehyde requires B vitamins, especially B_3, and B_6, magnesium, and EFA (essential fatty acids), for its metabolism. B_1 is also frequently depleted in this process. On a deep cellular level, acetaldehyde disturbs normal cellular activity. It interferes with the ability to absorb nutrients and the transport of metabolic factors, electrolytes, and hormones across the cellular membrane. Protein synthesis and EFA production are likewise affected, in addition to the formation of false neurotransmitters. Lymphocyte function is impaired due to membrane abnormalities. The production of these non-end product metabolites (toxins, oxidants, and free radicals) increases the body's need for the antioxidant vitamins, vitamin A, vitamin C, vitamin E, selenium, and possibly the sulfur-forming amino acids cysteine and methionine.

In addition, persistent Candida destroys the parietal cells of the stomach mucosa, inhibiting the production of hydrochloric acid (HCL). HCL is vital to the breakdown of all foods in the stomach and the first major step in digestion and the assimilation of nutrients. Prolonged stress weakens the pancreas, producing blood sugar problems and digestive disturbances. Food and chemical sensitivities increase and are manifested in both physiological and mental/emotional symptoms.

During recovery from Candida, die-off symptoms will occur. Die-off symptoms are sometimes confusing; they will reproduce or enhance the symptoms that the person started with. Stick to your program of rotated foods, supplements, and other guidelines and eventually you will succeed. If the old lifestyle and diet is returned to, Candidiasis symptoms and problems will return. Moderation, based upon experience and knowledge, will be the key to continued success.

Epstein-Barr Virus (EBV)

Epstein-Barr is caused by the same virus that is responsible for mononucleosis. It is a member of the herpes family of viruses including the ones that cause genital herpes, shingles, and chicken pox. Most people develop antibodies to EBV, but once contracted will remain in the body. Many people are carriers of the virus and do not manifest any symptoms. Often people who have had mononucleosis as a child or teenager will develop

EBV as an adult. A correlation between chicken pox exposure or a real case of it as a youth has been linked to people suffering from shingles as an adult. Women contract the EBV syndrome three times as often as men.

The Epstein-Barr virus is extremely contagious and is easily contracted from kissing, sharing food, coughing, or sexual contact. Because it is a viral disease, antibiotics and other conventional drugs are ineffective. The extent of the infection throughout the body overwhelms the immune system and the stress load upon the adrenals increases proportionately. An autoimmune reactive condition results. No vaccine for this virus has been developed, and at this time there is no known cure. The disease may be arrested but not cured.

Some experts believe that the Epstein-Barr virus causes chronic fatigue syndrome.[3] Others assert that they are two separate disease states.[4] Tests are available that will confirm if the EBV is present in the body. However, it will not tell you that is your problem because you may have developed antibodies. If all other symptom-related illnesses have been eliminated and elevated antibodies to EBV exist, and if symptoms persist for two to three months, then EBV is the primary suspect to any discomfort.

Other doctors feel that the symptoms, especially fatigue, must persist for at least six months before a diagnosis can be made. EBV is a difficult disease to pin down. It can be misdiagnosed as depression, psychosomatic illness, or even hypochondria. After a while the person with EBV can begin to doubt themselves or become desperate for a treatment of any kind. Epstein-Barr is a real disease. Anyone believing they suffer from this disease should continue to seek for help and guidance.

The symptoms associated with Epstein-Barr closely resemble other disease states like Candida, AIDS, viral infections, endocrine imbalances, anemia, or even parasites. Among the symptoms are swollen lymph glands, fever, sore throat, loss of appetite, severe fatigue, respiratory infections, intestinal problems, headache, aching muscles and joints, muscle spasms, anxiety, depression, sleep disturbances, memory loss, irritability, and mood swings. Candida albicans overgrowth usually accompanies EBV and the presence of Candida should always be checked for when EBV is suspected. If Candida is not responding to treatment as it should, then EBV is a possibility.

The destruction of the immune system by the Epstein-Barr virus and the accompanying weakening of the adrenal system will also produce digestive disturbances and food intolerances. Many of the same procedures which are implemented for a Candida recovery program can be applied to EBV. Build the immune and adrenal systems, correct nutrient deficiencies, and follow a rotation plan to alleviate food and chemical sensitivities.

Chronic Fatigue Syndrome (CFS)

Chronic fatigue syndrome is often called the yuppie disease. Some experts believe that chronic fatigue syndrome is caused by the Epstein-Barr virus. It is possible that the virus damages, on a cellular level, the ability to generate energy. Other probable causes of CFS are Candida albicans, anemia, chronic mercury poisoning (from dental amalgam fillings), hypoglycemia, hypothyroidism, prolonged stress, and sleep disturbances. From my own experience, drug and alcohol abuse, and chronic allergies and food intolerances, especially considering their cellular metabolism, also provide an environment for the development of CFS.

It is estimated that three million Americans suffer from chronic fatigue syndrome. The many symptoms associated with chronic fatigue syndrome can be debilitating. To the list of symptoms connected with Epstein-Barr, there is also carbohydrate intolerance, rash, nausea or vomiting, brain impairment (impaired neurotransmitter production) with sometimes loss in IQ, brain lesions, heart ailments, impaired energy metabolism, impaired central nervous system, and essential mineral deficiencies.

Key metabolic disturbances and imbalances are present in chronic fatigue syndrome. Magnesium and potassium levels are particularly low and several studies have shown that potassium and magnesium supplements significantly improve fatigue symptoms. Lactate levels are found to be two times, and pyruvic acid levels ten times, the normal, indicating suboptimal aerobic basic energy production (ATP) and the need for Krebs cycle vitamins: B_1, B_3, B_6, and the minerals potassium and magnesium. The amino acids phenylalanine and tryptophan are also found to be deficient. These amino acids are precursors to the neurotransmitters catecholamines and serotonin, respectively. Neurotransmitters are important for brain function and this organ is particularly susceptible to deficiencies. These two neurotransmitters are also helpful for depression and carbohydrate metabolism. Vitamins B_1, B_3, and B_6, and magnesium facilitate their proper conversion.

Chronic fatigue syndrome requires the same basic approach as Candida or Epstein-Barr: correct deficiencies, restore proper digestion, avoid offending foods and substances, implement a rotation plan, and build the immune and adrenal systems.

Environmental Illness (EI)

Activities a normal person would take for granted are no longer practical or pleasant for one with environmental illness (EI). An everyday trip to the store, with exposure to exhaust fumes, perfumes, packaging materials, cigarette smoke, and other irritants, can produce debilitating symptoms. The sensitivities are not limited to chemicals and also include food, animals, cosmetics, and clothing. Often those with EI are forced to move to remote areas away from urban sprawl and pollution. Their homes include bare floors, natural bedding and clothing, air filters, water purifiers, and organic food. Frequently and unfortunately, people with EI are diagnosed as having psychological problems.

Environmental illness is often caused by an acute or prolonged exposure to one or more chemicals. Working in a self-contained, airtight building with inadequate ventilation will cause contact with many possible pollutants: formaldehyde from formulated wood products, fumes from carpeting, upholstery, and textile-covered partitions, air fresheners in bathrooms, chemicals from copying machines, and the carbon dioxide that humans exhale. Other conditions which contribute to the development of EI are: severe stress, untreated Candida or other immune disorders, extensive food or natural allergies (like trees or animals), or being born with an impaired or missing immune system. The central nervous system toxicity (or toxic brain) of EI creates the classic symptoms of mental confusion, dizziness, inability to concentrate, and unfounded depression. The individual who suffers from these multiple sensitivities displays a wide variety of symptoms. Different organs in the body will respond and adapt or maladapt, depending upon the individual. Environmental illness is difficult to trace as symptoms and responses are so varied.

Sherry A. Rogers, M.D., of the Northeast Center for Environmental Medicine, discovered through research that zinc deficiency was prevalent among chemically sensitive individuals. Zinc-dependent enzymes are represented in every major metabolic pathway in the body. Zinc is a key nutrient that other nutrients are dependent upon for the detoxification process in the body. The other nutrients include B_6, B_3, EFA (essential fatty acids), cysteine, vitamin A, vitamin E, pancreatic enzymes for digestion, and the metabolism of acetaldehyde. In addition, the release of free radicals (xenobiotics) require an increased demand for the antioxidants: vitamin A, vitamin C, vitamin E, and selenium.

Many factors can contribute to zinc deficiency, even in healthy people. It is leeched from the soil by acid rain, and depleted by modern farming methods and refining of foods. If a person is addicted to processed foods, their diet will be low in zinc. Exposure to pollutants in air, water, and food increase the need for zinc. Medications, like diuretics, birth control pills, and steroids, and lifestyle habits, like alcohol and tobacco, also deplete zinc. A chronic illness, surgery, pregnancy, or a teenage growth spurt will also cause zinc deficiency. Zinc does not store well in the body and needs to be replaced daily. Repeated dieting or fasting, improper use of vitamins and minerals (which creates a loss of zinc and mineral imbalances), or simply eating too many carbohydrates (grains with phytates) inhibit the absorption of zinc.

Zinc alone is not the cure for recovery from environmental illness. Singular nutrient deficiencies are unlikely. Many factors have contributed to the development of the disease. The same whole body approach is just as important for EI as for any other immune disorder. Correct nutrient deficiencies, repair digestive problems, build the immune and adrenal systems, remove as many irritants and allergens as possible, use only clean water, and correct food sensitivities by implementing a rotation diet.

Acquired Immune Deficiency Syndrome (AIDS)
Acquired Immune Deficiency Syndrome is an epidemic of worldwide proportions. Those mainly at risk to develop a full blown case of AIDS are homosexual or bisexual men, intravenous drug users, recipients of blood or blood products, and heterosexual partners of these groups. The new Type A strain of the virus appears to favor heterosexual part-

ners. AIDS is also passed to infants during birth from infected mothers. It is also possible for dentists or medical workers to contract the disease from an infected person, or to pass it on to patients if the workers themselves are infected. Most AIDS infections are passed from infected blood, saliva, or semen.

Controversy is emerging as to the exact cause of AIDS. Most researchers believe that the HIV (human immunodeficiency virus) virus causes AIDS. It is estimated that 30 percent of those who become infected with HIV develop a full blown case of AIDS. A compromised immune system with a severely weakened nutritional status appear to be important factors in whether a person with HIV will contract AIDS. Dr. Jay Levy, a University of California at San Francisco researcher, reported at the International Conference on AIDS in 1992 that there is a key immune cell (CD8 cells—a white blood cell) that appears to block the virus from reproducing. General lifestyle factors during the incubation period, such as tobacco and alcohol use, drugs, environmental chemicals, and emotional stress, also play a role in the development of AIDS. In addition, 95 percent of all AIDS patients have Candida which manifests itself as thrush (the white hairy coat on the tongue). Usually by the time Candida is visible, it is systemic. Has Candida weakened the immune system to the point where AIDS can develop, or has the AIDS virus weakened the body so that Candida can run rampant? It's a question of who came first, the chicken or the egg.

The HIV virus suppresses the immune system and will kill T cells when it is replicating. In the body, HIV accumulates on lymphocytes in the lymph nodes and will infect susceptible cells as they pass through the lymph system. The purpose of the virus is to enter the genom of the cell. Once there the white cells cannot kill it, and the virus reproduces unchecked. At this point there is no cure for the disease. The individual may be stabilized, but not cured.

The classic symptoms of an acute infection with HIV include rash, malaise, fever, lymphadenopathy, and rarely meningitis. Brain disease, forms of cancer, and immunosuppression are consequences of AIDS. With the immune system weakened, the patient becomes susceptible to Kaposi's sarcoma (a rare skin cancer), Epstein-Barr virus, cytomegalovirus, herpes simplex virus, Candida, salmonella, tuberculosis, toxoplasmosis, and other diseases. Sixty percent of AIDS patients with a respiratory illness die from the complications of Pneumocystis carinii pneumonia, a parasite.

Not only the immune status, but also the nutritional status of those with AIDS, is compromised. Potassium and zinc levels are found to be particularly low in AIDS patients. In addition, the antioxidant vitamins A, C, E, and selenium, EFA (essential fatty acids), the B complex vitamins, especially B_5, B_6, B_{12}, folic acid, and the minerals magnesium, copper, and manganese are either low or supplements are required for proper immune and adrenal function, antioxidant and detoxification properties, and enhanced nutritional support. Research at the Linus Pauling Institute of Science and Medicine in California indicates that extremely high megadoses of vitamin C can ameliorate AIDS and other viral infections to a significant degree. Two important herbs which assist immune function and may be helpful for AIDS are echinacea (echinacea angustifolia) and mistletoe (viscum album). Recent pharmacological investigations and other studies are supporting the traditional supposition that echinacea contains immune-stimulating properties. Mistletoe has been used in France, Switzerland, and Germany for over 200 years and is still in use in clinics for the treatment of rheumatoid arthritis, autoimmune diseases, and cancer. Other herbs for immune support are: Japanese mushrooms, garlic, St. Johnswort, golden seal ginseng, and pau d'arco.

Emotional and stress support are important for any suffering from AIDS. Complete and absolute compliance to a prescribed treatment plan is essential. It is suggested that an aggressive, anti-Candida program be implemented along with an eradication of gastrointestinal parasites. Sugar, refined foods, salt, alcohol, and tobacco are to be avoided. Smoking will double and health risk. Animal fat and protein should be reduced. Drugs (especially immunosuppressive, cortisone, or radiotherapy), fluoridated water, chemicals, petrochemicals, and food additives, including the sulfites, MSG, colorings, preservatives, flavoring, emulsifiers, and any and all food allergens are also to be avoided. A rotation diet plan should be followed that includes whole grains, fresh fruits and vegetables, legumes, nuts and seeds, and perhaps a little fish to avoid the formation of additional food intolerances. Early detection of HIV is the best hope. Adhering to a complete program implemented with the help of a health practitioner or physician will assist in maintaining life, health, vitality, and enjoyment of life.

Most immune disorders contain a common theme. Candida albicans is connected with all of the disorders in one degree or another. Candida was the disease of the seventies and eighties. In the late eighties and the nineties, the emphasis changed to immune disorders. During the seventies and eighties information began to come forward concerning Candida; now researchers and practitioners are finding that it is a serious health problem of epidemic proportions. Candida can destroy the immune system and compromise metabolic integrity. It is connected with many disease states including immune disorders, alcoholism, eating disorders, allergies, arthritis, respiratory problems, female complications, and endocrine imbalances, digestive disturbances, and emotional and mental problems (including anxiety attacks). Health care practices, contemporary eating habits, high incidence of refined foods in the diet, and severe stress from modern living and pollution have all contributed to the prevalence of Candida.

The recovery process is similar for all the immune disorders. Correct nutrient deficiencies, supply vitamin and mineral supplements for building the immune and adrenal systems, support the digestive process, avoid chemicals and processed or refined foods, remove allergens from the diet and local environment, apply an appropriate rotation diet plan, learn stress management techniques, and seek emotional support when needed.

The most difficult part of the program is the realization that permanent changes in lifestyle are required. The disease can only be arrested if the changes are maintained. If a person returns to the former lifestyle that cause the disease, the problem will return. Moderation is the key— an occasional pizza or piece of birthday cake will undermine the whole program. No one is perfect all the time. One reason for this book is to provide people with interesting and delicious recipes of traditional type foods that can be made from nonallergic ingredients. As my husband said, when given an oatmeal cookie from whole grains and date sugar, "If I couldn't have any other cookie, I'd be perfectly satisfied."

Notes

1. *The Nutritional Supplement,* Volume 7, Number 1, 1992.

2. Natalie Angier, "Vitamins Win Support as Potent Agents of Health," *The New York Times,* March 10, 1992.

3. James F. Balch, M.D. and Phyllis A. Balch, C.N.C. *Prescription of Nutritional Healing* (New York: Avery Publishing, 1990).

4. *SIMILIA Newsletter,* Volume 1, Number 2, January-February 1992.

CHAPTER 4

Eating Disorders and Alcoholism and Drugs

TYPICAL TREND IN AMERICAN society is to isolate problems. In medicine, specialists are required for each bodily function. Medical, social, and psychological concepts separate the physical from the mental, emotional, and spiritual. Following this logic, eating disorders are separated from alcoholism and drug addiction. These addictions come from the same sources: biochemical, genetic, and psychological.

Eating disorders can be broken down into anorexia nervosa, bulimia, and compulsive overeating. Eating disorders are complex and dynamic and often life-threatening. They involve the entire individual: mental, emotional, spiritual, and physical. Chemical dependency is much more than an addiction to alcohol, mind-altering drugs, or food. Abstinence by itself will only arrest the physical part of the illness, not heal it. Treating or addressing one aspect without the others while in recovery will effect little or no permanent change.[1]

Anorexia Nervosa

Anorexia nervosa is a disorder of starvation which manifests itself in an extreme aversion to food. Anorexia predominately affects adolescent, white females between the ages of 12 and 25 years. It can cause psychological, endocrine, and gynecological problems. Symptoms include a refusal to eat, weight loss of more than 25 percent of the original body weight, a bizarre preoccupation with food, an intense fear of becoming fat, hyperactivity, a distorted body image, cessation of menstruation, and no known medical illness leading to the weight loss.

Bulimia

Bulimia is a serious and distinct eating disorder. It involves episodes of bingeing on enormous quantities of food followed by purging with vomiting or laxatives, exercising, or compensatory fasting. Bulimia, more than anorexia, is a form of addictive behavior. Food is the bulimic's fix. The binge eating is accompanied by an awareness that the eating pattern is abnormal and a fear of not being able to stop eating.

Typically, the bulimic is slightly older than the anorexic (usually 18 to 29 years old), female, and tends to maintain her weight. She is more sociable and conforming, and often appears to be the ideal student, working woman, or married woman. Underneath she is acutely disturbed with impaired impulse control, fear of obesity, low self-esteem, and depression. Approximately 23 percent of bulimics attempt suicide. A substantial proportion of recovering anorexics and alcoholics develop bulimia patterns because of the highly addictive nature of the foods they ingest and the ignorance of this basic physiological principle. While the psychic pain can be lethal, so can the physiologic effects of binge/purging with severe dehydration and electrolyte imbalances. Hypoglycemia, digestive disturbances, and genito-urinary tract problems are also common.

Compulsive Overeating

Compulsive overeating is found in the male and female population through all age groups, usually manifesting itself in varying degrees of overweight, from slight to obese. The underlying cause of compulsive overeating is food addiction. Kay Sheppard, vice president of the Food Addiction Program at Humana Hospital in Florida and a recovering food addict, says, "Food addiction is characterized by an obsession with specific foods and the compulsive use of those foods." The obese person has no idea that their daily food cravings or eating habits, are based on a physiological need to stop withdrawal symptoms caused by food allergy addiction. Compulsive overeaters crave and continue to eat the allergenic foods to which they are addicted. Like any biological system, the body can only take so much. Compulsive addiction weakens the immune and adrenal systems and can influence any organ system of the body, including the brain, with multiple symptoms and metabolic problems.

Alcoholism And Drugs

One definition of alcoholism or drug addiction is having lost the ability to control one's drinking or using, usually accompanied by a noticeable personality change. Alcoholism and drug addiction affects all age groups including the very young (alcohol fetal syndrome in newborns or crack babies). It crosses all social, economic, and ethnic distinctions. It is a physical disease with mental, emotional, and spiritual manifestations. Physiologically and biochemically, alcoholism and drug addiction have the same common foundation as eating disorders; they are based upon a genetic predisposition, common nutrient dependencies, addiction to the substances from which it is made, and hypoglycemia.[2]

It is not uncommon for the alcoholic or drug addict to become clean and sober and develop bulimia. This is called problem switching. When a person forces themselves to give up one substance, alcohol for example, they may dramatically increase consumption of coffee, cigarettes, and addictive foods to compensate. In this manner, the stimulated state is maintained and withdrawal symptoms are avoided. Father Joseph Martin says, "Addiction is a single disease with Siamese twin children: alcoholism and food addiction."[3]

In my practice, I have found that bulimia and compulsive overeating especially, are distorted forms of alcoholism. For most of my cases, alcoholics are in the family history (parents, grandparents, uncles, brothers, sisters). Many are children of alcoholics, directly suffering from the emotional damage of being an adult child of an alcoholic (ACA). All come from dysfunctional homes. The biochemical and genetic components establish the predisposition to the addictive process while the environment establishes the form of addiction: drugs, alcohol, or eating disorders.[4]

The most noticeable dynamic of an ACA, or an individual from a severely dysfunctional home, is an almost total lack of self-worth or self-esteem with a tremendous load of shame. Individual identity, self-knowledge, and healthy boundaries are absent and there is a compelling desire to people please, to gain the approval and love they never had as children. This lack of self-worth can be devastating. They often feel they have no right, because they are so "bad," to occupy space on this planet.

Patterns are often deep and familiar; as an ACA matures, they uncon-sciously choose the familiar in order to continue to fulfill their role as they understand it. Self-destructive behavior, to punish their "badness," is a strong characteristic manifesting itself in the various eating disor-ders, severe depression, and even suicidal thoughts and attempts.

Control, or the lack of it, is also a major issue for an ACA. Eating dis-order victims frequently fulfill their role as codependents in the social structure. A strong characteristic of codependency is the need to con-trol in an uncontrollable environment by trying to please or fix a prob-lem. This process compromises the sense of self and value. If only I could do more, if I didn't do that or this, or if I didn't exist, are often repeated mental patterns. In the attempt to rescue, an ACA becomes used. The pattern develops in youth. Children of alcoholics develop a strong sense of responsibility that they are the cause of the situation or problem, not realizing that they are powerless to change people, places, or things. Often they become tightly controlled by an abusive parent or spouse. Their bodies and the ability to use them are their only sense of power left. Overeating or not eating are means of blotting out the rage at being used.

Similar to the alcoholic, eating disorder victims do not have the tools for living. There is a sense of isolation, loneliness, and not belonging. They have poor social skills in interpersonal relationships because of dysfunctional relationships and poor examples in parenting and basic family living. In addition, there is a genetic predisposition to both alco-holism and overeating with common biochemical imbalances. The envi-ronmental stimuli (dysfunctional home) can cause the complex to develop. The alcoholic chooses alcohol. Those with eating disorders usu-ally avoid alcohol, sensing they would become an alcoholic, and obtain the desired euphoria from bingeing on food instead. The guilt, similar to alcoholic remorse and guilt, triggers exercising, fasting, and purging with vomiting or laxatives.[5] They frequently binge on foods containing sugar, yeast, and refined grains (the substances from which alcohol is made), and salt and fat (because of mineral and hormonal imbalances).[6]

Eating disorders are psychologically more complicated than alco-holism because of the need to eat to live and being surrounded every day by food choices. Common addictive and allergic foods are everywhere: sugar, yeast, wheat, corn, dairy, peanut, and soy are commonly found in everyday foods, especially convenience and processed foods. Sugar or yeast are rarely found in recipes for homemade soup, yet are often found in canned soups. Almost all social functions are centered around food, from family meal time and dining out with friends to pizza, ice cream or other fast foods. The contemporary busy lifestyle does not lend itself to spending time in the kitchen putting much thought into the preparation or planning of nutritious menus. We want the meal on the run so we can get to our next business. Ethnic backgrounds and traditions will also influence certain food choices and ideas.

Psychologically, the addictive foods are used to physiologically block discomfort. Food can seem to make one feel high, nurtured, comforted, loved, rewarded, revengeful, release anger, and suppress emotions. Food can suppress the real feelings, keeping you on the merry-go-round of denial, the same way that alcohol can. It keeps the person from seeing and feeling what is really going on in their life. There are definite reasons for this phenomenon. Researchers are finding that some foods may trigger the production of endorphins. Endorphins (produced by neurotransmitters) are the natural, morphine-like painkillers in the brain that ease stress and discomfort.[7]

Neurotransmitters, such as norepinephrine, neuropeptide Y, dopamine, or serotonin, regulate our appetites for the main components of our diets: fats, proteins, and carbohydrates. The ingested foods can greatly affect the balance of the neurotransmitters that the brain produces. In eating disorders, a neurotransmitter imbalance causes binge eating, which then causes further brain chemistry imbalance by the production of false neurotransmitters. If a single macronutrient, such as fat, is eliminated, the neurotransmitters begin producing erratic eating signals. A food addiction abnormally increases or decreases the amount of neurotransmitters in the brain, the chemicals responsible for determining most behavior.

The food addict is usually physically and psychologically addicted to their food of choice, with many actual food allergies and food intolerances. A chronic food allergy is really a food addiction, with allergy or allergic-like sensitivities nearly always accompanying addiction. Allergy may occur without addiction but generally addiction is accompanied by allergy. Alcoholics, drug addicts, and coffee drinkers are concomitantly allergic to the very substances which they crave. Food addicts experience actual withdrawal in the first days of abstinence from the addictive substances, with the same physical cravings familiar to the alcoholic and drug addict.

Like alcoholism, food addiction is a progressive disease with predictable symptoms. It begins at eating for pleasure, which leads to problem eating, and finally to an addiction to specific foods. When the addiction is established, control is lost and the ability to choose what or when to eat is gone. Early signs of food addiction echo those of its alcoholic twin: stealing food and lying about it; extreme concern at being deprived of a favorite food (food addicts and alcoholics hoard and hide their favorites); use of food to relieve tension, boredom, or frustration; and the use of food to relieve uncomfortable feelings.

Overeaters Anonymous can assist in the mental, emotional, and spiritual side effects of eating disorders. The program of abstinence is great, but usually the program chooses only sugar, which is not the only binge food of choice. Abstinence from an addictive food is as serious for the food addict as alcohol is for the alcoholic. The recovery program for food addiction, which emphasizes the acceptance of the addiction, has much in common with Alcoholics Anonymous. Father Martin says. "It speaks of a return to sanity. Insanity is not when an alcoholic is drunk, but when he is sober and picks up that drink." The same thing happens with sweets and it happens in every diet system except the one which is based on total abstinence from addictive foods.

The common addictions are sugar, yeast, refined grains, dairy, salt, and fat. Salt is chosen because of adrenal insufficiency and loss of potassium due to laxatives, stress, vomiting, and excess salt. Fat and protein sources such as meat, mayonnaise, and cheese (dairy), are usually high in sodium. Dairy is a fairly high source of tryptophan. Tryptophan requires B_6 for the conversion to NAD (niacin) and dairy is low in both magnesium and B_6. The resulting imbalance creates false neurotransmitters which enhance the addictive quality of dairy particularly when accompanied by its salt, protein, and fat content. Endorphins will boost the hunger for fat and protein further promoting the addictive state, with diets low in fresh fruits, vegetables, and EFA (essential fatty acids).

Finding all the addictive and allergic foods, eliminating them from the diet, and then rotating the remaining natural, unprocessed foods on a five-day rotation plan, helps to control the physical aspects of the disease of eating disorders. It is important to discern the hidden sources where various foods can be found to eliminate unknowingly sustaining the addiction. For instance, tobacco is laced with sugar and cocaine is cut with milk sugar (lactose). Sugar, yeast, and grains are indigenous to alcohol. Prescription and street drugs are frequently diluted with dairy forms, sugar, and other food substances. Caffeine is often used with dairy or sugar. The drugs nicotine and caffeine help maintain the food addictions, enhance the addictive qualities of the substances, and can draw the addict back into their original substance of choice. Unmasking all of the addictions is extremely important. The understanding of these principles provides a foundation for the client to make intelligent and knowing choices.

In addition to discerning all the addictions, the nutrient deficiencies and individual biochemical imbalances must be simultaneously corrected. There is a genetic predisposition to both alcoholism and eating disorders with common biochemical imbalances and similar nutrient dependencies. Because of the lack, or dependency on, the key nutrients that are amine donors for the neurotransmitters, alcoholics and addicts are born in imbalance. These nutrients are also responsible for energy production, blood sugar regulation, and other metabolic functions. When the addicted individual discovers their substance of choice, whether drugs, alcohol, or food, they feel normal and in balance due to the creation of false neurotransmitters.

Alcoholics are usually B_3, B_6, and magnesium dependent; food addicts are likewise, with B_6 being the most dominant.[8] Alcoholics and overeaters are also commonly deficient in B_{12}, potassium, zinc, EFA, and iodine, with potassium and zinc being the most deficient in eating disorders. Many neurotransmitters are amines and B complex vitamins, such as B_1 (thiamine), B_3 (NAD, nicotinamide adenine dinucleotide), B_6 (pyridoxamine), and B_{12} (cyanocobalamin), are amine donors in the transanimation reactions in the brain. A deficiency of one or more of these amine donors creates false neurotransmitters and disturbs metabolic pathways, especially in the Krebs cycle. This bind-ing and misuse throughout the body, especially the brain, can have serious effects on metabolism.

Zinc and potassium are poorly stored in the body and their losses need to be replaced daily. Fasting, repeated dieting, stress, many malabsorption disorders, sugar, diuretics, and irregular eating schedules promote development of these deficiencies. Zinc, magnesium, B6, and EFA (essential fatty acids) have a strong metabolic relationship to each other. Zinc is needed for proper immune function and fast cell replication. It is also a requisite for the metabolism of other nutrients that the detoxification system depends upon. When zinc is inadequate, vitamin A cannot be utilized. Zinc plays a role in the conversion of pyridoxine (B_6) to pyridoxal-5-phosphate, which is necessary in over 50 enzymes, including the synthesis of most neurotransmitters. Vitamin B_6 becomes active after oxidation to pyridoxal-5-phosphate (P-5-P). Vitamin B_6 is also necessary for the conversion of tryptophan to nicotinamide (NAD), and the synthesis of anti-inflammatory PGE 1. The anti-inflammatory PGE 1 series is a part of the EFA. The micronutrients most important for fatty acid metabolism and the synthesis of anti-inflammatory prostaglandins include zinc, B_6, C, E, magnesium and the fatty acids EPA (fish oil) and GLA (evening primrose oil). EFA deficiencies have been shown to suppress immune function and low levels of EFAs inhibit an important co-factor in the availability of B_6. Vitamin B_6 is required for transport of magnesium into the cells. Deficiencies of B_6 have also been shown to suppress immune function. B_6 is one of the important amine donors for the transanimation reactions in the brain and is also associated with PMS.

In both the alcoholic and food addict, malnutrition and biochemical imbalances are common, with a breakdown of the digestive, immune, and adrenal systems. All nutrients are likely to be deficient, especially those used for immune and adrenal response, including vitamin C, B_5, iodine, potassium, vitamin A, magnesium, vitamin B_6, zinc, and EFA. Vitamin C is needed in any illness or infection and is important for the immune and adrenal systems. Another important vitamin for the immune system is vitamin A. It is essential for the epithelial cells in the body, which line the stomach mucosa, the small intestine, and the respiratory membranes. The main function of B_5 (pantothenic acid) is adrenal support for stress response. Prolonged stress weakens the immune system. Iodine is the hormone for the thyroid gland, and the thyroid is vital to proper immune function. The mineralocorticoids, a hormone from the adrenal cortex, help to control electrolyte homeostasis, particularly the concentrations of sodium and potassium. Aldosterone is responsible for about 95 percent of the mineralocorticoid activity. It increases the reabsorption of sodium and decreases the reabsorption of potassium, so that large amounts of this ion are lost in the urine. With urine loss there is a depletion of such important minerals as magnesium, potassium, and zinc. These minerals are vital to the maintenance of fluid balance and to many chemical reactions in the cells, including muscle contraction.

The internal fermentation of refined sugars and grains produces acetaldehyde, which is also a by-product of alcohol metabolism and Candida albicans. Acetaldehyde requires zinc, vitamin B_6, vitamin B_3, magnesium, and EFA for its metabolism.[9] Because of the deterioration of the immune and adrenal systems, widespread use of antibiotics or cortisone to treat the systemic complications of both disease states, and the internal production of acetaldehyde, Candida albicans frequently becomes a predominate complication of alcoholism and eating disorders. Authors William Crook, M.D. and Orian Truss, M.D. both implicate Candida albicans in the development of behavioral disorders. Anorexics may adhere to the consumption of only a single acceptable, low-calorie, good food, nutritionally restricting their diet and setting up an allergic-addictive response to that food. The good food is likely to provide a good host environment for Candida. On the other hand, the bulimic binges on carbohydrates and becomes allergic-addicted to these foods. Candida albicans loves refined carbohydrates, feeds on them, and in the process of the disease creates additional allergies. Another less common side effect of both disease states is anxiety neurosis/agoraphobia which requires special consideration.

For the addict and alcoholic, the food substances from which their drug of choice is made react as allergens and raise blood sugar levels. The pure ethanol alcohol and the active ingredient in drugs lower blood sugar levels. When alcoholics initially encounter the first drink, they frequently feel in balance. A sense of homeostasis has occurred. As the disease progresses, this is no longer true. When the alcoholic enters recovery and continues in the food portion of the disease, hypoglycemia is a major problem. Food addicts suffer with this imbalance throughout the course of the disease and during recovery until all addictions are unmasked. It is important that all allergic-addictive foods be discovered.

In working with clients and those attempting recovery, it is important to stress that recovery is possible. Recovery requires understanding of the principles involved, education, and willingness to implement the program and make the commitment. Education provides clarity and motivation. Knowing what is going on inside the body leads to understanding the problem and helps make the mind-body connection. The program presents clear information regarding addiction and related addictive foods, setting specific goals and objectives. Treatment is definitive and complicated but recovery is possible. It requires a full program to address the mental, emotional, spiritual, and physical aspects of the disease and the rigorous honesty, open-mindedness, and willingness of the individual.

Notes

1. "The conventional therapeutic mode, which is psychotherapy, is so unsuccessful in the rehabilitation of the anorexic or bulimic patient that even classical psychoanalysts are looking for alternatives. The biomedical model based on mechanistic hypotheses is not generally successful in the treatment of eating disorders because it is based on the theory of 'one cause, one effect, one treatment.' However, if the therapist perceives that the eating disorder is based solely or primarily on an abnormal family situation, the actual biochemical predisposition will be overlooked." Margaret Nusbaum, "Food for Thought: The Problem of Anorexia Nervosa and Bulimia." *Journal of Orthomolecular Medicine,* Volume 1, Number 4, 1986.

2. Orbach mentions the problem of symptom switching, such as "from alcoholism to bulimia, from anorexia to heroin addiction, and from eating disorder to phobic responses." Susie Orbach, *Hunger Strike: The Anorexic's Struggle as a Metaphor for Our Age* (New York: W.W. Norton, 1986).

3. Lynne Dowling, *Food Addiction as Crippling as Alcohol, Drugs: Father Joseph Martin's Story* (Boston, MA: 1985).

4. "The psychoanalytic approach ignores these differences and feeds the vulnerable patient ideas about the origin of her problem that very likely had little or nothing to do with it, except perhaps to establish anorexia (as opposed to bulimia, obesity, alcoholism, or drug abuse) as the symptom." Margaret Nusbaum, "Food for Thought: The Problem Anorexia Nervosa and Bulimia." *Journal of Orthomolecular Medicine,* Volume 1, Number 4, August, 1986.

5. "Endorphin levels are elevated by fasting and exercising; the patient may become addicted to her endogenous opiates.

   "Bingeing not followed by induced vomiting in the patients may involve some other abnormal behavior, such as depression, fasting, or excessive exercise." Margaret Nusbaum, "Food for Thought: The Problem of Anorexia Nervosa and Bulimia." *Journal of Orthomolecular Medicine,* Volume 1, Number 4, l986.

6. "There is a physical need for carbohydrates by the food addict. The typical addict will rarely eat nutritious foods but feels compelled to consume sugary and flour-based foods. The latter is a matter of dark irony for Father Martin, who notes that sugars and grain are also the basic ingredients in alcoholic beverages." Lynne Dowling, *Food Addiction as Crippling as Alcohol, Drugs: Father Joseph Martin's Story* (Boston, MA: 1985).

7. Paul Raeburn, "The Pistachio Ice Cream Neurotransmitter," *American Health,* December 1987.

8. Roger J. Williams, M.D., *Prevention of Alcoholism Through Nutrition* (New York: Bantam Books, 1986).

9. Orian Truss, M.D., "Production of Acetaldehyde by Candida Albicans and Its Toxic Effects." *International Clinical Nutrition Review,* Volume 5, Number 2, April 1985.

CHAPTER 5

The Five-Day Rotation Diet

THE ROTATION DIET CREATES space between the ingestion of the same food; the same food is not eaten for a specific length of time. If you had carrots on Monday, you would not have carrots again until Saturday, establishing a five-day rotation. There are different time spacing for rotation plans, usually three or four days. The information presented here is based upon the work of Theron Randolph, M.D., Stephen Levine, Ph.D., and Marshall Mandell, M.D., whose research has proven the value of the full five-day plan. As a clinical nutritionist, I have found that an expanded rotation using the five-day plan as a base is an excellent way to allow for increased variety and diversity in the diet. Other leaders in the clinical nutrition field, such as Jeffrey Bland, Ph.D., Robert Buist, Ph.D., Russel Jaffe, M.D., Ph.D., and James Braly, M.D. support my research and work.

Why A Rotation Diet?

For those individuals with allergies, Candida, environmental illness, chronic fatigue syndrome, and other immune disorders, the rotation diet plays a major role in recovery and maintaining an acceptable level of wellness. Rotating allows both the immune and adrenal systems to rest from the effects of the offending food and to prevent the formation of additional allergies. The greatest cause of stress comes from what is ingested: air, water, food, and other substances like alcohol or coffee. The accumulative effect of these stressors weakens the immune system, depleting the basic metabolism of essential nutrients, causing more stress reactions in the body. The repeated use of a good food (such as tomatoes, apples, or any whole grain) can create an allergic reaction or intolerance, especially for those who already have allergies or other immune disorders. With food sensitivities or intolerances, it takes three to four days for the offending substance to leave the body. The fifth day acts as a buffer zone and respite for the immune, digestive, and adrenal systems.

The rotation diet can seem overwhelming. However, the purpose of this chapter is to empower and assure the reader that deprivation is not an issue. The extended rotation plan allows for richness, interest, variety, and the moderate use of partly offending foods. A food to which you are not fully allergic can be included in the diet.

It is important to leave out the major offending or allergic foods for a time. Following a full rotation plan will relieve the immune system and allow it to heal. Upon retesting, offending foods can often be reintroduced into the diet. You may find that you are not allergic to an entire food family. For example: there is a reaction to yellow onions, but not to green onions; to red potatoes, but not to russet potatoes; to cantaloupe but not to watermelon. Very few allergies are fixed or permanent allergies. It is not the end of the world to refrain from a few, or more than a few, foods for a time. In the sample menus on page 162, different varieties within food families have been alternated and incorporated to provide many delicious and interesting ideas for creating rotation diets.

🦋 How to Start a Rotation Diet

Beginning a rotation diet can be overwhelming and difficult. Support is extremely important! Substitution is the key for implementing the rotation diet plan. You honestly look at the foods you can have, remain open-minded regarding new choices and be willing to try them. The delicious recipes with their substitutes are the focal point in this book to support you in this process.

Definition of Terms

Acceptable Foods
Acceptable foods are ones that show no reaction on the allergy test.

Addiction
Addiction is the obsession or compulsion with one or more foods. If a

person feels that they simply can't live without a specific food, then there is a problem with that food. The compulsive food cannot be avoided for more than two or three days.

Allergy
Normally associated with a fixed response to a food or substance which elicits the same reaction each time (hives, asthma, or others). An individual's reaction to a food never changes, even if the food is avoided for a period of time.

Avoided Foods
Avoided foods have shown a definite allergic reaction when tested. Whether it is a fixed allergy or an intolerance may not be known at the time of testing. Retesting will establish the category. Also, if you have not had an allergy test, avoided foods include any that are suspected at this time to cause a problem or are highly addictive.

Basic Five-Day Plan
The rotating of all foods in a diet, with a five-day space between the ingestion of the same food.

Extended Plan
The extended plan incorporates a seven-day rotation and is used for those with extensive allergies and/or many foods in the Questionable category.

Food Diary
A food diary keeps a record of the foods, including liquids, which are eaten on a daily basis. It can be simple or elaborate.

Intolerance (Sensitivity)
Intolerances are more subtle and difficult to trace than allergies. Allergies directly correlate with the foods consumed. With an intolerance, the body is tired of having to use the same substance for metabolism. Stress and other reactions occur in the body creating confusing responses and symptoms.

Plan of Rotation

After choosing a five- or seven-day plan, make up a set of menus for the five or seven days (one cycle of rotation) and recreate it every five or seven days. A two, three, or more weekly plan based on the five- or seven-day rotation can be devised. A three weekly plan based on five-day rotation would include 15 days of menus (a seven-day plan would be 21 days of menus). The entire plan can then be rotated again.

Questionable Foods

Questionable foods show a low scale reaction to on the allergy test. These foods are potential problems and some may cause reactions. They are not entirely safe and are rotated on a double extended basis.

Rotation

A specific length of time between the ingestion of the same food.

Substitution

Exchanging one food for another.

Symptom Diary

A method of recording reactions to foods and substances. It should be used in conjunction of the food diary.

Ideas for Beginning

If available in your area, join a support group. Simply knowing that it is not all in your head can be very reaffirming. Besides the support, very helpful suggestions and interesting recipes are often exchanged. Another idea is to find someone who understands the problem and ask them to for help in putting together your rotation plan. It is much easier for two people to sort through the extensive information. Finally, keep a food and symptom diary to identify problem foods (see the example). Any food in the questionable foods category can be a potential problem.

It is important to write down your menu plan in advance. Use a large calendar, a notebook, or any creative method to keep track of what you are eating. It is also helpful to leave room for notes. You may rotate any 24-hour period that you want. Rotation can go from breakfast to breakfast, lunch to lunch, or dinner to dinner. You can also have dinner for breakfast or lunch for dinner. It does not matter as long as the rotation is maintained.

How to Create a Rotation Plan

If you have already had an allergy test, make a list of all the major allergens. These are known as avoided foods.

Break foods into two categories: those that are acceptable foods (no indication of an allergic reaction to these substances), and those that are questionable foods (foods which had a partial reaction when tested). If there has not been an allergy test, follow a basic five-day rotation. If any foods are suspected to bother you or be an obvious addiction, eliminate them from the diet for now.

Break food groups into the following categories: grains, fruits, vegetables, legumes, nuts and seeds, proteins (flesh foods), and miscellaneous (includes oils, herbs, and spices).

List the foods that are acceptable foods under the various foods categories. Grains, like barley and corn go under grains; do the same for the other categories.

List separately the foods that are questionable foods under the same food categories.

Establish the number of your rotation days. If you are highly sensitive, then a seven-day rotation plan will be more beneficial and used for all acceptable foods. Questionable foods will be introduced every 14 days. On a five-day plan, questionable foods are introduced every ten days.

Decide how you want to establish a plan of rotation, whether for one week, two weeks, or more depending if you are on a five-day or seven-day schedule. This will create a base for your rotation. Maintaining a menu plan frees your energy for other interests and simplifies your life. The rotation diet creates your shopping list. You can then re-rotate the entire plan eliminating the need to recreate menus on an ongoing basis. Menus for up to a month or more can be rotated indefinitely. Other recipes can be substituted using the same ingredients.

🦋 Food Selection

Write down each of the following on a temporary schedule allowing for the number of days or weeks selected for your rotation plan:

One grain for each day. Example: Monday—barley, Tuesday—millet, Wednesday—wheat

One main course (flesh food, legume, or other vegetarian dish) each day.

The vegetables included in the main course. Example: Lentil soup—lentils, onion, carrots, tomatoes, parsley. These vegetables will be your vegetables for the day and will be included in other dishes, used as snacks, or served individually.

One nut or seed for each day which will complement the main course and also be served as a nut milk for cereal or a snack.

One to two fruits for each day which will complement the other foods chosen. Examples: a fruit juice on your cereal, a fruit jam melted for pancakes, or lemon for your fish or salad.

From the miscellaneous list, select the oils, margarine or butter, and herbs that will complete your selections. Space them as far apart as possible on your rotation plan. Oil, herbs, and lemon/lime are used more frequently in recipes. If allergies are severe, then strict rotation is necessary.

Adjust selections according to taste, variety and interest. If you are allergic to onions, this does not mean that you are allergic to everything in the same food family. Explore the possibility of shallots, chives, green onions, or leeks.

Example

Following is Samantha's allergy test results and the rotation plan developed based on the results. Samantha had extensive food allergies. Substitutions will be used for the menu to provide interesting choices and options for daily meals, considering that it could otherwise be bland and boring, especially with her limited selection.

Example Allergy Test
Steps 1 and 2

Avoided Foods	Questionable Foods	Betweens	Acceptable Foods
Acorn squash	Accent	Blackberry	
Anise	(seasoning)	Broccoli	Almond
Apple	Avocado	Cantaloupe	Artichoke
Apricot	Banana	Celery	Asparagus
Aspirin	Black pepper	Clove	Boysenberry
Banana squash	Black-eyed pea	Curry powder	Brown Rice
Barley	Butternut squash	Green bell	Brussels Sprout
Basil	Cashew	pepper	Buckwheat
Bay leaf	Cauliflower	Lamb	Canola Oil
Beef	Chili	Lima bean	Carob
Black beans	Chocolate	Mustard	Cucumber
Blueberry	Clam	Nutmeg	Egg Replacer
Brazil nut	Coconut	Oats	Eggplant
Butter	Cod	Papaya	Ginger
Butter lettuce	Corn	Poppy seed	Grape
Carrot	Fennel	Pork	Grapefruit
Chicken	Fig	Raspberry	Green Bean
Cinnamon	Garlic	Scallop squash	Honeydew
Coffee	Goat cheese	Spaghetti squash	Kale
Egg	Goat parmesan	Thyme	Kiwi
Garbanzo	cheese		Leek
Green onion	Green cabbage		Lemon
Honey	Halibut		Lentil
Kidney bean	Jicama		Millet
Macadamia	Molasses		Mushroom
Mango	Nectarine		Orange
Milk	Olive oil		Orange Roughy
Olives	Parsnip		Paprika
Oyster	Peach		Peppermint
Peas	Peanut butter		Pinto Bean

Example Allergy Test, *Continued*

Avoided Foods	Questionable Foods	Betweens	Acceptable Foods
Radish	Pear		Plum
Rosemary	Pecan		Potato
Sesame	Pineapple		Pumpkin Seed
Shrimp	Red bean		Quinoa
Soybean	Red cabbage		Red Onion
Split pea	Snow pea		Red Plum
Strawberry	Sole		Romaine lettuce
Tuna	Tomato		Rye
Turkey	Veal		Safflower Oil
Turnip			Sage
Walnut			Scallops
Yellow squash			Spelt
Yogurt			Spinach
Zucchini			Sunflower
			Sweet Potato
			Vanilla
			Water Chestnut
			Watermelon
			Wheat

Food Categories

Steps 3, 4 and 5

Grains

Brown rice	Oats	Spelt
Buckwheat	Quinoa	Wheat
Millet	Rye	

Questionable Foods

Corn

Food Categories, *Continued*
Steps 3, 4 and 5

Fruit

Blackberry	Honeydew	Papaya
Boysenberry	Kiwi	Raspberry
Cantaloupe	Lemon	Red plum
Grape	Lime	Watermelon
Grapefruit	Orange	

Questionable Foods

Banana	Nectarine	Pear
Fig	Peach	Pineapple

Vegetables

Artichoke	Green bean	Romaine lettuce
Asparagus	Green bell pepper	Scallop squash
Broccoli	Kale	Spaghetti squash
Brussels sprout	Leek	Spinach
Celery	Mushroom	Sweet potato
Cucumber	Potato	Yam
Eggplant	Red onion	

Questionable Foods

Butternut squash	Jicama	Snow pea
Cauliflower	Parsnip	Tomato
Green cabbage	Red cabbage	

Legumes

Carob	Lima bean	Sunflower seed
Lentil	Pinto	

Questionable Foods

Black-eyed peas	Pecan	Red bean

Food Categories, *Continued*
Steps 3, 4 and 5

Nuts And Seeds

Almond   Pumpkin seed
Poppy seed   Water chestnut

Questionable Foods

Cashew   Coconut

Protein

Goat cheese   Orange roughy
Lamb   Pork

Questionable Foods

Clam   Halibut   Veal
Cod   Sole

Miscellaneous

Canola oil   Ginger   Peppermint
Clove   Mustard   Safflower
Curry   Nutmeg   Thyme
Egg Replacer   Paprika   Vanilla

Questionable Foods

Accent (seasoning)   Chili   Fennel
Black pepper   Chocolate   Olive

Sample Food Diary
Steps 6 and 7

Because of the extensive amount of allergies and foods in the questionable foods category, a seven-day rotation plan was selected and established with a 14-day schedule of menus. The plan will then be re-rotated with some changes in the individual dishes using the same ingredients.

Breakfast	Morning	Lunch	Afternoon	Dinner	Evening

Sample Symptom Diary				
	Time of Day				
Symptoms	Before Breakfast	After Breakfast	After Lunch	After Dinner	During Night
Tired or Drowsy					
Irritable or Overactive					
Headache					
Respiratory (stuffy nose, cough)					
Digestive (bellyache, nausea)					
Muscle and joint symptoms					
Other					

CHAPTER 6

Help and Recovery

MANY REASONS HAVE LED you to this book: an interest in self-help; studying and reading about the subject; a suspicion that you have food allergies or Candida; being in recovery from an eating disorder, alcoholism, or drug addiction and discovering that food is the main drug of choice in your addictions. Perhaps you have worked with an alternative health practitioner or an allopathic physician, but have not fully recovered as you think you should have. You sense more clearly the complexities of the problem and need more help. What do you do now?

Health continues to be the new fad. Self-help books abound, experts appear frequently on popular talk shows. There is an abundance of new diets and other practitioners are suddenly experts in nutrition. The weight-loss diet business is an approximately 40 billion dollar industry. So how do you find help?

One way is to become educated by reading this and other books in the field. Another avenue of information is to attend lectures and seminars. Ask questions, then ask more questions. Take notes. Health, or wellness, requires self-responsibility. You are responsible for preventative health care and for your ultimate well-being. Knowledge will empower you to make healthy choices.

If you are sick (especially with immune disorders, allergies, eating disorders, alcoholism, or addictions), your best source of help is from someone whose major focus, experience, and education is in the field of clinical nutrition. That person could be an M.D., a clinical ecologist, or a clinical nutritionist. Do not be afraid to ask them questions. A quality health practitioner should be willing to answer your questions in a preliminary consultation before an initial appointment. Some important questions to address are:

What is their background, experience, and training?

Do they understand biochemical individuality?

Do they understand allergies/addictions and rotation diets?

Do they have knowledge regarding the various forms of allergy testing?

Do they have knowledge in others areas of nutrition and health?

If you asked about a diet for gout, would there be a practical answer?

Will they correct nutrient deficiencies and supply nutrients to build the immune and adrenal systems?

Do they use supplements to treat symptoms?

Do they sell supplements, or do they suggest and give guidance on the brands and types available?

Are they published? Are there any available articles or books by them?

Do they present lectures or seminars that you can attend?

Are they willing to explain their program?

Is their manner supportive?

Will they return your phone calls?

Is their approach holistic? Will they recommend other health care practitioners who will complement and support their work, such as a chiropractor or acupuncturist?

Are they familiar with 12-step programs?

Do they offer a support group as a part of their program?

Are they familiar with local support groups or therapists who understand your condition and problems?

Will they recommend additional books?

Major health care providers for immune disorders, allergies, addictions, eating disorders, alcoholism, and drug addiction are usually M.D.s, clinical ecologists, and clinical nutritionists. There are doctors in the field who have specialized in nutrition and will understand the above problems. Clinical ecologists are normally M.D.s who will have their own private practice or clinical ecology unit at the local hospital. Their main focus is immune disorders and allergies. Frequently, they will use intradermal (like a scratch test on back or arm) allergy testing, which may include neutralizing doses for discovered allergies as a part of their program. For some people it is effective.

A clinical nutritionist can be either an M.A. or M.S., a Ph.D., or an M.D. that has received certification through the International and American Association of Clinical Nutritionists (IAACN). The IAACN is presenting legislation so that clinical nutritionists will be organized and recognized as a separate field, like chiropractors. A clinical nutritionist should have a background and working knowledge of biochemistry, anatomy, and physiology, and knowledge of the application of nutritional principles. If your clinical nutritionist is not an M.D., they should work closely with your physician. Check for a health care professional who will specialize in your particular problem or call Immuno Services at (800) 231-9197 and ask patient services for a list of references. Not all practitioners are familiar with eating disorders, alcoholism, or drug addiction. Remember to ask questions.

General Recovery Guidelines for Health Practitioners

Treat the most life-threatening problems and stabilize (detox alcoholics, stop dehydration in eating disorder victims).

When stable, begin a comprehensive program by evaluating individual biochemical needs by assessing vitamin, mineral, protein, or hormonal imbalances.

Reestablish proper digestion with hydrochloric acid (HCL) or appropriate pancreatic enzymes.[1]

Supply nutrients and supplements to correct deficiencies and provide adequate adrenal, digestive, and immune support based on individual needs.

Test for allergies using the IgE immuno assay test, RAST, cyto-toxin testing, or applied kinesiology. Do not use avoidance and challenge testing unless under in-hospital supervision as it can be a problem for those with eating disorders, resulting in severe allergic reactions.

Set up a five-day rotation diet and/or extended plan with remaining nonallergic foods, introducing unfamiliar and healthy foods slowly.

Use fresh, natural, unprocessed, unrefined foods and include raw nuts and seeds as they are tolerated. Keep the diet light and free of heavy protein (meat, dairy). If protein levels are low, use a complete amino acid complex to raise the amino acid pool.

If Candida is present, use a yeast-free, no sugar, restricted (or non fruit) fruit diet with a comprehensive program of natural yeast inhibitors, such as garlic, pau d'arco, black walnut, pumpkin, caprylic acid, Para Micocidin, and lactobacillus acidophilus, depending on allergy restrictions.

If anxiety neurosis is present, prohibit caffeine use, restrict exercise, avoid biguanides drugs, use only whole grains, and increase thiamine, pyridoxine, niacin (B_1, B_6, B_3) and magnesium.[2]

Provide an exercise program dependent on individual needs.

Provide private counseling with someone that understands the dynamics of immune disorders, alcoholism, drug addiction, or eating disorders.

Suggest attendance at outside support groups where appropriate: OA (Overeaters Anonymous), AA (Alcoholics Anonymous), NA (Narcotics Anonymous), ACA (Adult Children of Alcoholics), Alateen (Teenagers of Alcoholics), Alanon or CODA (for those living with a practicing alcoholic), PU (Parents United—past or present sexual abuse), EI (Environmental Illness), AIDS, CFS (Chronic Fatigue Syndrome), and other groups.

Give lots of tough love and support.

🦋 A Client's Epilogue

It was late winter in 1990 when I walked into the conference room where Liz Reno was giving a lecture on nutrition and women's health issues. I had for two months been in constant pain from an unclear reproductive disorder that followed several years of increasing discomfort and troubling symptoms. When the crisis hit, my doctors gave me drugs and when that didn't work, they recommended surgery, though it wasn't certain it would relieve the pain. Something happened to my feelings about responsibility when I found myself robbed of my quality of life. Facing surgery or drugs, I had to decide to commit myself to finding another way back to a life worth living. I was at a crossroads and then I met Liz.

Listening as she eloquently described the delicate workings of the female body, I began to hear another more important message: that my suffering was not hopeless and I would heal myself. Liz spoke of her own experience and how she recovered her health through nutrition. I found I had a new and exciting option. After the lecture, I made an appointment to see her.

It was during the first appointment that I learned about the connection between Candida albicans, food allergies, food addictions, a genetic background of alcoholism, stress, and a host of physical problems, including the ones I was experiencing. I was surprised to find that I had an allergic response to many foods, especially my favorites.

In the process of digesting this new information, I had to reconsider my relationship to food. What were my eating habits? When did I eat for nourishment or for emotional comfort? Had I created my food allergies by limiting my diet to certain convenient dishes (a common habit which turned out to be very strong)? Where did my attitudes about food come from and how could I improve them?

I jumped into my new regimen with enthusiasm. I stuck to the cleansing diet, learned to rotate my foods, took my supplements and was overjoyed when the constant pain disappeared after two weeks.

But that was only the beginning. My problems, though of increasing intensity over the previous three years, had been going on since the age of 12. While the immediate crisis was relieved, I still had a chronic cycle of menstrual pain and migraine headaches to contend with. However, as I got to know Liz, I learned that more was possible. I had a chance to recover from the chronic pain cycle and be healthier than I had ever been before. And that possibility was going to take time and commitment.

Something happened to my feelings about responsibility when I found myself robbed of my "quality of life." Facing surgery or drugs, both of which exact an irreplaceable price, I had to decide either to pay the price or commit myself to finding another way back to a life worth living.

Three years prior to the crisis of 1990, I had begun putting together an informal health program for myself. Like a jigsaw puzzle, there were many pieces in my program. First I learned to ask for help and to keep asking. I discovered how important it is to have a supporting and skilled team of health care providers to guide me and give me options. I made lifestyle changes. I purchased a stationary bike and used it. I worked with a chiropractor and an acupuncturist, and drank Chinese herbal teas. I constructed a daily exercise and diet schedule to live up to. I stopped taking my health for granted and started to support my well-being with new habits.

I consulted my allopathic doctors and did research on the possible causes that they suggested. I worked with a medical advocate and health care consultant, learning how to clarify my problems, prioritize my needs, research my options, and find sources of help, including the services of a good nutritionist. I became my own medical detective, tracking down any possible connection or solution.

During this process, I learned to trust my intuition about my health care providers. Was I comfortable with the communication between us? Did we work as a partnership? Was I being taken seriously? Was I getting results?

I learned to ask lots of questions, take notes at appointments, send letters stating my concerns and questions when necessary, to preface an appointment, and request extra appointment time for discussion. It became clear, the responsibility for finding answers was mine. Ultimately, I was the one who would put the whole picture together, make the decisions, and live with the results.

Finally, I realized that my recovery was going to take time and persistence. This was not a broken bone or skinned knee. My whole body needed to be brought back into balance and allowed to heal with daily support. To do this I needed to ask new questions.

How will I know I am making progress when the recovery period could last several years? How do I stay motivated to continue over the long term? For me the answers came when I set goals for diet and exercise, learned how to gauge the symptom level on a scale of 1 to 10, kept records, and looked for patterns and results. I used a chart where I recorded the basic components of my program and a profile of the symptoms so I could see relationships between them. In a sense, it was a return to earning gold stars in school as a child and the stars began to multiply. Then in April of 1991, I entered a new world without chronic menstrual and headache pain. I had my first normal period. And the next month, another normal period, and then another. I felt like I should be wearing a sign, Miracle in Progress. For the first time in my life I felt free.

Several months after my breakthrough, I sustained a back injury in a car accident. The shock to my body was so great that many of the old symptoms returned. Frustrating and disappointing though it was, I brought to this new challenge the knowledge that healing comes with good care, persistence, and patience.

It is easy to forget in our fast-paced, high-tech world that the natural powers of healing are constantly at work, repairing, rebuilding, renewing. With the help and support of such people as Liz Reno, we each have the opportunity to choose and create our own optimum well-being. It is only a matter of time and commitment.

—Chris Cone, April 1992.

Notes

1. "A low gastric pH, a slightly alkaline duodenum, and active gastric and pancreatic enzymes are necessary prerequisites for the digestion of food antigens. Undigested peptides or proteins that escape this first line of defense are subsequently digested by the lysozomal enzymes in the intestinal epithelial cells or are phagocytosed and digested by macrophages in the lamina propria. Hence the patients with potential food sensitivities

must have optimal functioning of the digestive system and the immunological defense system." Robert Buist, "Food Intolerance—A Growing Phenomenon: Current Concepts in Development, Manifestation and Treatment." *International Clinical Nutrition Review,* Volume 6, Number 1, January, 1986.

2. Robert Buist, "Anxiety Neurosis—The Lactate Connection." *International Clinical Nutrition Review,* Volume 5, Number 1, January 1985.

PART II

The Healthy Diet and Tools for Change

Being motivated to change your diet and understanding the importance of change is the first step. Applying the tools for change is the next step. In this section you will discover the hidden sources and names of common allergens and ways to avoid them. In this section you will find straight answers on a healthy diet; practical substitutions for dairy, sugar, and eggs; ways to shop to save money and buy the foods you need; ways to eat out and still maintain the diet; practical rotation menus; and much more.

CHAPTER 7

What is a Healthy Diet?

THE MODERN LIFESTYLE OF holding down career, family, community, or church responsibilities, plus individual needs for exercise, recreation, and personal growth creates stress! Pollution in the air, water, and food supplies, and depletion of the ozone layer increases the stress load on the immune and adrenal systems, demand a more supportive diet and healthy food and lifestyle choices.

The typical American diet includes dairy, refined sugar, heavy proteins (meats and poultry), refined and enriched flours, grains and cereals, and a small amount of fruits and vegetables, usually frozen or canned. In terms of percentages, approximately 40 percent of daily calories are derived from fat, 30 percent from refined carbohydrates (including sugar), and 30 percent from animal protein sources (meats and dairy).

Most of the American diet is processed: too many convenience foods are consumed, loaded with chemicals, preservatives, and additives and void of vitamins and minerals. Agribusiness is a major industry with huge food producers, packagers, and supermarket chains. Food is considered a product rather than as food. Key factors influencing marketing decisions are long shelf life and advertising. Foods can be spoiled or damaged from harvesting to shelf, and wanting to minimize the loss is good. But the overuse of chemicals and additives in increasing shelf life can change the basic structure of the food, destroy valuable enzymes for digestion, and add substances the body cannot use, or that can be damaging. Foods have been stimulated with hormones, hybridized for color, size, and shelf-life, and have been sprayed, waxed, or gassed for uniformity of appearance. Appearance has become a major factor in food choices, and the taste of real food, or even knowing what that is has been lost. Products are designed for impulse buying. Most snack foods (soda pop, chips, processed cheese, and dried soup) did not exist until recently. They are heavily advertised on TV, weekly food ads, magazines, and displayed extensively in the stores, from the supermarket to the corner market. These products are designed for high-profit, high-volume sales and have little or nothing to do with true nutritional value. We have been led away from fresh natural foods toward the preserved, manufactured foods which are under the control of the processors, producers, advertisers, and manufacturers.

Grants are given by the U.S. Department of Agriculture in amounts ranging from as little as a few hundred dollars to millions of dollars, to major companies like McDonald's, Campbell Soup Company, Joseph E. Seagram and Sons, Burger King, M&M-Mars and Hershey Foods, Del Monte, Welch's and Ocean Spray Cranberries, Nabisco, and Quaker Oats to promote their products to potential customers around the world.[1] Representative Dick Armey said, "You go down the list of companies and it's hard to imagine they need a handout from the American taxpayer to market their products abroad."

There has been extensive congressional lobbying by the meat and dairy industry. The original four basic food groups wheel was developed by health officials and the dairy and livestock industry in the 1940s and 1950s with an emphasis on getting enough essential nutrients and protein. In a *Washington Post* article by Malcolm Gladwell, "Nutritional Advice Overhaul," Bonnie Liebman of the Center for Science in the Public Interest said, "Nutrition thinking has turned around 180 degrees since then. Since then we recognized that the major killers threatening Americans are linked to excesses, not deficiencies, in our diet. We are more likely to die of too much fat or cholesterol than too little vitamins or protein." In the early April 1991, the Agriculture Department announced they would replace the four basic food groups wheel with an "eating right pyramid" which called for a diet that centered around fruits, vegetables, and grains.[2]

The proposed change, hailed by many nutritionists as a long overdue improvement in the way the government encourages good eating habits, represented the four basic groups as layers of a pyramid. By putting vegetables, fruits, and grains at the broad base and meat and dairy products in a narrow band at the top, government health experts had hoped to create a more effective visual image of the proper proportions each food group should have in a healthful diet. But in meetings with agriculture officials, representatives of both the dairy and meat industries complained that the pyramid 'stigmatized' their products. By the end of April, the Agriculture Department capitulated to pressure and abandoned its plans.

One year later in April 1992, the Department of Agriculture released a new version of the "eating right pyramid" reflecting the influence of the lobbying groups. Basically, it is the four food groups now arranged in a pyramid. Nothing has changed. Senator Patrick Leahy, chairman of the Senate Agriculture Committee, said, "USDA's delay cost nearly $1 million and the administration ended up right where they started."

🦋 The Healthy Diet

Forget about a food wheel or "eating right pyramid." Let's examine the elements basic to life and metabolism: air, water, sunshine, vitamins, minerals, carbohydrates, amino acids, lipids, and fiber.

Air

We require air to survive. Air supplies us with much-needed oxygen. Aerobic exercise means increasing oxygen intake. If sufficient oxygen is not present, then the basic human energy cycle (Krebs cycle) will not function properly, depositing non end-product metabolites (like lactic acid) in body tissues, resulting in soreness, fatigue, and eventually disease. Unfortunately, the air that we breathe cannot always be controlled. Pollution and smog are constant problems and indoor air quality can sometimes be worse than the outside. (See page 130 for what you can do about indoor air quality.)

Water

Our bodies are 57 percent water. Drinking six to eight glasses a day cleanses impurities from the system and provides moisture for body tissues. Water also supplies some hydrogen and oxygen for basic metabolism. The quality of our water is not always good (see page 129 for more information).

Sunshine
It would be a sad, dark, and dreary world without the sun. The sun provides heat, photosynthesis for plants, stimulates growth of all things, gives light and beauty, and is the major source of vitamin D, needed for the assimilation of minerals. As the ozone layer is being depleted, the sun also can be an enemy. Dangerous ultraviolet rays contribute to skin cancer, eye damage, weakened immune system, and other problems. Common sense when exposed to sunlight is important: use sun screen, dark glasses, or wear clothing, but do continue to enjoy the sunshine through moderate exposure. A beautiful sunny day can be a real mental lift!

Vitamins
Vitamins are found in living things and are absolutely essential for proper growth and health. They must be supplied by the diet or in supplements, because the body cannot synthesize vitamins. Vitamins bind with protein molecules to produce enzymes. Enzymes are then responsible for the oxidation process in the body, transporting the oxygen into the cell and in exchange removing the waste products, like carbon dioxide. Vitamins (enzymes) work on a cellular level and are a major factor in biochemical processes such as growth, metabolism, cellular reproduction, repair, and digestion. A lack of one or more vitamins can impair function and cause many different symptoms.

Vitamins are either water soluble or fat soluble. Water soluble means that they will dissolve in water and when an excess amount of a vitamin has been ingested, it will be eliminated, usually through the urine. The B complex vitamins and vitamin C are water soluble. Eleven factors comprise a complete B complex. B_1, B_2, B_3, and B_5 play a major role in the Krebs cycle (the basic energy cycle in the body—energy for heat and function and all activities). The B complex vitamins work synergistically. Any B vitamin deficiency should be addressed after a complete B complex is taken. B_{12} is the only B vitamin that is stored in the body for any length of time. It is stored in the liver.

The fat soluble vitamins, A, D, E, and K are stored in the liver and fatty tissue in the body. Vitamin A is an important antioxidant and provides basic prevention against cancer. Vitamin A from animal sources (dairy, fish) can accumulate, and when used in high doses can become toxic. Beta-carotene (provitamin A), which is from plant sources, is rich in antioxidant properties and nontoxic to the system. At the Health By Choice conference held in Atlanta in 1991, experts stated that less than five percent of the U.S. population received enough vitamin A in their diet to prevent cancer. Vitamin D, which is necessary for the assimilation of calcium, phosphorus, and magnesium for strong bones and teeth, can be toxic in amounts over 800 international units (I.U.). Vitamin E, another important antioxidant, is known as the reproductive vitamin, and is useful for the treatment and prevention of heart disease. Little-known vitamin K helps with the basic matrix production for strong bones and teeth. It is more famous for its blood clotting properties. Major sources for vitamins are fruits, vegetables, legumes, nuts, seeds, and whole grains.

Vitamin B Complex

Vitamin B_1 (thiamine)

Vitamin B_2 (riboflavin)

Vitamin B_3 (niacin/niacinamide)

Vitamin B_5 (pantothenic acid)

Vitamin B_6 (pyridoxamine)

Vitamin B_{12} (cyanocobalamin)

Folic acid

Choline

Inositol

Biotin

PABA (Para-aminobenzoic acid)

Minerals

Approximately seventeen minerals are essential for metabolism. Minerals are found in organic and inorganic combinations in food and in the body. Minerals interact with vitamins and their work in the body is interrelated. They act as catalysts for many biological functions. Although minerals are only four to five percent of our weight, they are responsible for many physiological processes: skeletal structure, teeth, muscle contraction (including the heart), and nerve responses. Minerals must be maintained in a delicate balance in the bloodstream or else the body goes into crisis. They also help preserve water balance in the tissues that are essential to proper mental and physical processes.

All the minerals are essential and must be supplied from the diet. Any mineral deficiency should be added on the base of a good, balanced mineral complex. In order for the minerals to be properly absorbed and assimilated into the body, they need to be broken down by sufficient HCL (hydrochloric acid) in the stomach during digestion and bind with a substrate (an amino acid). Minerals are broken down into macrominerals (large), microminerals (small), and trace minerals (minute).

Minerals

Macrominerals	Microminerals	Trace Minerals
Calcium	Chromium	Arsenic
Chlorine	Copper	Cadmium
Magnesium	Iodine	Cobalt
Phosphorous	Iron	Fluorine
Potassium	Manganese	Molybdenum
Sodium	Selenium	Nickel
Sulfur	Zinc	Silicon
		Tin
		Vanadium

Phosphorus is usually found in abundance in the diet, especially if meats, dairy, grains, and sodas are being consumed. It is not necessary to take additional phosphorus as a supplement, whether alone or in combination with other minerals. Potassium, important for fluid balance, muscle and nerve function (including the heart muscle and hypertension), and a foundation for stress support, can easily be lost in the urine with stress, excess salt consumption, caffeine, diuretics, alcohol, sugar, drugs, and laxatives. Approximately 5000 mgs. of potassium are needed for every teaspoon of salt sodium that is consumed. Potassium is found mainly in fresh fruits and vegetables. Magnesium is often a missing ingredient for strong bones and teeth, and for nerve and muscle function. It is not abundant in foods and can be lost in freezing (up to 40 percent) and cooking. If someone has diarrhea or misuses laxatives, they can develop a magnesium deficiency. Important sources for the minerals are fruits, vegetables, nuts, seeds, fish, sea weed (kelp), whole grains, legumes, blackstrap molasses, and raw cow's milk or goat dairy.

Carbohydrates

Carbohydrates are the main fuel and energy source for all metabolic functions, including muscular exertion, and assisting in the digestion and assimilation of other foods. They also help regulate fat and protein metabolism. Carbohydrates are metabolized more efficiently than other fuels. Due to biochemical individuality, there are some people who are carbohydrate intolerant and function better with fatty acids or protein. The intolerance is usually caused by nutrient imbalances, and/or allergy reactions to refined carbohydrates, or individual ones (like wheat or corn). The main types of carbohydrates are refined and complex; these are present in foods as sugars, starches, and cellulose.

Simple sugars (monosaccharides), such as those found in honey or fruit, are easily digested. Even though they are not complex in nature, neither are they refined. Other disaccharides, like table sugar, are highly refined. The refining process strips the product of essential nutrients. Chemicals frequently are involved in the manufacturing of these products. Refined sugar products (sucrose, corn syrup, fructose) are not enriched in any way to restore nutrition that has been lost. Refined grain products are usually enriched or fortified with some of the missing nutrients. Not only are necessary vitamins and minerals lost in the process, but also essential fiber. Refined white flour acts very much like sugar does in the system and will aggravate blood sugar levels.

Starches are composed of polysaccharides and may be either refined or complex. White flour is a refined starch; whole wheat is a complex carbohydrate. A complex carbohydrate has not been processed and is whole and unchanged from the way nature intended it to be. It contains the vitamins, minerals, fiber, oils (if present), and enzymes.

Carbohydrates

Mono-saccharides	Disaccharides	Polysaccharides (complex carbohydrates)
fructose	maltose (two glucose molecules)	grains
fruit	sucrose (glucose and fructose)	legumes
galactose	lactose (glucose and galactose)	vegetables
glucose	mostly refined sugar	nuts and seeds
honey	milk sugar	

Amino Acids

Proteins are constructed and broken down into amino acids. All foods contain one or more amino acids. Some amino acids can be produced by the human body; some cannot be produced in the body and are called essential amino acids. When a protein contains the essential amino acids, it is referred to as a complete protein. It is the amino acids we are after and not necessarily protein (meat) itself. After digestion (the breaking down of food from a protein or vegetable source to obtain the amino acids), the reformed polypeptide chains of amino acids, now called proteins, become building materials for muscles, blood, skin, hair, nails, internal organs, hormone production, immune function, water balance, and acid/alkaline balance. Proteins can also be used for basic heat and energy production when there are insufficient carbohydrates or fats. It is not the most efficient method of producing energy, and may even draw amino acids from muscle tissue to be processed in the Krebs cycle. Some excess protein is converted by the liver and stored as fat by the body.

The human body requires far less protein than is usually thought. Between 25 to 45 grams a day is normally sufficient, depending upon a person's size, weight, and activity levels. This converts to three to four ounces of uncooked meat, fish, or poultry per day, or the equivalent amount of protein derived from proper food combining of legumes, whole grains, nuts and seeds, vegetables, and raw cow's or goat milk dairy.

The body contains an amino acid pool. Unused amino acids are stored and drawn upon when needed. It is not necessary to make sure you consume all the amino acids at every meal, or even every day. However, they should be ingested within a fairly short time span.

Beware: the amino acid balance in the body is very tricky to maintain. Individualized amino acids, whether in a weight building program, a vitamin/mineral supplement, or to address a specific problem (lysine for herpes), taken for an extended length of time (several months) will cause an imbalance and upset the proper proportions. Side effects will occur (impaired immune function, nerve damage, depression). Heavy proteins from meat sources will slow down elimination, and contribute to putrefaction in the intestinal tract.

Lipids

Lipids, or more commonly known as fats, provide energy, help to transport the fat soluble vitamins (A, D, E, and K) into the cells, protect and hold in place major organs like the kidney, heart, and liver, insulate the body from environmental temperature changes, and preserve body heat. Excess fats in any form, especially from saturated or potential carcinogenic sources, are major contributing factors related to heart disease, diabetes, cancer, and obesity. They are also high in calories; one gram of fat yields approximately nine calories.

Different terms are associated with lipids: polyunsaturated, fatty acids, essential fatty acids, triglycerides, phospholipids, cholesterol and sterols, LDL, and HDL. Following is a brief explanation. Saturated, unsaturated, polyunsaturated, hydrogenated, and mono-unsaturated are explained in page 143.

Fatty Acids

Two main types of fatty acids are saturated and unsaturated. The substances in fatty acids give fats their different flavors, textures, and melting points. Biochemically, fatty acids are composed of long chains of carbon atoms with hydrogen atoms attached and with an acid group at one end (oxygen, carbon, and hydrogen atoms). Their position on the chain determines their qualities.

Essential Fatty Acids

Essential fatty acids cannot be manufactured in the body. There are three essential fatty acids: linoleic, arachidonic, and linolenic. Linoleic is the only one that is absolutely essential, because arachidonic and linolenic acids can be synthesized from linoleic acid if sufficient quantities are present in the diet. Arachidonic acid is inflammatory in nature and is derived mainly from animal sources. Linoleic and linolenic acids are anti-inflammatory and are supplied from vegetable, fish, nut, and seed sources. Essential fatty acids are important for normal growth; healthy blood, nerves, and skin; magnesium and B6 metabolism; the immune system; PMS; and the transport and breakdown of cholesterol. The average diet supplies far too much arachidonic acid, creating an imbalance and cellular deficiencies.

Triglycerides
Triglycerides is another name for lipids. Almost 95 percent of the lipids in the diet are triglycerides.

Cholesterol and Sterols
Sterols are compounds composed of carbon, hydrogen, and oxygen atoms arranged in rings with any of a variety of side chains attached. Cholesterol is one of the sterols. Cholesterol is needed metabolically, but is not essential because the body is capable of manufacturing its own in the liver from glucose and fatty acids. Cholesterol is transported through the bloodstream and is an essential building block for hormones (like testosterone or cortisone), cell membranes, the sheaths that protect nerve fibers, and the manufacture of vitamin D. It should comprise less than five percent of the diet.

After cholesterol is manufactured in the liver, it is either transformed into related compounds or leaves the liver to be excreted, deposited in bodily tissues, or accumulated in the arteries. Most of the cholesterol that the liver makes becomes bile salts and the bile in turn is stored in the gallbladder. A healthy gallbladder is an important part of the proper digestion, distribution, and elimination of cholesterol.

Phospholipids
Less than five percent of the lipids in the diet are phospholipids. Phos-

pholipids are found as the protective part of the cellular membrane. Lecithin is an example of a phospholipid.

LDL

LDLs, or low-density lipoproteins, are usually referred to as bad cholesterol. LDLs are responsible for depositing the excess cholesterol on the arterial walls.

HDL

HDLs, or high-density lipoproteins, are known as good cholesterol. HDLs remove excess cholesterol from the bloodstream. It is then returned to the liver for processing or elimination. The higher the proportion of HDL in the bloodstream, the lower the risk of heart disease.

Fiber

Fiber does not supply nutrients and is not digestible. It is a loose term for the indigestible substances in plant food. Pectin, cellulose, hemicellulose, crude fiber, and dietary fiber are all names for fiber. The skin of an apple or oat bran are examples of fiber. The normal and healthy functioning of the intestinal tract depends upon adequate fiber in the diet. The fiber attracts water into the digestive tract, softening stools and preventing constipation. It helps to exercise the muscles of the colon, helping to prevent diverticulosis. In addition, it speeds up the transit time through the digestive tract, reducing the exposure to cancer-causing agents. Fiber binds lipids and assists in the elimination of excess cholesterol. Approximately six grams daily of fiber, supplied by fresh fruits, vegetables, and complex carbohydrates, is adequate.

❧ A Well-Balanced Diet

How do we put all this information together so it can be easily understood? Divide foods into three main categories—fats, carbohydrates, and proteins—with the correct percentages that would represent a healthy diet. Placing the foods under their appropriate category would look like this:

Fats (10 to 15 percent)	Carbohydrates (70 to 80 percent)	Proteins (10 to 15 percent)
avocado	fruits	dairy
butter	legumes	fish
dairy	nuts	legumes
fish	potatoes	meats
meats	seeds	nuts
nuts	vegetables	poultry
oils	whole grains	seeds
poultry		vegetables
seeds		whole grains

The best supply of vitamins, minerals, fiber, carbohydrates, lipids (including essential fatty acids), and amino acids is under carbohydrates. This covers all the nutrients needed for a healthy diet. Many items listed in the carbohydrate column are also listed in the other two. If you incorporate 70 to 80 percent of your diet from the middle column, it will supply adequate amounts of vitamins, minerals, fiber, lipids, amino acids, and basic carbohydrates for energy metabolism. Fish or another animal protein could be added in moderation, if desired, about two to three times a week. Additional lipids and amino acids would then be supplied and you could still stay within the 10 to 15 percent levels. The trick to the above is to maintain a balance, stay away from known allergens, and explore for variety and new taste treats. Expand and explore; variety is the key. Different foods contain different nutrients even if it is from the same food family (spinach has a good deal of vitamin A, while chard has many B vitamins).

🦋 Food Combining for Amino Acids

The following food groups complement each other to provide the essential amino acids in balance. Other amino acids will also be present in these foods. The proper combining of these food groups form complete proteins. Potatoes, yams, sweet potatoes, and seaweed (micro algae) by themselves are very high in amino acids and provide complete protein.

Food Families

---

legumes and dairy (goat)   nuts or seeds and whole grains
legumes and whole grains   nuts or seeds and legumes
legumes and nuts or seeds   nuts or seeds and dairy (goat)

whole grains and dairy (goat)   mushrooms and peas
whole grains and legumes   mushrooms and cauliflower
whole grains and nuts or seeds

❧ Food Combining for Digestion

Food combining can be either simple or complex. Some people appear to benefit from careful combining of foods. For most, a simple approach is usually adequate. I recommend that all fruits, especially melons, be eaten separately from other foods. Fruits digest quickly (from thirty minutes to one hour) and can putrefy if they have to wait around for the digestion of other foods, which can take much longer to digest (pork takes up to nine hours).

A more complex version suggests that:

All vegetables together combine well.

All fruits together, except melons, combine well.

Whole grains combine with leafy vegetables.

Legumes combine with leafy vegetables.

Protein (flesh foods) combine with leafy vegetables.

Nuts and seeds combine with leafy vegetables.

Starchy (sweet) vegetables like carrots and beets do not mix well with fruits or protein foods such as whole grains, legumes, nuts and seeds, or flesh.

🦋 Digestive Enzymes

The digestive juices which cause the chemical breakdown of food contain complex proteins called enzymes. These enzymes induce changes in other substances without being changed themselves. Each digestive enzyme has a specific action and is capable of breaking down only one substance. Amylase breaks down carbohydrates; protease helps to digest protein; and lipase aids in fat digestion.

Digestion and this enzymatic action occurs in the four major areas of the salivary glands, stomach, pancreas, and the wall of the small intestine. Amylase in found in the saliva, or the mouth, and works on carbohydrates. The stomach contains protease; and the protease, along with another enzyme pepsin (found in the gastric juices), assists in the digestion of proteins. When the partially digested food (chyme) enters the small intestine from the stomach, the pancreas secretes additional enzymes (amylase, protease, and lipase) and a substance that neutralizes the digestive acids.

Fat digestion is more complicated. It begins in the acid environment of the cardiac portion of the stomach where the enzyme lipase is found. Additional lipase is also released by the pancreas when the fat reaches the small intestine. Bile, an enzyme produced by the liver and stored in the gallbladder, aids in the digestion of fats. Other enzymes that you may hear about, or see listed on a supplement are the proteolytic enzymes. These work exclusively on proteins and are called pepsin, trypsin, rennin, pancreatin, and chymotrypsin. Hydrochloric acid is secreted by the partial cells in the stomach muscosa and is necessary for proper digestion and assimilation. Cooking destroys these enzymes in the foods. An adequate amount of raw food in the diet will supply usable digestive enzymes, and prevent the depletion of the body's store of enzymes.

Even though a food is a good food (like whole wheat), does not mean that it is good for you. Any wholesome food can be a potential allergen. I have discovered clients that were sensitive to many usual vegetables and fruits, like cucumber, lettuce, zucchini, banana, apple, and plum. Do not assume anything; any and all food can be suspect. Complete allergy testing can be extremely important.

Notes

1. Jennifer Dixon, "USDA Boosts Big Food Companies." *Associated Press,* February 3, 1992.

2. Malcolm Gladwell, "Nutritional Advice Overhaul." *The Washington Post,* April 17, 1991.

CHAPTER 8

How to Shop

O MAKE LASTING CHANGES in your lifestyle and increase your awareness of the food industry, read! Reading labels in the supermarket and the health food store is a major keys to your health. Consumer demands for more information has led to changes in labeling procedures. The following chapter will add even more clarity for conscious buying, especially for those with allergy concerns. As an added bonus, you will discover that eating healthy is not expensive.

This information will assist you in deciphering the new nutritional information labels and enable you to identify potential problems. Support and hints will help guide you through the maze of shopping, especially if you are unfamiliar with health food products. With this new knowledge, you can make healthy, conscious choices regarding your health and the health of your family.

Where to Shop

Many of the things necessary for a healthy diet can be purchased at the supermarket, even the super store where one can buy anything from food to clothing, from drugs to oil for the car. Supermarkets often contain health food sections, or health foods scattered in several different departments.

If you have not yet discovered your local health food store, do so. The employees are usually helpful, friendly, and willing to spend time explaining products and answering questions. But just because it is a health food store does not mean that everything in it is healthy. There are several different types of health food stores. The supplement variety, usually found in malls, sells mainly supplements. The most common type of health food store sells supplements, herbs, grains, flours, pastas, canned foods, oils, juices, cosmetics, and has a refrigerator or freezer section with juices, soy or goat dairy products. The larger health food stores carry all of the above, plus a produce section featuring organic produce. The super health food store, the supermarket of health food stores, includes all of the above and a complete selection of organic poultry, meat, and fish. Frequently, the health food stores will have a delicatessen or small restaurant available.

For those who live in the country or even the suburbs, you may be familiar with the farmer's market, a local produce stand, or a farm where you can go once a week or so to purchase produce and other products like honey, herbs, or dairy. These can be a delightful adventure for everyone, especially for those who live in the city, a feast for the eye, and an inspiration to your cooking. Often growers will share their favorite recipes. It can be educational and fun, especially for children. To locate the nearest farmer's market, local produce stand, or farm, contact your county or state Department of Agriculture. In Northern California, we have Farm Trails, which lists the local farms, their produce, when to buy their products, and the locations. Contacting your local organic gardening club can be an additional source of information.

Another resource is the food co-op. A co-op is formed by a group of individuals and can be operated from a home or store, and will have various products available depending upon the size of the group. Frequently, they will carry the bulk items like grains, legumes, nuts, and other basic foods. This is an excellent place to buy long-term storage items. The prices are good and often the health food store has already purchased the products through the co-op.

🦋 Where to Buy

Not everything needed for a healthy, allergen-free diet can be purchased in the supermarket and it is not necessary to buy everything at the health food store. The following guidelines will be helpful:

Whole grains, cereals, flours, pastas are usually not available at the supermarket. The health food store or co-op are your best sources.

Real, whole grain bread can be found in supermarkets, health food stores, and local, whole grain bakeries, depending upon your area. In order for bread to be real, whole grain bread the label must read 100 percent stone ground whole wheat plus salt, water, yeast, oil, and a natural sweetener like honey. Even if the label reads whole wheat it may not be whole grain, as white flour is wheat. Food coloring, dough conditioners, and other additives are frequently added. If you cannot read or pronounce the ingredients listed on the label, forget the product.

Legumes can be purchased at the supermarket unless organic foods are required. Depending upon your area, only certain varieties will be available. The health food store will carry both organic and regular types of legumes and have more choices.

Nuts are available in their shells during the fall season at the supermarket, the farmer's market, and local farms or produce stands. Raw, shelled nuts and seeds should be found in the refrigerator section of the health food store all year round. Packaged, plain nuts are also available at the supermarket all year, but may be treated in some way. Some vending machines provide packaged nuts (other than peanuts) and seeds.

Juices can be found in both the supermarket or health food store. Plain juices without added sugar or fillers, like frozen orange juice, unfiltered apple juice, frozen or bottled grape juice, pineapple juice, prune juice, grapefruit juice, and others are available at the supermarket. Often the supermarket will include health store brands mixed in with their other juices. Explore the health food store for delicious different ideas, like boysenberry, cranberry, and papaya.

Goat and soy dairy products will be found at the health food store and sometimes at the farmer's market. A full-range co-op store may also carry these items. Tofu is frequently available at the supermarket. Specialty cheese shops or sections, may carry goat, soy, or even sheep cheese.

Different items like rice milk, are purchased at the health food store.

Miscellaneous products, like natural peanut butter, fruit juice-sweetened jams (no sugar), and good crackers without yeast (rye mainly, but also rice cakes), can be found at the supermarket, often at a savings over health food store prices.

Frozen fruits and vegetables are acceptable if there is no corn allergy. The packaging material is treated with corn. Freezing, however, destroys some nutrients; as much as 40 percent of the magnesium in peas can be lost in freezing. Health food stores, if they have a freezer section, will carry organic frozen fruits and vegetables. Frozen berries are a better buy than fresh because they will be free of molds and you only use what you need.

Meat, fish, and poultry can be obtained from several sources. The supermarket stocks all of these, but from a nonorganic source, usually containing antibiotics, hormones, chemicals, pesticides, artificial flavoring, artificial coloring, or tenderizers. Organic, or clean meat or poultry, can be found at a health food store or local ranch. Sometimes stores that sell specialty or ethnic foods will feature clean meat or poultry. A gourmet shop is also another possibility.

Fresh fruits and vegetables can be found at the supermarket, health food store, produce stand, farmer's market, local farm, and the co-op. Organic produce is sometimes available at the supermarket. It can be purchased at a health food store that carries organic produce.

🦋 Taking the Frustration Out of Shopping

Shopping can be an overwhelming experience, especially for those with Candida, CFS, EI, or severe allergies. The number of products, the seeming chaos, the energy of the other shoppers, and the harsh lighting can all contribute to the drain of your low energy and ability to cope. Once you are in control of your shopping needs and making informed decisions, shopping will become a new and more pleasant experience. It can be fun and something to look forward to. The challenge may be especially rewarding as you find that you will also be saving money.

There is a definite pattern to the floor plan and arrangement found in the supermarket. Understanding the plan and shopping from your list will eliminate unnecessary purchases and impulse buying. It is true that it is a bad idea to go shopping when you are hungry. When you are new at this method of shopping, allow plenty of time for your first visit to the stores to explore and to read labels.

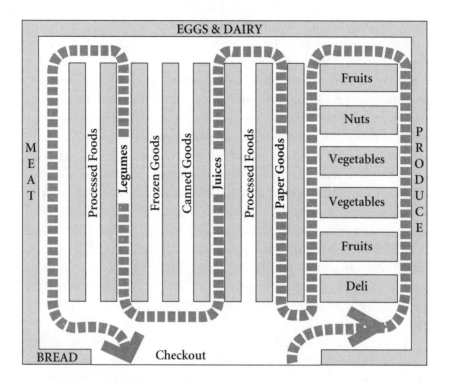

The basic arrangement found in the supermarkets are designed to draw attention to the high profit items with bright colors, snappy phrases, and addictive appeal. Candy, magazines, and other last minute items are available at the check-out counter. The products that are attractive to small children—the sugared, popular, advertised cereals or fruit drinks—are placed at their eye level. Snack foods, like chips or cookies, may be scattered throughout the store. It can become a confusing maze.

Make a shopping list of healthy foods and allergy restrictions. Shop for the basics and staples (see page 125). Leave the boxes, mixes, and processed foods alone. Not only will you improve your health, but you will also save money. Processed foods cost more per serving and frozen vegetables are more expensive than fresh. Cake mixes contain flour, sugar (usually first on the label), salt, leavening, and flavoring plus a long list of chemicals and additives. You have to add the eggs and oil, which are the expensive items. A cake mix will run anywhere from 89 cents to $1.49; using ingredients in your cupboard will cost approximately 25 cents. Packaged foods do not require less time. To make the mix, you have to measure the oil and water, assemble pans, mixer, eggs, flour and butter the pans, preheat the oven, and then mix it together. Making the cake from scratch includes all of the above plus measuring the flour, salt, leavening, and flavoring, like vanilla. The amount of time saved using the cake mix is about five minutes, not nearly enough time to justify the added expense and questionable nutritional quality.

The supermarket is usually laid out with the basic, good food items located on the perimeter of the store: dairy, eggs, meats/fish, and produce sections. Start shopping around the outside areas where these foods are found. Only go into the aisles when you know there are things you need, like legumes, juices, and toilet paper. Leave the other aisles alone. Read all the labels and do not assume anything; check the label first and search all the fine print. Remember to leave sufficient time for your first few visits to the stores in order to read the labels and discover where the good, basic products are located. Subsequent trips to the store will become easier and faster.

This information should empower you to see that you do have choices and control over your life. The empowerment will come from the sense of self-reliance achieved by doing things for yourself, making informed decisions, and rediscovering connections with the earth and the people growing food, getting closer to the source of our nourishment. Shopping can then become an interesting challenge and an enjoyable experience as you explore the various stores and other places for finding food.

❦ Labels

It is very important to read labels and all the fine print on any food purchase. The information is a key that will enable you to make informed decisions about the food you eat. This can literally mean the difference between life and death, or at least a trip to the emergency room, for individuals with severe allergies.

In May 1993, a new U.S. law went into effect regarding the information printed on labels regarding contents and nutritional information for food items. Consumer desire for clearer, more understandable, and easier to read labels led to the implementation of this new law, but the new labeling still leaves much to be deciphered. In December 1991, humorist Erma Bombeck wrote in her nationally syndicated column, "I don't trust the government to simplify anything. For example, the FDA food-labeling proposal will include definitions of terms. Here's a sample: "A word like 'more' means that food contains more of a desirable nutrient, such as fiber or potassium, than does a comparable food. To use the term, a food must contain at least 10 percent more of the nutrient than the comparable food." See what I mean? American housewives want to buy healthy. They just don't have three days to stand around over a shopping cart reading labels, looking up definitions and separating fat from saturated fat." For even more confusion, a soup label may state that it is low fat but neglect to say that it is high in sodium. Low fat cottage cheese is higher in sodium than regular cottage cheese. The low calorie desserts are frequently as much as 50 percent fat. But there is some positive, wonderful news for those with allergies. Umbrella terms such as "natural flavoring," "food coloring" and "vegetable oil" must list their sources. Caseinate, a milk derivative,

Nutrition Facts

Serving Size 1 cup (228g)
Servings Per Container 2

Amount Per Serving

Calories 90   Calories from Fat 30

	% Daily Value*
Total Fat 3g	**5%**
Saturated Fat 0g	**0%**
Cholesterol 0mg	**0%**
Sodium 300mg	**13%**
Total Carbohydrate 13g	**4%**
Dietary Fiber 3g	**12%**
Sugars 3g	
Protein 3g	

Vitamin A 80%	•	Vitamin C 60%
Calcium 4%	•	Iron 4%

* Percent Daily Values are bsed on a 2,000 calorie diet. Your daily values may be higher or lower depending on your calorie needs:

		Calories:	2,000	2,500
Total Fat	Less than		65g	80g
Sat Fat	Less than		20g	25g
Cholesterol	Less than		300mg	300mg
Sodium	Less than		2,400mg	2,400mg
Total Carbohydrate			300g	375g
Dietary Fiber			25g	30g

Calories per gram:
Fat 9 • Carbohydrates 4 • Protein 4

has to be identified in foods that claim to be nondairy, such as coffee whiteners. Vegetable oil must be identified as soy or peanut or corn and others. Certified color additives must be named. Drinks that claim to contain fruit juice must say what percentage is juice. The specific ingredients lists are a great help to people with food allergies and sensitivities, or are vegetarians.

🦋 Tips For Label Reading

Main ingredients are listed in descending order and comprise 98 percent of the product.

All natural means the product ingredients were produced solely by nature. It does not mean that it is healthy; sugar begins from a natural source, white flour starts with whole wheat.

"Lite," means ⅓ fewer calories, or 50 percent less fat, than the regular product.

Cholesterol free means fewer than 2 milligrams of cholesterol and 2 grams or fewer saturated fat.

Low cholesterol means 20 milligrams or less cholesterol and 2 grams or less saturated fat.

Low fat means three grams or less of fat per serving.

Fat free means less than ½ gram of fat per serving.

Low calorie means 40 calories or less per serving.

Reduced calorie means at least 25 percent fewer calories than the regular product.

Reduced sugars or less sugar means at least 25 percent less sugar than the regular product.

Sugar free means less than ½ gram of any sugars.

Low sodium means 140 milligrams or less of sodium.

The term organic means that it is grown without the use of chemicals, pesticides, or drugs.

The phrase "80 percent fat free" may refer to the weight of the fat in the food not the percentage of calories from fat.

Not everything that is in the product has to be included on the label.

Enriched means that the manufacturer has replaced nutrients that have been destroyed during processing. The replacement only includes those nutrients that have been determined to cause severe deficiencies in the diet if not added, like vitamin D, B_1 (thiamine), B_3 (niacin), B_2 (riboflavin). Whole wheat contains the eleven B factors that comprise the B complex. Processed white flour contains none. Enriched white flour has B_1, B_2, and B_3 added usually in the form of malted barley which is both a sugar and a yeast.

Fortified means that the manufacturer has added more than the bare minimum required to enrich the product. Usually, the vitamin sources are synthetic and artificial.

Real, pure, fresh, no added sugar, no preservatives added, and fiber rich are designed to attract your attention and draw you to the product. Watch out for these. With no added sugar they neglect to inform you that sugar may already be in the product not listed as sugar but with another name for it. I found a juice spritzer with no added sugar written on the label. When I finally found the fine print, I discovered that the first ingredient was sucrose, which is nothing more than regular, white, refined sugar.

As of May 1994, foods made in the United States must utilize the new standardized form for labeling, "Nutrition Facts" (see example on page 109). This new label form with larger print, and logically arranged information will be helpful. Problem areas to watch out for are those that are exempt from the labeling law: foods served in restaurants, cafeterias, airports, and ready-to eat foods from bakeries and delicatessens; bulk foods; food vendors such as mall cookie counters; foods produced by small businesses; medical foods—specially formulated for people with medical or metabolic disorders; foods sold in very small packages. If the product is regulated by the FDA, a telephone number or address for consumers to get the information must be provided.

Fat percentage on a label is a nightmare. This information may be helpful. Each gram of fat contains 9 calories (each carbohydrate contains 4 calories). If the product has a total of 160 calories and 9 grams (9 x 9 = 81) of total fat, the product is 50 percent fat. Another labeling problem resulting from the new legislation is that the fat percentage is based upon a 2000 calorie diet, not what is the actual percentage for that product. One product I noticed listed 90 calories total and 30 fat calories (3 grams of fat, 3 x 9 = 27), the percentage for fat listed was 5 percent. The actual percentage is 33 percent or ⅓ fat.

The following are lists of the most frequently used common allergens that are found in food and other products. Quite often they are discovered under another name or hidden in a common food.

Sugar

Sugar refers to refined products whether from sugar cane, corn, or beet (see page 133 for more information).

Also Known As

Beet sugar
Brown sugar
Cane syrup
Confectioner's sugar
Corn syrup
Dextrin
Dextrose
Fructose/levulose
Galactose
Glucose
Jaguary sugar
Lactose
Malt syrup
Maltodextrin
Maltose
Molasses
Raw sugar
Sucanat

Sucrose
Turbinado
Xylose

Artificial Sugars

Aspartame
Cyclamate
Maltitol
Mannitol
Saccharin
Sorbitol
Xylitol

Hidden Food Sources

Bakery goods
Bouillon
Bread/rolls
Breaded fish
Breaded vegetables

Canned beans
Canned clams
Canned soups
Canned and frozen fruit
Carob treats
Cereals
Chinese food
Chips, flavored
Cigarettes
Condiments (catsup, mustard)
Desserts (cake, pie)
Frozen entrees
Frozen juice
Frozen potatoes
Ham
Hot dogs
Hundai rice
Liquor

Over-the-counter drugs
Pizza
Prescription drugs
Processed meats
Recreational drugs
   (cocaine)
Salad dressings
Salt

Sauce and gravy mixes
Sauces (barbecue,
   tomato, chili)
Sweetened mineral
   water
Tomato sauce
Toothpaste
Turkey

Weight loss products
White flour
Yogurt, flavored

This list is NOT all
   inclusive!

Yeast

Also Known As

Baker's yeast
Brewer's yeast
Fermentation
Fungus
Malted barley
Molds
Sourdough starter

Hidden Food Sources

Ale and beer
Antibiotics
B vitamins (yeast
   source)
Bakery products
Berries (molds)
Bouillon
Bread
Breaded fish
Breaded vegetables
Canned soups
Catsup
Cereals
Cheeses (molds)
Chili peppers, pickled

Cookies
Cottage cheese
Crackers
Dressings
Dried fruits (molds)
Extracts, vanilla and
   others
Fortified or enriched
   products
Frozen entrees
Gerber's oatmeal (baby)
Ginger ale
Gravy and sauce mixes
Herb tinctures
Horseradish
Malted products (milk)
Mayonnaise
Milk, fortified
Minced pie, commercial
Mushrooms
Mustard, commercial
Olives
Pickles
Pizza
Pretzels

Processed foods
Relish
Root beer
Salad dressings
Sauces (barbecue, chili,
   tomato)
Sauerkraut
Soft-shelled melons
   (molds)
Sourdough bread
Soy sauce
Stuffing mix
Truffles
Vinegars
White flour
Wine
Yeast-free sourdough
   starter (sourdough
   not listed on the
   label)

Peanut

Also Known As

Goober

Hidden Food Sources

Candy
Cereal mixes
Chocolate
Granola
Indian cooking
Margarine
Mixed nuts
Oriental cooking
"Party" mix
Peanut butter
Peanut oil
Salad dressings,
    commercial
Thai cooking
Vegetable glycerin
Vegetable oil

Dairy

Also Known As

Acidophilus milk
Beef
Bovine serum albumin
Breast milk (mother
    drinks cow's milk)
Butter
Buttermilk
Casein
Cheese
Condensed
Cottage cheese
Cow dairy products
Cow's milk
Cream
Cream cheese
Evaporated
Hydrolyzed casein
Keifer
Lactose
Milk
Nonfat
Parmesan cheese
Powdered/dry
Ricotta
Skim
Sour cream
Whey
Yogurt

Infant formula

Nutramigen
Progestimil

Hidden Food Sources

Au Gratin dishes
Bread products
Candy
Chocolate (except
    bitter)
Chowders
Cocoa (all forms)
Cocomalt
Cream pie
Cream sauces, commer-
    cial
Cream soups
Custards
Donuts
Fritters
Frozen yogurt
Gravies, commercial
Hamburger mixes
Hard sauce
Hot dogs
Ice cream
Ice milk
Instant cereals
Junket
Lunch meats
Macaroni
Malted milk
Mixes (muffin, Bisquik,
    pancake)
Nondairy substitutes
Noodles

Nougat
Omelets
Ovaltine
Pie crust
Pizza
Potato mixes (box or frozen)
Prescription drugs

Pudding
Quiche
Rarebits
Recreational drugs (cocaine)
Salad dressings
Salami
Sausages

Sherbet
Soda crackers
Soufflés
Soy cheese products (some)
Spaghetti
Timbales
Zwieback

Wheat

Also Known As

Bagels
Bran
Bulgur
Couscous
Durham
Gluten flour
Self-rising flour
Seminola
Unbleached
Wheat germ
White flour
Whole wheat

Hidden Food Sources

Baked beans
Baked goods
Barbecue chips
Beer
Beverages
Biscuits
Bouillon
Bread crumbs
Breaded fish

Breads
Cakes
Cereals
Chili
Chips
Chowders
Cocomalt
Cones
Cookies
Corn flakes
Crackers
Custards
Donuts
Dumplings
Farina
Frozen entrees
Gin
Graham
Grapenuts
Gravies
Hamburger
Hot dogs
Lunch meats
Macaroni
Malted milk

Matzos
Mayonnaise
Mead's cereal
Meat loaf
Meats
Muffins
Noodles
Ovaltine
Pablum
Pancake mixes
Pancakes
Pastry
Pies
Pizza
Popovers
Postum
Potato chips
Pretzels
Pudding
Ralston's Pep
Ravioli
Rice Krispies
Rolls
Salad dressings
Sauce mixes

Sausage   Synthetic pepper   Waffles
Soups   Teething biscuits   Whiskey
Spaghetti   Vermicelli
Stuffing   Vitamin E

Corn

Also Known As

Corn cereal
Corn chips
Corn flour
Corn oil
Corn on the cob
Corn sugar
Corn syrup
Corn tortillas
Cornmeal
Cornstarch
Dextrin
Dextrose
Fructose
Glucose
Hominy
Kernel corn
Margarine
Polenta
Popcorn
Sorbitol

Infant formulas

Advance
Enfamil
Isomil
Lofenalac
Nursoy (powder)

Pedialyte
Portagen
Prosobee
Similac
Soylac (except I-Soylac)

Hidden Food Sources

Ale and beer
Bacon
Baking mixes
Baking powders
Batters for frying
Beets, Harvard
Bleached white flour
Body building products
Bread, commercial
Brown sugar
Cake mixes
Candied fruits
Candy
Canned fruits
Carob (CaraCoa)
Catsup
Cereals
Cheeses
Chewing gum
Chili, canned
Chinese food

Chips
Chocolate
Coffee Rich
Confectioner's sugar
Cookies
Cottage cheese
Cranberry juice
Cream pies
Cream puffs
Custard, commercial
Dates, confection
Donuts
Dried fruits
Eggnog
Frosting, commercial
Frozen fruit, sweetened
Fruit desserts
Fruit juice drinks
Fried foods
Fish (batter, frozen,
    fresh)
French dressing
Gelatin (mixes and
    desserts)
Gin
Ginger ale
Graham crackers
Gravies and mixes

Grits
Ham
Hot dogs
Ice cream
Jellies and jams
Jell-O
Karo syrup
Leavening agents
Lemonade
Lunch meats
Metrical
Mixes
Monosodium glutamate
Orange juice
Pablum
Paper milk containers
Pastries, commercial
Peanut butter
Peas (canned)
Pickles
Pie fillings
Pizza
Pork and beans
Pudding
Puretose syrup
Ravioli
Rice (coated)
Root beer
Salami
Salad dressings
Salt
Sandwich spreads
Sauces (mixes and
    bottled)
Sausages
Sherbets

Soft drinks
Soups (canned)
Soy milk (some)
Spaghetti (some)
String beans
Succotash
Sweetose
Tea (instant)
Vanillin
Vegetables (canned,
    creamed, frozen)
Vinegar, distilled
Waffles, commercial
Weight loss products
Whipped cream,
    commercial
Whiskey
Wieners
Wines
Yeast
Yogurt, flavored

Nonfood Products

Adhesive tape
Aspirin
Bath and body powders
Breath spray and drops
Capsules
Cough syrups
Dentifrices
Deordorant soap
Envelopes
Excipients
Hair spray
Hand soap
Labels

Laundry soap
Lozenges
Ointments
Paper products (boxes,
    cups, plates)
Plastic wrap (some)
Stamps
Starch
Starched clothing
Starching products
Stickers
Suppositories
Tablets (medicine)
Talcum powder
Toothpaste/powder
Vitamins (some)

Soy

Also Known As

Bean sprouts
Cellulose
Glycerin
Hydrolyzed vegetable
    protein
Lecithin
Miso
Nitroglycerin
Soy beans
Soy dairy products
Soy nuts
Soy oil
Soy pastas
Soy sprouts
Soy sauce
Tofu

Infant formulas

Advance
Alimentum
Good Start
Infamil
Isomil
Nursoy
Portagen
Prosobee
Similac
SMA
Soyalac/I-Soyalac

Hidden Food Sources

Baby food
Baked goods
Butter substitutes
Candy
Cereals
Coffee Rich
Coffee substitute
Crisco
Custard
Dry lemonade mix
Hamburger mixes
Ice cream
Joyanna
Lea & Perrins sauce
Liquid protein foods
Lunch meat
Margarine
Mayonnaise
Mull-Soy
Pam
Puritan Oil
Reezon (seasoning)
Salad dressings
Sausage
Sobee
Soups
Spry
Vitamin E
Weight loss products
Worcestershire sauce

Nonfood Products

Adhesive tape
Animal fodder
Automobile parts
Blankets
Candles
Cloth
Cosmetics
Enamels
Envelopes
Fertilizer
Labels
Linoleum
Lubricating oils
Massage creams
Paper sizing and finish
Pet food
Printing ink
Stamps
Stickers
Soap
Textile dressing
Varnish

Eggs

Also Known As

Albumin
Dried egg
Egg white
Egg yoke
Powdered egg

Hidden Food Sources

Baby food (some)
Baked goods
Baking powders
Bavarian cream
Batters for frying
Bouillon
Bread crumbs
Candy
Coffee
Custards
Cakes
Creamed foods
Croquettes
Crusts (shiny)
Cookies
Consommés
Donuts
Deviled egg
Dumplings
Fritters
Frostings
French toast
French ice cream
Glazed rolls and pastry
Hamburger mixes
Hollandaise sauce
Ices
Ice cream
Icings
Laxatives (Agarol)
Meringue
Macaroons
Malted cocoa drinks
Meat loaf
Marshmallows
Noodles
Omelets
Pancake mixes
Pie fillings
Pudding
Pretzels
Quiche
Quick breads (muffins, banana)
Root beer
Salad dressings
Sauces
Sausages
Sherbet
Soufflé
Soups (some)
Stuffings
Tarter sauce
Timbales
Waffle mix
Wine (cleared with egg white)

Cottonseed

Also Known As

Cottonseed flour
Cottonseed meal
Cottonseed oil
Linters
Xylose (sugar)

Hidden Food Sources

Baked goods, commercial
Barbecue sauce
Chocolate
Cheese pizza mix
Crisco
Donuts
Dry lemonade mix
Fried foods, commercial
Margarine
Mayonnaise
Milk (animals fed with cottonseed oil)

Olive oil
Polish on fruit
Popcorn, commercial
Popcorn oil
Potato chips
Salad oils
Sardines
Sweet and sour dressing,
    commercial

Tartar sauce,
    commercial

Nonfood Sources

Animal feed
Camphorated oil
Cosmetics
Cotton batting:
    Comforters

Cushions
Mattresses
Pads
Upholstery
Fertilizer
Miner's lamp
Varnish

Flaxseed

Also Known As

Bi-flax
Flaxlinum
Flaxolyn
Flaxseed meal
Flaxseed oil
Flaxseed tea
Kremel
Linen

Hidden Food Sources

Beef (animals fed with
    flaxseed)
Cereals
Milk (animals fed with
    flaxseed)
Poultry (animals fed
    with flaxseed)

Nonfood Sources

Art linen
Bird lime
Cambric
Carron oil
Collars and cuffs
Cough remedies
Damask
Depilatories
Dress linen
Fiberboard
Flaxseed poultices
Furniture polish
Hair products
Handkerchief
Insulating material
Laxative
Linoleum
Linseed oil
Lithographic ink
Oil cloth
Paints and varnish
Paper

Plaster
Printer's ink
Refrigerator
Rugs
Sewing thread
Sheeting
Soft soap
Straw mats
Table linen
Upholstery (cushions)
Wax paper

Bisulfites

Also Known As

Metabisulfites
Potassium
Sodium Metabisulfite
Sulfites
Sulfur dioxide

Hidden Food Sources

Ale and beer
Beet sugar
Cheese pastes
Chicken loaf
Cookies
Cordials
Corn sweeteners
Crackers
Dairy products
Fruit yogurt
Dessert toppings
Dried fruit
Dried vegetables
Food starch
Mushrooms, fresh
Fried potatoes
Frozen pizza
Fruit
Fruit bars
Gelatin
Hot dogs
Instant potatoes
Jams
Juice
Maraschino cherries
Olives
Pastry
Pickles
Relish
Restaurant foods
Sauerkraut
Sausages
Shellfish
Sodas
Tomato paste and puree
Vegetables
Vinegar
Wines

Nonfood Sources

Adrenaline ampoules
Antibiotics
Antiemetic drugs
Asthma drugs
Cardiovascular drugs
Compazine
Gerovital
GH-3 (supplement)
I.V. solutions
Novocain (dentist)
Psychotropic drugs
Smog
Steroids

Monosodium Glutamate

The following information is condensed from *In Bad Taste–The MSG Syndrome* by George R. Schwartz, M.D. (Santa Fe, NM: Health Press, 1988).

Also Known As

Accent (seasoning)
Ajinomoto
Chinese seasoning
Flavorings
Glutacyl
Glutavene
Gourmet powder
Hydrolyzed vegetable
   protein (12 to 20
   percent MSG)
Hydrolyzed plant
   protein
Kombu extract
Mei-jing
Monopotassium
   glutamate
Monosodium glutamate
   (MSG)
Natural flavorings
RL-5

Subu
Vetsin
Wei-jing
Zest

Hidden Food Sources

Accent (seasoning)
Alfredo sauce,
   commercial
Bacon (cured, smoked)
Basted turkey, frozen
Beef, canned
Beef (smoked, jerky)
Beef stew, canned
Bouillon
Breaded fish
Breading mixes
Chicken (canned,
   smoked, cured)
Chicken salad,
   commercial
Chili, canned
Chinese food (canned,
   frozen, fresh)
Chowders
Corn chips
Crab or clam, canned
Crackers
Croutons
Delicatessen items
Diet foods (Lean
   Cuisine, Weight
   Watchers)
Dips (for chips)
Dried soup mix
Freeze dried food (Back

Packers Pantry,
   Mountain House)
Fried chicken, frozen
Gefilte fish
Goya All Purpose
   (seasoning)
Gravy mixes
Italian dishes, frozen
Lawry's garlic salt
   (seasoning)
Manischewitz Fishlets
Manischewitz Pike
Manischewitz Whitefish
Meat entrees, frozen
Mexican food, frozen
Noodles, canned
Pasta salad, commercial
Pizza, frozen
Potato chips
Potatoes, frozen
Poultry injected with
   broth
Ravioli, canned
Rice mixes
Salad dressings
Salad toppings,
   commercial
Salads, commercial
   (Suddenly Salad)
Sausage (smoked,
   cured)
Schilling Savor Salt
Schilling Season All
Seasoned lite salt
Seasoned vegetables,
   frozen

Seasoning mixes (flavor
   packs)
Seasoning salt
Soups, canned
Soy sauce
Spaghetti, canned
Spike All Purpose
   (seasoning)
Steak sauce
Stuffing mixes
Tater Tots, frozen
Tobacco
Tortellini, canned
Tuna
Tuna salad, commercial
Turkey, canned
White or red clam
   sauce, commercial
Worcestershire sauce

Other Sources

Airline food
Cafeterias
Fast food
   Wendy's
   Jack-in-the-Box
   Burger King
   McDonald's
   Arby's
   Denny's
   Dairy Queen
   Kentucky Fried
   Chicken
Restaurants
Passenger ships
Passenger trains

Chapter 9

Helpful Hints

MANY QUESTIONS ARISE SURROUNDING the preparation, use, cooking, storing, and buying of unfamiliar foods and products. Will I need to buy different cooking equipment? Where can I purchase these foods or products? Which is the most economical? How to store them? Will I always be cooking or thinking about food? What is my time factor and involvement? What should I have on hand or do I have to go to the store every day? This chapter will answer these questions and others you may have.

Whether you are a health food lover, a gourmet cook taught in Paris, or a basic home cook, you all have one thing in common. All food preparation begins with fresh, whole, natural foods and uses no packaged mixes or artificial ingredients.

Healthy eating does not have to be bland, restrictive, boring, or strange. A healthy lifestyle can be creative, stimulating, and fun, yet simple, and does not have to be restrictive or dull. Some change in habits will have to occur in order to be successful. Change is more about your perception and approach, rather than an enormous upheaval in daily living. The approach is to help you see things in a different way—the how of change: honesty, open mindedness, and willingness.

Included in this chapter are an equipment list, a staple list, storage and preparation of foods, the why of organic, a discussion of water and air quality, basic cooking hints, and a simple cooking dictionary. Many items that will be discussed you may use already. No mysterious or complicated items are mentioned. Practicality and simplicity is the guideline.

Equipment List

Blender or food processor

Cast iron frying pans, muffins tins, Dutch oven, or griddle

Egg beater or hand mixer

Glass baking dishes or casseroles

Grater

Kitchen knives

Measuring spoons and cups

Mixing bowls and spoons

Rolling pin

Sifter

Spatulas

Stainless steel cookware (*do not* use aluminum)

Strainers and colander

Vegetable peeler

Vegetable steamer (steamers from a cookware set, the fold-up variety, or an oriental bamboo steamer basket)

Wire whisk

Optional Equipment List (see page 464 for manufacturers, brands, and addresses)

Sprout jars or basket
Sprouting jars can be made from any wide mouth jar with screening or cheese cloth as a covering. Fresh, homemade sprouts can ease the worry of mold and mildew forming.

Grain mill
A grain mill is a fun addition to your kitchen, especially if you do not have the different grain flours available in your area. A good mill will grind any grain into a flour. The whole grains will store for a long time.

Juicer
A wonderful piece of equipment for extracting the juice from fruits and vegetables. The juice is loaded with nutritional value. A juicer does not have be overly expensive or complicated. The Krups juicer makes an excellent product, is easy to clean, reasonably priced, and can be found at major department stores.

Wok
An excellent tool for cooking oriental dishes and stir frying vegetables.

✤ Staples

Staples are items used often in cooking and baking that will keep over a long period of time. Having a supply of frequently used products on hand will eliminate unnecessary shopping trips. Cooking will be more fun and less time consuming.

Certain foods definitely belong on the staple list. Your list will depend upon your allergy restrictions and taste preferences. The following suggestions may be helpful: grains (whole, pasta, cereals, crackers, flour), legumes (whole, pasta, flour), and nuts and seeds (butters and whole). Vegetables like potatoes, onions, carrots, garlic, and celery also keep and store well.

Cooking Basics

Baking powder

Baking soda

Black pepper

Extracts (vanilla, almond)

Gelatin (agar)

Herbal teas

Herbs (oregano, rosemary, tarragon)

Margarine or butter

Oils (olive, canola)

Powdered broth (vegetable bouillon)

Sea salt

Spices (nutmeg, cinnamon)

Sweeteners (honey, rice syrup)

Thickeners (cornstarch, arrowroot, egg replacer)

Vinegars

Canned goods are also important and convenient for cooking. Choose carefully and be sure to read all labels. Some ideas are tomato sauce or paste, fruits in their own juice, beans, whole tomatoes, fruit juices, jams and jellies, coconut milk, and fish.

🦋 Storage and Preparation of Foods

Some people have never used fresh produce and other foods which require some preparation. For many people, the box, can, and microwave have been a way of life. There is a mystery surrounding fresh produce, especially that it will be a time consuming or more expensive. This is not necessarily true. It may take a few more minutes to prepare for cooking, but it frequently costs less, and the rewards are great. Remember the taste of tomatoes right off the vine or garden fresh corn? Rediscover those tastes through the use of fresh produce.

In support of a healthy and allergy-free diet, the proper storage and preparation of foods is important. Specific information for grains, legumes, nuts and seeds, and oils are found in their individual chapters. The following general guidelines will be helpful.

Storage

All basic staples should be stored in a cool, dark, dry place away from direct sunlight.

Store potatoes and onions in a cool dark place. They do not require refrigeration. Store potatoes away from sunlight in a paper bag.

Vegetables need to be refrigerated. Storage time will depend upon variety. Leafy types do not last long and should be used fresh. Root vegetables like carrots, beets, and turnips will last for a long time. Head varieties like cabbage, broccoli, cauliflower, and artichoke have a longer shelf life than leafy types and less than root vegetables. Do NOT wash vegetables until ready to use.

Hard fruits, like apples, will keep for a period of time and do not require refrigeration. If you have room, storage time will increase with refrigeration. Citrus fruits will store for about a month in a cool place. Soft fruits, like peaches, should be eaten right away. Berries can pose special problems; they are delicious fresh, but molds and mildew form quickly. Frequently, when you purchase berries in the store, you will discover moldy berries in the basket. One solution is to buy the previously frozen varieties. There are many varieties available frozen without sugar. Better yet, find a source of fresh berries from your own garden or a local berry farm.

A freezer should be kept at 32 degrees F for the most efficient storage of foods. Rotate the stored foods and be sure not to keep them too long.

Meats, fish, and poultry, if purchased fresh, should be used as quickly as possible. Depending upon the recipe, meats can be cooked while still frozen. It merely adds to the cooking time. If the meat has defrosted, then it needs to be cooked immediately.

Preparing Food for Storage

Choose fresh, firm, unbruised fruits and vegetables. Refrigerate if necessary until ready to use; washing is not needed.

When ready to use, wash vegetables in cool water. There is no need to soak them: they will loose nutrients. Washing with a special solution will not remove pesticide residue or chemicals. If chemicals have been used, they have been applied periodically during the growing season and have penetrated the plant. Use only running water for leafy vegetables, and a vegetable brush for mushrooms and potatoes to remove surface dirt. Discard coarse stems or any bruised looking areas. Peel produce that has been waxed as a preservative. For those with severe allergies or chemical sensitivities, use purified water for rinsing.

Wash poultry, fish, and organ meats. Make sure that any surface which comes into contact with these items are thoroughly cleaned afterward.

Fresh fish should be used the day it is purchased. If not, then rinse the fish with cold water, pat dry, wrap in plastic, and store in coldest section of the refrigerator for no more than 48 hours. If frozen, use within two months. Thaw in refrigerator before cooking, not at room temperature, or cook while still frozen, allowing extra time.

Rinse and sort through the legumes to make sure there are no stones or other foreign matter in them.

🦋 Why Organic?

For those with severe allergies and chemical sensitivities organic products are essential. In my practice, I have found clients allergic to a store-
bought egg, but have no reaction to an organic egg. This can also apply
to other foods, especially if you are chemically sensitive. For those who
desire to improve the quality of their health, organic foods play an important part. The delicious taste of organic produce is well worth any extra
effort involved. Good, fresh produce can be obtained in the local supermarket, farmer's market, local produce stands, yours or a friend's garden, a community garden, the local chapter of an organic gardening
club, and health food stores. Be aware: not all produce available in a
health food store is organic, and organic produce can even be found in
some supermarkets. Unless the product says certified organic, it is not
truly organic. Foods in health food stores are rated according to their
degree of organic purity. They are frequently labeled on packages, bins,
and in the produce department. In a full service health food store, organic
meat and fish are also available.

🦋 Water

One of the frequently overlooked aspects of health is the quality of water.
Water makes up 57 percent of the human body. Considering the high
percentage of water in the human body, we should evaluate the amount
and quality of the water we drink everyday. It is one area of life in which
you can have some control; for those with allergies and chemical sensitivities it is essential. People are often allergic to the water they use and
can be one of the biggest problems they will face in recovery. If you say,
I can't stand water, perhaps you have allergy to it. I have found this to
be true for my clients.

Water helps to cleanse and purify the body. Drinking 6 to 8 glasses
of clean water everyday will detox your system of impurities, remove
toxins, waste, and chemicals, also help you to lose weight. Most weight
loss programs encourage drinking lots of water everyday. In obese people, fat has replaced the water in the body. Water may comprise only 45
percent of their bodies, instead of the 57 percent they should have.

The water from most municipal water systems is neither free from contaminates, nor does it contribute much that is worthwhile to health. You may be trying to solve this problem by only drinking bottled water, but the bottled water may not be necessarily pure, clean, or safe. If you buy bottled water for the home in 5 or 6 gallon containers, the dispenser for the water must also be clean. Molds and mildew will easily form in the dispenser and spigot and both should be cleaned every time the bottle is changed. Chlorine bleach will kill the mold and mildew, but then there is the problem of successfully removing all traces of the chlorine. Chlorine readily mixes with other chemicals to form carcinogenic compounds. Chlorine and chlorine compounds (such as chlortrihalomethanes) have been identified in studies to be directly related to colon cancer.

Water should not be stored in soft plastic containers, like the water or milk gallon jugs that are often used. The plastic in these containers leeches chemicals into the water and combines with the contents to form other chemical compounds. Water can be stored safely only in glass, stainless steel, or hard plastic like two-liter pop bottles. It should not be placed in strong light or direct sunlight.

The best way to solve the water safety problem is a good water purifier. We personally and professionally endorse the Multi-Pure Corporation and its selection of products. Whether you live in a city, or in the country on a well, Multi-Pure has a solution to your problem. There are products for home, office, or travel. The patented Multi-Pure filter will remove lead, asbestos, pesticides, chemicals, bacteria, and microscopic impurities, but will retain the natural minerals essential for good health. For about seven cents a gallon, Multi-Pure will provide delicious clean water from your tap for drinking, cooking, and rinsing of food. Another reason we have confidence in this company, is that clean pure water is their only business.

Multi-Pure has been in business for over twenty years and has been tested and approved by NSF (National Sanitation Foundation). The MPC500 drinking water system is one of the first to be certified by the California Department of Health. It has recently been registered or certified in Iowa, Wisconsin, and Massachusetts. Multi-Pure will be more than happy to send you copies of the independent laboratory tests. For more information regarding Multi-Pure products or for a distributor near you, please call their toll free number (800) 622-9205. There are other companies on the market. Investigate and compare for yourself. Remember when you are considering other products, good, safe, quality drinking water is your concern.

🦋 Improving Air Quality

We cannot do very much to control our outside environment, but we can do something about our living space. The Environmental Protection Agency (EPA) has found that indoor sources of air may expose home dwellers to levels of toxic air polluted to ten times that of outdoor air. There are plants and products that can filter and clean the air inside the home. Filters range in size from small table units to a complete house system. For those with severe allergies and chemical sensitivities, a complete house system may be your solution to formaldehyde, combustion gasses, household chemicals, household odors, and excess humidity.

Many people already have air purifiers in their homes in the form of house plants. The plants exchange the carbon dioxide people exhale for the oxygen they produce. According to B. C. Worlverton, an environmental engineer and research scientist of NASA, some plants will absorb specific chemicals. The following is a partial list of these plants:

Spider plant—Formaldehyde

Golden pothos—Formaldehyde

English ivy—Benzene

Gerbera daisy—Trichloroethylene

Chrysanthemum—Trichloroethylene

🦋 Basic Time-Saving Cooking Hints

Easy cooking starts with good organization and planning ahead. Incorporate your methods and create your own solutions to the time problems surrounding cooking. The following ideas may be helpful and simplify the experience.

Keep your staple supply current.

Purchase vegetables for the week.

Work from a rotation plan or weekly menu.

Shop from a list.

Bake extra potatoes for hash browns or cottage fries.

Cook enough grains at breakfast for use the rest of the day.

Cook an extra entree (like bean soup) and freeze for next time on the rotation.

Leftover complementary vegetables can be pureed in a blender for use as a gravy or sauce on grain and nut loafs.

Use leftovers for lunch the next day (rotating from dinner to dinner, or for snacks).

Prepare extra dishes while fixing dinner for use the next day (like a baked apple for breakfast).

Make enough nut milk for the day.

When shelling or chopping nuts, do extra for later use. Store in the refrigerator or freezer.

Soak beans overnight to shorten cooking time.

Prepare slow-cooking pot in the morning.

Use a thermos to cook grains or beans overnight .

Cooking time-savers:
  Prepare all vegetables before stir frying.
  Assemble ingredients and utensils before baking.
  Sift the dry ingredients together first.
  Beat egg whites at the beginning of recipe.
  Melt necessary ingredients before assembling.
  Begin with chopping or grating items to be used.

Cooking tips:

Peel onions under water to save eyes.

To prevent discoloration of apples or potatoes, place them in lemon water.

To keep parsley and watercress fresh, wash, then place in glass jar.

To keep cornmeal from lumping, moisten with cold water before adding to boiling water.

Cooking Terms

Blanch: Drop food into boiling water, leave one to two minutes. Drain and rinse in cold water. Blanching is used for freezing vegetables, blanching almonds, or to remove skins of peaches or tomatoes for canning.

Chop: To cut into medium-size pieces.

Dice: To cut into small pieces.

Dissolve: To allow to slowly combine in a liquid, like dissolving gelatin in juice.

Fold: Gently and carefully combining an ingredient into a mixture by scooping and lifting, like adding egg whites.

Marinate: Placing a food into a sauce or liquid for a period of time (used for meats, or salads). Enhances the flavor.

Melt: To liquefy by heating slowly.

Peel: To remove the outer skin of a fruit or vegetable.

Sauté: To cook slowly and briefly with a small amount of oil, butter, or water, stirring frequently over medium heat.

Slice: To cut into even pieces. Slices can be thin or thick, round or oblong.

Steam: To cook in the steam generated by boiling water. The food is placed in a steamer. After the pot comes to a boil, it is turned down to simmer for the remainder of the cooking time.

Stir Fry: To cook quickly over high heat with a small amount of oil.

CHAPTER 10

Sweeteners, Thickeners, Dairy, Oils

🦋 Sweeteners

MOST PEOPLE HAVE A sweet tooth. Any dietary change usually implies that those goodies you used to indulge in can no longer be enjoyed. Don't give up hope—there is life after sugar! There are other natural sweeteners which retain their vitamins, minerals, and enzymes, have nutritional value and are good for you in moderation.

Table sugar is a dead product which contributes to many health problems. In the United States at the turn of the century, the average consumption of white, refined sugar was seven pounds per person per year. Today the average consumption is between 120 to 170 pounds per person per year. As far as we know, there is no such thing as raw sugar. There may be some products on the market that are unbleached and slightly less refined than regular table sugar, but none are raw unless you are eating the sugar cane itself. One highly touted alternative is Sucanat (sugar cane natural), made by processing the juice of the sugar cane. If you are allergic to sugar, you will be allergic to any form, refined or less refined, from sugar cane or sugar beets. Even if you are not physically allergic to sugar, the seductive taste of sugar is very addicting. A small amount of it can cause the addiction to reoccur. For those in recovery, the use of alcohol or drugs is actually feeding a sugar addiction. The alcohol passes the blood/brain barrier and gives the user the sugar immediately. Drugs like nicotine act is a similar manner; tobacco is cured with sugar or other refined sweeteners, and the smoker gets the sugar first. Recent media advertising says that sugar does not relate to hyperactivity in children. The child may not react directly to the sugar, but to the food(s) with which it is combined. The sugar takes the food across the blood/brain barrier effects the brain and nervous system.

"Sugar is a major carbohydrate source but is completely devoid of protein, vitamins, and minerals and is not considered nutritious. Refined white sugar, in granulated or powdered form, and brown sugar, are made from either sugar cane or sugar beet. White sugar contains no vitamins or minerals. The B vitamins needed for the assimilation of sugar are robbed from other parts of the body. Sugar leads to an imbalance in the calcium-phosphorus relationship. Sugar may also be a contributing factor in the development of overweight, diabetes, arthritis, tooth decay, pyorrhea, asthma, mental illness, nervous disorders, and low blood sugar."[1]

In some products, fructose is used to replace white sugar. The name fructose implies that it is derived from fruit. Some of it may be manufactured from a combination of fruit and honey. However, most of the fructose available is even more refined than white sugar. White sugar, or sucrose, is composed of glucose and fructose. During the refining process, the glucose molecule is dropped off and the fructose remains. Glucose is the type of sugar that is broken down from other carbohydrates by the body for use in glycolysis and the Krebs cycle for basic energy metabolism. There is research which suggests that it is the fructose in sugar which is fattening. Other researchers feel that fructose may contribute to elevated cholesterol, and that it contributes to retinopathy in diabetics. Another name for fructose is levulose. Other forms of refined sugar, besides sucrose (white sugar) and fructose, include glucose (corn syrup), maltose (starches), lactose (dairy), dextrose (corn syrup), galactose, Turbinado sugar, jaguary sugar, and sorbitol.

A number of sugar substitutes have been developed over the years hoping to find a low-calorie replacement, especially for those with blood sugar problems and weight issues. However, none of the replacements are free of health problems and side effects. Mannitol, sorbitol, and xylitol are natural sugar alcohols which produce gastric side effects and kidney disease. Both cyclamates and saccharin (which is manufactured from toluene, known as methyl benzene) have been linked to cancer and birth defects. Aspartame (from methanol from methane gas), which has been developed in the last few years, is not totally safe either and has

been linked to brain dysfunction. The sad illusion for dieters and diabetics in particular is that the use of sugar substitutes may actually encourage the overeating of sweets. It reinforces the taste for sweet foods and
does nothing to change lifestyle and eating habits, nor does it provide
adequate education.

Where there is bad news, there is also good news! Following is a list,
explanation, and conversion table for the various alternative sweeteners. Depending upon allergy and Candida restrictions, select and experiment with the new sweeteners. Recipes which include these sweeteners
can be found on pages 201 and 359.

❦ Safe Sweeteners

Barley malt
A sweetener made by combining sprouted whole barley with barley
enzymes which converts the starch to sugar. It is both a sugar and a yeast.
It has a strong flavor and a consistency similar to honey.

Blackstrap molasses
This thick, dark syrup is derived from the last sugar cane refining process.
The refining process leaves behind a wealth of nutrients, including an
excellent source of iron and potassium, B vitamins and calcium, and
other minerals. Blackstrap molasses is safe for those with either diabetes
or hypoglycemia and can be tolerated by those with Candida. The only
problem with blackstrap molasses will be if you have an allergy to the
sugar cane or beet sugar itself, or simply cannot abide the taste of it. The
taste is extremely strong. To some people it has a taste similar to licorice.
Mixed with honey in the right proportion it tastes like brown sugar and
in recipes, you cannot tell the difference. Make sure that you purchase
blackstrap molasses, which is normally found in health food stores. Regular molasses is a refined product, may contain sulfites, and will be lack-
ing in nutrients.

Brown rice syrup
Similar to barley malt in sweetness, this syrup is made from brown rice,
water, and a cereal enzyme (one percent barley malt). There is no yeast

in it. Though similar to barley malt in sweetness and consistency, the flavor is not as strong.

Concentrated fruit juice
An innovative and new form of sweetener is the use of concentrated fruit juice. Apple and white grape juice are the two main sources. It makes an excellent sweetener for jams and jellies, fruit juice mixes which need a little sweetness, such as lemonade, and even cookies or other baked goods. The flavor is subtle and does not seem to overpower the product. For information on how to make your own concentrated juice, see page 437.

Date sugar
Date sugar is dehydrated dates which are ground into a course sugar. It can be used to replace sugar and works well with grains (quick breads, brownies, and cookies). It does not dissolve in liquid and that limits its uses. The flavor is mild and not quite as sweet as sugar.

Fruit juice
Fruit juice is not as sweet as the other sweeteners, nor as versatile. In moderation it can usually be tolerated by those with Candida and sugar metabolism problems, depending upon allergy restrictions to the various fruits. It is best used on hot cereal replacing both the dairy and the sugar. Other uses are in salad dressings, muffins, pies, and desserts. For ideas on how to use fruit juice, see Food and Recipes.

Grape/rice granular concentrate
This concentrate has a taste, texture, and a sweetness similar to sugar. It is made from grape juice concentrate and whole rice syrup. It reacts in a manner like sugar in recipes, but requires high heat to fully dissolve it. This product is also available in liquid form.

Honey
Honey has been known since before the time of the first pharaohs of Egypt. In ancient days, honey was regarded as the food of the gods. It is the original sweetener! Honey is manufactured by bees from the nectar they so diligently collect. It is stored in the cells of the hive for food.

There are many different flavors and colors of honey, from very pale to very dark. The flavor depends upon the season, the species of flower, and when it was collected from the hive. It is easily assimilated by the body and contains trace amounts of B vitamins, especially B_5 (pantothenic acid), and minerals, especially chromium, required by the system for sugar metabolism. Honey needs to be cooked for infants and the elderly because it can contain trace amounts of botulism which their digestive systems cannot handle. It is quite sweet and should be used in moderation.

Maple syrup and sugar

Nothing compares to real maple syrup. It is absolutely delicious. Maple syrup is the sap collected from the sugar maple tree which grows mainly in New England. For individuals highly sensitive to chemicals, maple syrup may contain residues of harsh chemicals that are used to increase the flow of the sap. The flavor is unique and strong. Concentrated maple syrup produces the sugar. Unfortunately, real, pure maple syrup is very expensive.

Rice syrup. *See* brown rice syrup.

Sorghum

Sorghum is typical sweetener familiar to those who live in the southern United States. Sweet sorghum is a plant which closely resembles the grain sorghum. The crushed stalk produces a golden syrup and the flavor is like refined molasses.

Vegetable glycerin

Glycerin is recommended as a safe sweetener for those with allergies and Candida. It is a refined, manufactured product composed of fatty acids (not sugar based) derived from various vegetables or grains, including corn, peanuts, or soy, depending upon which crop was most abundant at the time. Herb Craft (see page 464) makes a vegetable glycerin from coconut which is safe for those with Candida or blood sugar problems. The flavor does not resemble sugar or any other sweetener. Experiment with it before using in a recipe.

Conversion Table for White Sugar

1 cup of white sugar equals:

1 cup barley malt syrup	1 cup concentrated fruit juice
1 cup brown rice syrup	½ cup honey
1 cup date sugar	¾ cup maple syrup
1 cup grape, rice granular concentrate	1 cup sorghum
	3 tablespoons vegetable glycerin

A good alternative to the brown sugar flavor and for use in most baked goods, use a mixture of honey and blackstrap molasses. Blackstrap molasses has a powerful flavor and honey's flavor will frequently overpower a recipe. But the two together in the right proportions is amazing. You cannot tell the difference between this mixture and brown sugar. If your recipe calls for one cup sugar or brown sugar, put a full ⅓ cup honey in a ½ cup measuring cup and add blackstrap molasses until it is full, resulting in ½ cup of the mixture.

The above proportions for the conversion of the sweeteners are guidelines and will work nicely in various recipes. Since tastes may vary, experiment according to your desired degree of sweetness. Besides honey and blackstrap molasses, other possible combinations in the same proportions are barley malt and honey, sorghum and honey, and brown rice syrup and barley malt.

For those with Candida and other conditions which require little or no use of sweeteners, fruit juice is a good replacement for sugar and liquid in a recipe. See Food and Recipes for ideas on making muffins, quick breads, dressings, and other recipes.

🦋 Thickeners, Egg Replacers, and Rising Agents

For those with allergy restrictions or who wish to experiment, the following information will be important. There is a large variety of products available whose properties are similar to the ones we already know. Do not be afraid to try them; remember, this is an adventure!

Agar (powder and flakes)

Agar is derived from an algae and acts as a gelling agent similar to gelatin. It needs to be cooked to dissolve. It can be used in desserts and salads, or any recipe that calls for unflavored gelatin. Another name for agar is kanten. For directions on using agar, follow the instructions on the package or see page 441.

Arrowroot

Arrowroot is a thickener which originates from the root of a tropical plant. The substance can be used to replace cornstarch and looks and tastes similar. It is excellent substitute for flour in making sauces and gravies.

Baking powder

Baking powder is a leavening agent consisting of bicarbonate of soda and cream of tartar mixed with flour or starch. Baking powder can have aluminum in it; be sure to check the label. The baking powder in health food stores normally does not have the aluminum in it (see Sources). Check the date on the jar or can and be sure it is fresh. There are several types of baking powder: double action, phosphate, and tartrate. Tartrate is the healthiest choice and you have to use twice as much as the double action.

Baking soda

Bicarbonate of soda is baking soda, an alkali that readily combines with acid to produce carbon dioxide, and has many household uses besides a leavening agent. Unless a specific recipe calls for baking soda, it does not work well with water or fruit juice because the flavor will be far too salty.

Corn starch

Corn starch is a very refined form of corn flour and is a traditional thickening agent.

Egg replacers

Eggs are a familiar ingredient in many recipes. Eggs help to both bind and lighten in recipes. For people with an egg allergy, the following serve well as a substitute for eggs: Commercial egg replacer, tofu, gelatin, baking powder, vinegar, soy flour, flaxseed, and psyllium seed. Duck eggs can be used to replace chicken eggs in cooking and baking. The conversion list below is completely egg free and from the *Freedom From Allergy Cookbook* (Vancouver, BC: Blue Poppy Press, 1990).

Conversion Table For Egg Replacers

Commercial egg replacer usually contains potato starch, tapioca flour, and baking powder. Add more water to recipe when using it. Use for leavening or as a binder. Check labels, some may contain egg.

Substitute ¼ cup tofu for each egg. Good as a binder.

Soften 1 teaspoon of gelatin in 3 tablespoons boiling water. Stir until dissolved, then place in freezer. Take out when thickened and beat until frothy. Equals one egg. Use as a binder.

One teaspoon baking powder for each egg substituted for leavening.

One teaspoon vinegar (if tolerated) for each egg in a cake recipe, for leavening.

Cornstarch, arrowroot, tapioca flour, potato flour, and soy flour act as thickening agents. See chart on page 142.

⅓ cup soy flour and ⅔ cup water. Blend and heat in double boiler for 1 hour. Whip in 1 tablespoon oil and ¼ teaspoon salt. Store in refrigerator. Use as a binder for making cookies.

Boil ⅓ cup flaxseed in 1 cup water for 15 minutes. Add to muffins and other baked goods as a binder.

Combine 1 tablespoon psyllium seed husk with 3 tablespoons water and let sit briefly. This makes an excellent binder.

Gelatin
Unflavored gelatin is wonderful for making your own Jell-O salad with pure juice and fruit. It is a gelling agent extracted from the bones and cartilage of animals, mainly cattle. See page 272 for exciting and delicious recipes.

Conversion Table for Gelatin

To gel 1¾ cups of liquid:

1 tablespoon gelatin equals 1 tablespoon granulated agar or 2 tablespoons flaked agar

½ stick of agar also equals 1 envelope of gelatin

1 tablespoon gelatin equals ½ tablespoon low-methoxyl pectin

Kuzu

Kuzu is from a town of the same name in Japan. It is a flour made from the kuzu root and is interchangeable with arrowroot. This product is often used in macrobiotic cooking.

Methoxyl

Methoxyl or methoxate (low-methoxyl pectin) will gel honey and other nonsugar products, like jams and jellies, aspics, and puddings using concentrated fruit juice. The methyl atoms of carbon and hydrogen are activated by oxygen and the addition of calcium. Methoxyl is made from citrus. Follow package directions carefully for excellent results. It is available in packages and also in bulk in health food stores. If purchased in bulk, you may have to add the calcium. See page 00 for more information.

Potato starch (flour)

Potato starch is a fine flour prepared from cooked, dried, and ground potatoes. It is useful for thickening soups and sauces.

Tapioca

Tapioca flour is finely ground flour from the cassava plant. It is available in the health food stores and used as a thickening agent.

Yeast

Yeast is a leavening agent formed from common fungus organisms which are found even in the air. Yeast is often put into products that one would never suspect, such as canned soup. There are three main types of yeast available for commercial use: baker's yeast, brewer's yeast, and sourdough.

Baker's yeast is found in breads and other baked goods. It is the agent which causes bread to rise.

Brewer's yeast is used in the manufacture of alcoholic beverages. It is also sold in health food stores as a food supplement and contains varying trace amounts of B vitamins, chromium, and other minerals. Its overuse has contributed to the proliferation of Candida, a major health issue of our time.

Sourdough is a yeast! Yeast organisms are absorbed from the air into a flour and water mixture. It has a delicious sour taste and is leavened similar to baker's yeast. Technically, as nothing is added to the product except the flour and water which comprises the sourdough starter, companies will advertise the product as yeast free. Be careful, because it is not yeast free!

Conversion Table for Using Thickeners in Sauces and Gravies

1 tablespoon of white flour equals:

1 tablespoon whole wheat

1 tablespoon brown rice flour

1 tablespoon soy flour

1 tablespoon flour of choice

½ tablespoon kuzu

½ tablespoon cornstarch

½ tablespoon potato starch

½ tablespoon arrowroot

2 teaspoons tapioca flour

NOTE: 1 tablespoon cornstarch equals 1 tablespoon arrowroot or 1 tablespoon kuzu.

🦋 Oils (Fats)

Fats and oils are a major energy source and very satisfying, helping us to feel full. Some of the sources of fats and oils contain essential fatty acids which are important to health and proper metabolism. They are essential because they are not manufactured within the body but must be supplied from outside sources. Fats and oils can be listed as saturated, unsaturated, mono-unsaturated, polyunsaturated, and hydrogenated.

Saturated fats are from animal sources, except for coconut and palm oil. They are solid at room temperature. Unsaturated fatty acids are derived from vegetables, nuts, and seeds. They are liquid at room temperature, and are quite volatile and unstable. Their flavors can be a delightful addition to a recipe, but they become rancid and carcinogenic easily. Only small amounts of oil should be purchased at a time.

The best form of oil available is the *cold pressed* variety. The cold pressed process extracts the oil at the lowest possible temperature to prevent the spoilage of the product. Cold pressed (unsaturated) oils should be refrigerated and used only in dressings or in a recipe, not for cooking or frying.

Mono-unsaturated oils are the healthiest forms of oil available. Studies have found that the use of olive and canola oil lowers the unhealthy forms of cholesterol (LDL). People who live in countries that use a lot of olive oil have a lower incidence of heart disease. The mono-unsaturates have both saturated and unsaturated properties. They are liquid and stable at room temperature. There is no need to store them in the refrigerator and they will keep for a long time. The rancidity, or heating point, on them is quite high and they are safe for cooking and frying.

Polyunsaturated fatty acids have the same properties as unsaturated fatty acids. They are found mainly in oils and margarines. *Hydrogenated* oils are to be avoided! Hydrogenation of the unsaturated oils occurs during the manufacturing process when the hydrogen atom is split and repositioned on the fatty acid chain. The result is a product that will harden at room temperature. Although it seems like an innocent process, it renders the product carcinogenic and produces what are termed "trans fats." The metabolism of hydrogenated oils interferes with the uptake of calcium and other minerals, contributes to unhealthy cholesterol, and is a free radical in the body using stores of the antioxidant vitamins (A, C, and E). The most common sources of hydrogenated oils are shortenings and margarines.

Butter is a saturated fat from animal sources. It is delicious and found in two forms, regular salted butter and unsalted sweet butter. Both can be found in the raw form in your local health food store. Butter is fat and can often be tolerated by those with dairy allergies; be sure to ask or have it tested first. Butter is safer at higher heats than margarine. It can become rancid, producing free radicals, but not carcinogenic. Regular salted and unsalted sweet butter have the same amount of calories. Clarified butter eliminates the milk sugar which might feed Candida. Heat the butter in a pan and skim off the white foam. Place the clear yellow liquid in a tight container and store in a cool place. Once clarified it will keep for a long time.

Monosaturated	Saturated	Polyunsaturated
Olive oil	Coconut oil	Corn oil
Canola oil	Lard (not to be used)	Sesame oil
Grape seed oil	Cottonseed oil	Peanut oil
	Palm oil	Safflower oil
	Butter	Soybean oil
		Walnut oil
		Sunflower seed oil

Conversion Table for Fat

In baking, one cup of pureed fruit (banana, apple, pear, prune, peach) can be substituted for one cup of butter, oil, or margarine in an appropriate recipe, such as muffins.

In cooking, several options are available. For a marinade or dressing, cut the oil in half and substitute water for the other half. To sauté, either use the minimum required to prevent sticking or use water. In soups, skip the sautéing of the vegetables and add directly to the pot.

🦋 Dairy

Dairy is one of those foods most people feel they simply cannot live without. Most of this is related to upbringing, culture, and advertising.

Dairy is not good for everybody. Approximately 70 percent of the population is allergic to dairy either as lactose intolerant or casein allergic (protein intolerant), or addicted to its mind-altering properties. It is mucus forming, can cause constipation, and is a major contributing factor in sinus and migraine headaches and osteoporosis. The latest findings from the July 1992 issue of *The New England Journal of Medicine* links cow's milk with juvenile diabetes. According to author of the study, Dr. Hans-Michael Dosch, strong evidence suggests that the diabetes occurs when the body confuses cow milk proteins with a protein found on the surface of insulin-producing cells in the pancreas.

Regular cow's milk from the supermarket is a manufactured product. It has been pasteurized, homogenized, and fortified. Milk is pasteurized in order to destroy the bacteria which cause many diseases like typhoid, tuberculosis, and salmonella that can be found in milk. Homogenization of milk suspends the fat molecules and distributes them evenly. Homogenization also contributes to the buildup of cholesterol. Milk samples in various parts of the United States have revealed contamination by antibiotics, sulfamethazine, chloramphenicol, and other chemicals. Milk is fortified because the other processes destroy most of the nutrients, and fortifying replaces the nutrients with synthetic substitutes, such as D-2. Other processes are involved which prolong the shelf life. If the milk goes beyond the date on the bottle, the result is an unusable product.

The latest unhealthy additive to milk is BGH (bovine growth hormone). BGH is a synthetic hormone which is used to double the amount of milk a cow can produce. According to researchers, the hormone is supposed to be safe—cows naturally produce some BGH in order to produce milk. But the overextention of their endocrine system weakens their immune system and the cows become sick more frequently, requiring an increase in medications. The medication traces are then passed on to the consumer. There are certified organic dairies which produce BGH-free milk products. However, BGH and medication traces could be present in any product which uses any form of dairy.

Bovine serum albumin is a surface antigen (named p69) shares a 17 amino acid sequence in common with cow's milk serum albumin. "The similarity of this 17 amino acid chain found on both bovine serum albumin and surface proteins on pancreatic cells confuses the immune system, causing the immune system by means of cross-reacting BSA-specific IgG antibodies to bind and attack both." (From the article "Insulin-Dependent Diabetes, an IgG-Mediated Cow's Milk Allergy?" by James Braly, M.D. in *The Immuno Review,* Volume 1, Number 2, Fall 1993.)

The study also finds that prevention of insulin-dependent diabetes is possible through careful monitoring of the immune system and lessening exposure to viral infections, exclusive breast feeding for at least the first four months, and the strict elimination of cow's milk, beef, and products containing any form thereof which would contain the bovine serum albumin.

Raw milk, on the other hand, retains the nutrients originally found in dairy. The milk and cream separate naturally. Raw milk must be tested frequently to insure that the cows are disease free. It is still high in protein, mucus forming, constipating, and can be an allergen. When raw milk goes beyond the date, buttermilk, or sour milk, is the result (excellent for pancakes and biscuits). If you drink milk, then a good clean source of raw milk is a better choice.

Because of allergies, sensitivities, or health concerns, you might decide to give up cow's milk. The change might be difficult, as you will be bucking tradition and your own attachment to this familiar food. Milk has been with you since you were a baby, and is associated with comfort and love. Remember that your new commitment to health is an adventure and remain open to new ideas will ease the transition. The following are some excellent substitutions for cow's milk dairy.

❦ Dairy Substitutes

Goat milk dairy

If you have never seen baby goats playing together in an open field, you have really missed something! Goats have been a healthy source of milk since biblical times. The milk is popular in the Middle East, Europe, and in other sections of the world. Even today there are far more people worldwide who consume goat's milk than cow's milk. Goats do not carry the diseases which cows do.

Goat dairy is frequently not a problem for those who are allergic to cow's dairy. Goat milk more closely resembles human milk in protein content and structure. It also contains anticancer properties, and supplies the antioxidant vitamins A, C, D, and E, and iodine and sulfur which are important for proper immune function. The minerals are also available in good balance.

One thing which seems to deter people from trying goat milk is the taste. If the milk is fresh and has been handled correctly, the flavor of raw goat's milk is even sweeter than cow's milk. On a blind test, it is difficult for people to tell one from another. Find a good source from your local health food store or a local dairy. Goat dairy products easily substitute for cow dairy so do not be afraid to try them. There are many wonderful products available for your enjoyment.

Goat Products

Butter	Goat Jack	Parmesan cheese
Cream cheese	Goat milk	Powdered milk
Evaporated milk	Goat mozzarella	Ricotta
Feta cheese	Other cheese	Yogurt, plain and
Goat cheddar	varieties	flavored

Soy

Soy is a very versatile product and the most popular dairy substitute. Soy can be a major allergen because of its high protein content, is relatively high in fat (35 percent), and can be difficult to digest. It is usually the protein molecules which cause the allergy reaction. Soy is a good source of vitamin A and B vitamins, especially folic acid, and potassium and other minerals. Soy milk has its own distinct flavor; taste it before you pour it on your cereal. There are many different varieties of soy milk in a multitude of flavors to choose from. They are found in your local health food store on both the shelf and in the refrigerator sections. The flavor of the soy cheeses are quite good, but they do not respond in cooking the same as cow or goat cheese. The texture and consistency of soy sour cream works well in dips, and in combination with other ingredients in cooking. The Parmesan cheese is an excellent substitute for the real thing; check the label because the soy Parmesan can contain casein, which is cow's dairy protein. Other soy products might also contain either casein, whey, or lactose—check labels.

Soy Products

American cheese	Parmesan cheese	Tofu
Cheddar cheese	Powdered soy milk	Toffuti (like ice cream)
Jalapeño pepper cheese	Sour cream	Yogurt, plain and
Mozzarella cheese	Soy milk, plain and	flavored
	flavored	

Brown rice milk

A wonderful and delicious new addition for a dairy substitute is now available. Brown rice milk has a sweet, smooth, light taste which is an excellent replacement for milk on cereals, whether hot or cold. If on a Candida diet, the sweetness of the milk is usually enough to satisfy. It is very low in fat and salt. For those not allergic to brown rice, it is easily digested. The consistency is thinner than regular milk, but substitutes well in recipes.

Basic Rice Milk

Makes 4 cups

In a blender, combine 1 cup cooked brown rice and 4 cups of water and blend until smooth. A little salt or 1 teaspoon vanilla extract may be added for flavor. Let sit for one hour, then pour through a sieve. Refrigerate and shake before serving.

Brown Rice Products

Brown rice milk, flavored	Rice Dream Ice Cream
Brown rice milk, plain	Puddings

Nut milk

Nut milk is milk made from nuts! Nut milk contains all the nutrition which is found in nuts, including essential fatty acids. The milk is high in calories, with a richness and fullness to the flavor and consistency of other milks. Almond, cashew, and hazelnut (filbert) are the best choices. Some nut milk is available commercially. Coconut milk can be found everywhere, or you can make your own, and is excellent for soups. Nut milks substitute well for regular dairy in desserts and cream sauces, and are excellent on cereals. They can be thinned to your desired taste to produce a texture compatible to any recipe and augmented with vanilla or other flavorings. Below is a basic recipe for making nut milk.

Nut Milk Products

Almondrella cheeses	Milk

Basic Nut Milk

Makes 3 cups

In a blender, grind 1 cup of nuts until powdered. Gradually add 2½ cups water to form desired consistency.

Coconut Milk

Makes 1¼ cups

In a blender, combine ½ cup shredded coconut and 1 cup hot water and blend until smooth. Refrigerate before serving.

Notes

1. Lavon J. Dunne, *The Nutrition Almanac,* third edition (New York: McGraw-Hill, 1990).

CHAPTER 11

Eating Out, Bag Lunches, and Snacks

O NE OF THE GREATEST challenges for anyone with allergies or just trying to eat healthy, is eating out. Some of the most frequently asked questions are Can I eat out? Can I maintain my social life, friends, business functions, and travel? Can I do this diet and still have a life? The answer is yes! All it requires is planning, asking questions, and awareness of challenges and food traps. Although eating out can be a challenge, we hope that this chapter will provide inspiration, helping you to make eating a more pleasurable and fun experience.

Contemporary living has created fast-paced eating. We are accustomed to eating on the run, and finding something quick to eat to satisfy hunger. Whether you are an active person, or you like to eat out socially, this chapter is for you. First of all, you deserve quality food and the time to eat and enjoy it. You deserve to be able to maintain the healthy lifestyle you have chosen. Despite social pressures, there are choices. Eating out can lead to lessening your resolve and self-discipline. It can be a trap of hidden food addictions and allergens. This can sabotage the best intentions: a seemingly innocent food contains a hidden addiction and soon the eater is on a downward spiral creating a momentum that keeps them lost in old, negative food patterns. Eating out should be an enjoyable and positive experience. The following guidelines and suggestions are presented to help you avoid the pitfalls and give support to your efforts.

❧ Psychological Traps

Often eating out becomes a focus for all the other ways we have not nurtured ourselves and many justifications and excuses surface.

I've been responsible to my family. I've worked hard. I've put up with all kinds of garbage. I deserve to eat out and eat exactly what I want! I'm going to treat myself!

If I follow my diet and ask for different food in front of others they will think I am odd. Oh, you think you're so special. Why can't you eat what everyone else eats? It will take too much time. The restaurant will never fix what you want. What's this, another strange diet you're on? Here she (he) goes again!

If I don't eat what is before me, I will offend my hostess.

They'll never understand. People will make fun of me. _____ did when I confided in her about the changes I need to make.

I've been good on this diet. I've lost weight and feel better. I'll reward myself and eat _____.

I've been doing this for a long time. I must be over it by now, and I can eat the way I used to.

Answers

Take the time to nurture yourself in ways that do not include food. Make a list of things that are nurturing to you, such as a hot bath, flowers, a phone call to a friend, a fire in the fireplace, a walk, and even smell the roses. Resolve to do one or more per day. Eat to live and don't live to eat.

Slow down. Allow eating time itself to be a place of nurturing. Enjoy the beauty of the food itself as it is presented for eating. Slowly savor the taste. Choose a quality place to eat with a good atmosphere, perhaps include music.

Restaurants are usually accommodating and are there to serve the public. A part of the fun of eating out is to be served, to have someone wait on you and be pampered. Part of healing is to learn to accept nurturing. Get over the shyness or embarrassment about asking for what you need. You have the right to ask questions about the content of the food and ask for something other than what is offered on the menu, like a steamed vegetable plate or salad without dressing.

Most people try to please their guests and are solicitous regarding their welfare. Depending upon the social situation, call ahead to your hostess (or host) letting them know of your special requirements. A good hostess is more than happy to provide an alternative for someone who doesn't drink alcohol. Approach the food with the same attitude. If it is a potluck, bring something that you know you can eat.

Unless someone asks what or why you are not doing something, do not volunteer information. Most people do not have enough knowledge or personal experience to understand what you are going through.

Say, "No, thank you," when offered a food you know you should not have, or put a small amount on your plate and leave it there.

If going to a social function where the food will be questionable, eat before you leave. The food will be less tempting on a full stomach.

Diet changes are for a lifetime. An unintentional or deliberate slip can quickly reestablish addictions, trigger allergy reactions, and be unpleasant. Think the first desire through to the full conclusion. Allow plenty of time to lapse and check with your health care professional before trying problem foods. And yes, you will probably be able to eat problem foods again in moderation.

Call ahead to your travel agent, airline, train, ship, or hotel when planning a trip. Special meals can be arranged. When asking for what you need, be matter-of-fact. You do not have to apologize, but a thank you is always appreciated. When traveling by plane, consider bringing your own food.

When traveling by car, bring a small cooler and your own supply of food, especially foods that may be difficult to obtain. Shop along the way from supermarkets or road side stands. Water is important item to include: consider investing in the Multi-Pure Travel Kit.

Hotel and motel rooms often have small kitchens or a small refrigerator and microwave oven in the room, sometimes centrally located in the facility. Shop at a local store and eat some of your meals in the room.

Join a local support group or form one yourself. Explore Overeaters

Anonymous. Look into the possibility of professional therapy; be sure the therapist understands the role of addictions or eating disorders. Try to have a supportive group of friends. Call a friend for support if you are having a difficult day or will be facing a stressful social situation. Addictions are isolating, so reach out to others. Love helps overcome addictions.

You are not trapped and victimized—you do have choices. You do have the right to take care of yourself. Don't load yourself with guilt and shame and try to please others: in the process you will only harm yourself. Don't succumb to peer pressure and then hate yourself for doing it. The people you try to please will not necessarily like you any better. In fact, they may even think less of you for having compromised your principles and for not keeping your word. You can choose to take care of your needs. You do have that right. You are not being selfish. You are practicing self-love.

❦ Restaurant Guidelines

A current trend is toward restaurants offering high-quality food made from organic produce. Gourmet restaurants with a chef usually prepare foods from scratch, reducing the chances of questionable ingredients or the use of MSG. Health food restaurants can be found across the country from Veggieland in Atlanta, Georgia to the Good Earth in Santa Rosa, California. Health food stores frequently have a small delicatessen or snack area as a part of their services. If none of the above are available, here are some suggestions.

Select fresh fruit, plain fruit salad, or fruit juice.

Try hash browns or cottage fries. Make sure they are not the frozen variety.

Have a soft-boiled egg or possibly scrambled.

Order cooked oatmeal and eat it plain.

Order a green salad, including spinach salad. Ask for oil and lemon or vinegar on the side. Ask to have left out anything you know you cannot have, like tomatoes.

Baked potatoes are usually safe. Leave the things alone you know you shouldn't have and ask for chives, chopped green onions, or perhaps mushrooms to dress it up.

The vegetables for the day are normally acceptable. Ask to have the butter left off, if necessary. A steamed vegetable plate is a good bet.

Broiled or grilled fish or poultry without sauce is a good choice for an entree.

Plain, steamed, white rice is safe. It is not as good for you as brown rice, but it should not cause an allergic reaction, providing your system can able to tolerate rice.

To avoid sugar and MSG, request that your food be prepared without the use of salt or seasoning salts.

A bottled mineral water (plain or with lemon), or salt/sugar free club soda, is a good choice for a beverage. Tap water is almost always contaminated in some form or another with chlorine or other chemicals. Herb tea can be acceptable, if sensitivity to water is not a major problem. Bringing your own tea bag will assure that you will get what you need.

What to Look Out For

Soups and soup bases often contain sugar, MSG, dairy, and other allergens.

Most pastas are made from white flour, and may contain eggs. The sauces are very questionable. Sugar, dairy, and MSG are the main hidden problems.

All desserts are to be avoided.

Breaded or fried foods in any form: batters contain oils, MSG, dairy, sugar, corn, wheat, and other allergens.

Sauces, gravies, and dressings on food, or even on the side, contain many common allergens and chemical additives.

Salted foods: salt contains sugar and seasoning salts also contain MSG.

When traveling, request low-salt meals. Read labels on packaged products presented to you for your consumption, like salad dressing or peanuts.

Seafood entrees, sauces, or cold cuts will contain MSG, sugar, and other allergens. Carry liquid chlorophyll with you in case of an allergic reaction.

🦋 Never Be Bored with Bag Lunches Again

For the school lunch box, a cold lunch at work, or the person traveling, some simple bag lunches ideas are listed below.

Variations for a Cold Lunch

Trail mix (nuts, seeds, dried fruit if not an allergen, and coconut), raw vegetables for the day, and a piece of fruit. Herb tea, juice, or water in an appropriate container.

Rice cakes or rye crackers with nut butter in between like a sandwich, raw vegetables for the day, and a piece of fruit. Herb tea, juice, or water in an appropriate container.

Rice cakes or rye crackers with tuna, salmon, tofu, or avocado spread, raw vegetables for the day, and a piece of fruit. Herb tea, juice, or water in an appropriate container.

Rye or other nonyeast bread with nut butter or chicken, egg, or vegetables (such as cucumber, tomato, sprouts, grated carrot, lettuce, onion, or avocado), raw vegetables for the day, and a piece of fruit. Herb tea, juice, or water in an appropriate container.

Corn or wheat tortilla wrapped around beans, lentils, or rice, with additional vegetables like lettuce, tomato, avocado, or a vegetable taco. Salsa is a great complement. Herb tea, juice, or water in an appropriate container.

Goat or soy yogurt, raw vegetables for the day, and a piece of fruit. Herb tea, juice, or water in an appropriate container.

Goat or soy cheese with crackers or rice cakes, raw vegetables for the day, and a piece of fruit. Herb tea, juice, or water in an appropriate container.

Leftovers that will not spoil. Herb tea, juice, or water in an appropriate container.

A green salad with vegetables in a container and dressing on the side, crackers, rice cakes, muffin, and a piece of fruit. Herb tea, juice, or water in an appropriate container.

Soup, grains, or beans in a thermos, raw vegetables for the day, and fruit. Herb tea, juice, or water in an appropriate container.

Muffins with nut butter or plain, fruit. Herb tea, juice, or water in an appropriate container.

Variations for a Hot Lunch

For those who have a kitchen or a microwave at work, the following ideas may be helpful.

Bring leftovers from the evening meal and heat in the microwave.

Bake a potato, squash, or yam.

Cook frozen or fresh vegetables.

Heat soup or beans.

Make or heat rice.

Grill goat or soy cheese on a cracker, or other appropriate bread.

Heat a tortilla with the beans and cheese in microwave for about 1 minute. Add salsa or other vegetables.

Make or heat Cream of Buckwheat, Bits of Barley, or other grain.

Steam, grill, sauté, or cook in the microwave a piece of fish or chicken. Add vegetables, fruit, nuts and seeds, and beverage as they may apply to make a full meal.

Other ideas for the office include: use the refrigerator to store nut butters, nuts or seeds, goat cheese or yogurt, raw vegetables, or rice milk. If there is space, keep crackers, cereals, chips, and canned fish on hand. Be as creative as you want!

❦ Snacks

Old Stand-bys

Fresh fruit, raw vegetables, nuts and seeds, chips, popcorn, crackers with nut butter, cheese or jam, rice cakes, yogurt, carob chips, herb tea, hot carob, hot cider, fruit or vegetable juice, muffin, toasted appropriate bread, slice of banana or other quick bread.

Something Different

Nut butter on apple, nut butter stuffed celery, mixed rice milk and amazaki, hummus or tofu spread in celery or on crackers, goat cheese melted on tortilla with salsa, tahini dip with vegetables, avocado or bean or salsa dip for chips, cashew butter dip with vegetables or crackers or chips, smoked salmon with crackers and/or goat cheese, creamy dip from soy or goat milk for vegetables or crackers or chips, shrimp with salsa or spicy tomato sauce cocktail on crackers, tuna spread on crackers or bread, soy milk drink, rice milk carob drink.

CHAPTER 12

Rotation Diet and Sample Menus

AMANTHA'S ROTATION PLAN IS an example of a seven-day, extended rotation plan. Samantha's rotation plan and menus are the result of a complicated allergy test and the alternatives that were presented to her. Included in this chapter is an example of a regular five-day rotation plan. For those who don't like to cook or don't have the time, an even simpler five-day rotation plan is also presented. The following information illustrates steps 8 through 14 discussed in chapter 5. Because each individual and their test results are different, follow the guidelines presented and create your own rotation plan. The following examples will be helpful. Be creative and have fun! Approach it as a challenge. The rewards will be well worth the effort.

Review your menu for the following day the night before. This will help you be efficient regarding food preparation and eliminate unnecessary work. If a grain salad, grain loaf, or grain stuffed vegetable is part of your lunch or dinner, prepare the grain in enough quantity as a part of your breakfast cereal. Substitution is the key principle for the success of your rotation plan. For examples of how substitutions work and for more information, see page 183.

Samantha's Rotation Plan
Recommended Foods

Day 1

Black-eyed peas	Kale	Rice bread
Broccoli	Kiwi	Sunflower butter
Brown rice	Lemon	Sunflower seeds
Cucumber	Oregano	
Honeydew melon	Plum	

Day 2

Brussels sprout	Lamb	Red grape
Coconut	Mushrooms	Romaine lettuce
Garlic	Poppy seed	Rosemary
Green bell pepper	Quinoa	Sweet potato

Day 3

Cashew	Leek	Potato
Crackers	Lima bean	Rye
Fig	Nutmeg	Rye bread
Jicama	Pineapple	Spinach

Day 4

Almonds	Egg Replacer	Pancakes
Blackberry	Green bean	Pork
Canola oil	Oats	Safflower oil
Celery	Onion	Thyme

Day 5

Asparagus	Lentil	Wheat
Cantaloupe	Papaya	Yam
Curry	Pumpkin seed	
Green onion	Raspberry	

Day 6

Chard	Marjoram	Pecan
Grapefruit	Millet	Red bell pepper
Green onion	Olive oil	
Lime	Orange roughy	

Day 7

Boysenberry	Mushroom	Romaine lettuce
Buckwheat	Oregano	Tomato
Garlic	Pasta	
Kiwi	Red potato	

Day 8

Brown rice	Lemon	Squash
Canola oil	Orange	Tarragon
Chive	Parsley	Water chestnut
Halibut	Scallop squash	
Honeydew	Spinach	

Day 9

Almond	Green bell pepper	Quinoa
Banana	Lamb	Red onion
Beets	Marjoram	
Grapefruit	Potato	

Day 10

Canola oil	Eggplant	Rye
Celery	Green bean	Sunflower seed
Cucumber	Green grape	Yam
Curry	Papaya	Yellow onion

Day 11

Boysenberry	Oats	Shallot
Cantaloupe	Pork	Sweet potato
Jicama	Red bell pepper	Thyme
Kiwi	Savoy cabbage	

Day 12

Cauliflower	Olive oil	Red potato
Garlic	Oregano	Romaine lettuce
Ginger	Pasta	Snow pea
Mushroom	Pumpkin	Wheat
Nectarine	Raspberry	

Day 13

Avocado	Orange	Poppy seed
Corn	Pear	Safflower oil
Green onion	Pinto bean	Spinach

Day 14

Blackberry	Chili	Plum
Broccoli	Groats	Red bean
Buckwheat	Leek	Spaghetti

For a list of Samantha's avoided foods, see page 71.

Samantha's Menus

Day 1

Breakfast	*Lunch*	*Dinner*	*Snack*
Honeydew melon	Black-eyed peas	Brown rice	Plum
Rice cereal	with	Broccoli with	Honeydew
Rice milk	Oregano	Lemon	Rice cake
Rice bread	Kale	Oregano	1 tablespoon sun-
Margarine	Rice bread	Margarine	flower butter
	Margarine	Cucumber	⅛ cup sunflower
	Plum		seeds

Day 2

Breakfast	*Lunch*	*Dinner*	*Snack*
Quinoa cereal	Romaine lettuce	Brussels sprout	Coconut
Coconut milk	salad with	Lamb with	Green bell pepper
Kiwi	Mushroom,	Rosemary	Kiwi
Orange	Green bell	Sweet potato	Red grape
	pepper		
	Stuffed green bell		
	pepper with		
	Quinoa, Garlic,		
	Mushroom,		
	Rosemary		
	Red grape		

Day 3

Breakfast	*Lunch*	*Dinner*	*Snack*
Rye cereal	Baked potato	Lima beans with	Fig
Cashew milk	Steamed spinach	Leek	Orange
Rye bread	with	Spinach salad	Cashew
	Nutmeg	with	Jicama
	Margarine	Leek	Rye cracker
	Fig	Jicama	1 tablespoon
		Poppy seed	cashew butter
		Orange	
		Rye bread	

Day 4

Breakfast	*Lunch*	*Dinner*	*Snack*
Oat pancakes	Nut loaf with	Pork with	Celery with
Blackberry jam	Celery	Thyme	Almond butter
melt	Almonds	Green beans	Blackberries
Blackberries	Onion	Celery sticks	Pineapple
Safflower oil or	Egg Replacer		Green beans
margarine	Thyme		
	Pineapple		
	Celery sticks		

Day 5

Breakfast	*Lunch*	*Dinner*	*Snack*
Wheat pancakes	Yam	Lentil curry with	⅛ cup pumpkin
Raspberry jam	Asparagus	Shallot	seed
melt	Pumpkin seed	Curry powder	Raspberries
Raspberries	Margarine	Canola oil	Papaya
Canola oil	Papaya	Whole wheat	Wheat bread
		bread	

Day 6

Breakfast	*Lunch*	*Dinner*	*Snack*
Millet cereal	Millet loaf with	Orange roughy	2 ounces rice
Rice milk	Red bell	with	milk
Grapefruit	pepper	Lime	8 to 10 pecans
Pecan	Green onion	Green onion	Cantaloupe
	Chard stems	Margarine	Grapefruit
	Margarine	Marjoram	Red bell pepper
	Millet flour	Red bell pepper	
	Cantaloupe	Chard	
	Chard with		
	Margarine		

Day 7

Breakfast	*Lunch*	*Dinner*	*Snack*
Buckwheat	Red potato	Buckwheat pasta	Kiwi
pancakes	Baked tomato	with	Boysenberries
Boysenberry jam	with	Tomato	Mushrooms
melt	Garlic	Garlic	1 pancake with
Boysenberries	Olive oil	Mushroom	jam
	Oregano	Oregano	
	Kiwi	Olive oil	
		Romaine lettuce	
		salad with	
		Mushroom	
		Garlic	
		Oregano	
		Oil and	
		vinegar	
		dressing	

Day 8

Breakfast	*Lunch*	*Dinner*	*Snack*
Rice cereal	Halibut with	Brown rice	Honeydew melon
Rice milk	Lemon	Scallop squash	Orange
Rice bread	Canola oil	Spinach salad	Water chestnut
Margarine	Green onion	with	1 rice bread
Honeydew melon	Parsley	Water chestnut	
	Tarragon	Orange	
	Spinach	Parsley	
		Green onion	
		Orange	
		dressing	

Day 9

Breakfast	*Lunch*	*Dinner*	*Snack*
Quinoa cereal	Quinoa salad	Lamb with	Grapefruit
Almond milk	with	Marjoram	8 to 10 almonds
Banana	Green bell	Baked potato	Beets
Almonds	pepper	Margarine	Green bell pepper
	Red onion	Beets	
	Marjoram		
	Beet greens		
	Grapefruit		

Day 10

Breakfast	*Lunch*	*Dinner*	*Snack*
Rye cereal	Yam	Eggplant curry	Papaya
Papaya juice	Green beans	with	Green grapes
Papaya	Celery sticks	Curry	Eggplant dip
Raisins	Rye bread or	Yellow onion	Rye crackers
Rye bread	crackers	Green beans	Celery
Margarine	Green grapes	Cucumber	Cucumber
		Celery	
		Canola oil	

Day 11

Breakfast	*Lunch*	*Dinner*	*Snack*
Oat pancakes	Pork with	Sweet potato	Kiwi
Boysenberry jam	Thyme	Savoy cabbage	Cantaloupe
melt	Savoy cabbage	stir fry with	Jicama
Boysenberries	stir fry with	Canola oil	Red bell pepper
	Canola oil	Red bell	1 pancake
	Red bell	pepper	
	pepper	Jicama	
	Jicama	Shallot	
	Shallot		
	Kiwi		

Day 12

Breakfast	*Lunch*	*Dinner*	*Snack*
Wheat pancakes	Pasta with	Red potato	Nectarine
Raspberry jam	Olive oil	Vegetable stir fry	Raspberry
Raspberries	Oregano	with	Snow peas
	Garlic	Pumpkin seed	Cauliflower
	Mushroom	Garlic	Mushroom
	Romaine lettuce	Mushroom	⅛ cup pumpkin
	salad with	Cauliflower	seeds
	Snow peas	Snow pea	
	Mushroom	Ginger	
	Oregano	Nectarine	
	Olive oil		
	dressing		

Day 13

Breakfast	*Lunch*	*Dinner*	*Snack*
Corn muffin or mush	Corn tortillas with	Pinto beans with Green onion	Pear
Margarine	Pinto bean	Paprika	Orange
Orange	Avocado	Spinach salad with	Corn muffin
	Green onion	Poppy seed dressing	Corn chips
	Spinach	Orange	
	Pear	Avocado	
		Green onion	
		Safflower oil	

Day 14

Breakfast	*Lunch*	*Dinner*	*Snack*
Buckwheat pancake	Groats with Leek	Red beans with Leek	Plum
Blackberry jam melt	Spaghetti squash with	Chili powder	Blackberry
Blackberries	Margarine	Rosemary	Coconut
	Nutmeg	Broccoli with Lemon	1 pancake
	Plum	Margarine	Broccoli

Five-Day Rotation Plan Example
Avoided Foods

Apple	Dairy/beef	Wheat
Carrot	Sugar	Yeast
Corn	Walnut	

Five-Day Rotation Plan Example
Recommended Foods

Day 1

Almond	Cilantro	Marjoram	Safflower oil
Black bean	Cumin	Oats	Strawberry
Chard	Egg	Plum	
Chili powder	Green bell pepper	Red onion	

Day 2

Banana	Chicken	Poppy seed	Spinach
Canola oil	Jicama	Potato	Thyme
Cantaloupe	Millet	Red bell pepper	
Cashew	Nutmeg	Sage	

Day 3

Asparagus	Dill	Pecan	Shiitake
Blackberry	Green onion	Romaine lettuce	mushroom
Brown rice	Lemon	Salmon	Sunflower oil
Cucumber	Orange		Sunflower seed

Day 4

Basil	Buckwheat pasta	Olive oil	Tomato
Blueberry	Butter leaf lettuce	Peach	Yam
Brazil nut	Garlic	Sesame	Zucchini

Day 5

Barley	Celery	Hazel nut	Pear
Canola oil	Green beans	Kiwi	Pumpkin seed
Cayenne pepper	Green cabbage	Parsley	Yellow onion

Day 6

Almond	Green onion	Pineapple	Sweet potato
Chard	Halibut	Safflower oil	Tarragon
Flax seed	Lime	Savoy cabbage	
Green bell pepper	Oats	Strawberry	

Day 7

Banana	Mint	Red onion	Spinach
Cashew	Mushroom	Red potatoes	Tangerine
Jicama	Olive oil	Rosemary	
Lamb	Peas	Rye	

Day 8

Broccoli	Green onion	Raspberry	Yellow bell
Brown rice	Orange	Red leaf	pepper
Canola oil	Oregano	Soy cheese	
Cucumber	Pecan	Sunflower oil	

Day 9

Blueberry	Lemon	Parsley	Sesame seed
Butter leaf lettuce	Lentil	Pear	Tomato
Celery	Marjoram	Pinenut	White onion
Garbanzo	Olive oil	Quinoa	

Day 10

Barley	Green bean	Red bean	Yellow onion
Bok choy	Kiwi	Soy margarine	
Cayenne pepper	Pistachio nut	Thyme	
Grapefruit	Pumpkin seed	White rose potato	

Five-Day Rotation Menu Example

Day 1

Breakfast	*Lunch*	*Dinner*	*Snack*
Oat pancakes	Nut loaf with	Black bean chili	Almonds
with	Almonds	with	Strawberry
Egg	Oats	Cilantro	Plum
Oil	Red onion	Green bell	Green bell pepper
Strawberry jam	Marjoram	pepper	
Egg	Chili powder	Red onion	
Green bell pepper	Chard with	Chili powder	
Plum	Red onion	Cumin	

Day 2

Breakfast	*Lunch*	*Dinner*	*Snack*
Millet cereal	Spinach salad	Chicken with	Cashews
Cashew milk	with	Thyme	Banana
Cantaloupe or	Cashews	Sage	Cantaloupe
banana	Jicama	Potato oven fries	Jicama
	Red bell	Steamed spinach	Red bell pepper
	pepper	with	
	Poppy seed	Nutmeg	
	dressing		
	Banana		
	Baked potato		

Day 3

Breakfast	*Lunch*	*Dinner*	*Snack*
Cream of rice	Romaine lettuce	Salmon with	Pecans
Rice milk	salad with	Lemon	Orange
Pecans	Sunflower seed	Green onion	Blackberry
Orange or	Green onion	Dill	Cucumber
blackberries	Cucumber	Brown rice with	Rice cakes
	Lemonette	Green onion	Sunflower seed
	dressing	Asparagus with	
	Rice cakes with	Eggless	
	Sunflower	mayonnaise	
	butter		
	Blackberry jam		

Day 4

Breakfast	*Lunch*	*Dinner*	*Snack*
Buckwheat	Yam	Buckwheat pasta	Peach
pancakes with	Zucchini with	with Tomato	Blueberry
Egg Replacer	Sesame seed	Garlic, Basil	Brazil nut
Safflower oil	Sliced tomato	Shiitake	Zucchini with
Blueberry	with	Mushroom	Tahini
Blueberry jam	Basil	Butter leaf lettuce	Cherry tomato
	Peach	with Tomato	
		Zucchini	
		Basil dressing	
		Sesame seed	
		Olive oil	

Day 5

Breakfast	*Lunch*	*Dinner*	*Snack*
Barley cereal with	Cabbage slaw	Barley soup with	Pear
Pear juice or	with	Celery	Kiwi
Nut milk	Celery	Yellow onion	Celery
Pears	Yellow onion	Parsley	Hazelnut
Hazelnut	Parsley	Green cabbage	Pumpkin seeds
	Eggless	Cayenne	Green beans
	mayonnaise	pepper	Barley muffin
	Barley muffin	Green beans	
	Kiwi	Barley muffin	
		Canola oil	

Day 6

Breakfast	*Lunch*	*Dinner*	*Snack*
Oat muffins with	Sweet potato	Halibut with	Pineapple
Pineapple	Savoy cabbage	Lime	Strawberry
Egg Replacer	with	Shallot	Green bell pepper
Flax seed oil	Green bell	Tarragon	Almonds
Pineapple	pepper	Green bell	Flax seeds
	Shallot	pepper	Oat muffin
	Almonds	Chard with	
	Strawberry	Toasted	
		almonds	
		Oat muffin	
		Safflower oil	

Day 7

Breakfast	*Lunch*	*Dinner*	*Snack*
Cream of rye	Spinach salad	Lamb with	Tangerine
with	with	Rosemary	Banana
Cashew milk	Mushrooms	Red potatoes with	Jicama
Banana or	Red onion	Rosemary	Cashew
Tangerine	Jicama	Olive oil	Mushroom
	Mint dressing	Peas	Peas
	Rye crackers with		
	Cashew butter		

Day 8

Breakfast	*Lunch*	*Dinner*	*Snack*
Rice waffles with	Brown rice with	Brown rice pasta	Raspberry
Egg Replacer	Green onion	with	Orange
Raspberry jam	Broccoli with	Yellow bell	Pecan
Raspberries	Soy cheese	pepper	Cucumber
	Cucumber	Green onion	Yellow bell
		Oregano	pepper
		Soy cheese	Broccoli
		Red leaf salad	Sunflower seeds
		with	Rice cakes
		Cucumber	
		Yellow bell	
		pepper	
		Green onion	
		Sunflower	
		sprouts	
		Canola oil	

Day 9

Breakfast	*Lunch*	*Dinner*	*Snack*
Quinoa cereal	Stuffed tomato	Lentil soup with	Grapefruit
with	with	Tomato	Pear
Pear juice	Hummus	Celery	Celery
Grapefruit	Garbanzo	Parsley	Pinenuts
Pinenuts	bean	White onion	Cherry tomato
	Lemon	Pear juice	Hummus
	Tahini	Marjoram	Tahini
	Parsley	Butter leaf lettuce	
	on Butter leaf	salad with	
	lettuce	Lemonette	
	Celery sticks	dressing	
		Pinenut	

Day 10

Breakfast	Lunch	Dinner	Snack
Barley blueberry	White rose potato	Red bean stew	Blueberry
muffins with	Green beans	with	Kiwi
Blueberry	Pumpkin seeds	Yellow onion	Pumpkin seed
Egg Replacer	Kiwi	Thyme	Pistachio nut
Soy margarine		Cayenne	Barley muffin
Blueberries		pepper	Green bean
		Bok choy with	
		Yellow onion	
		Pistachio	
		Barley muffin	

Simple and Quick Five-Day Rotation Plan Example
Avoided Foods

Barley	Broccoli	Dairy/beef	Soy
Black beans	Celery	Orange	Strawberry

Recommended Foods

Day 1

Basil	Goat	Plum	Wheat
Cucumber	Mushrooms	Romaine lettuce	Zucchini
Feta cheese	Pear	Sunflower seed	
Garlic	Pinenut	Walnut	

Day 2

Avocado	Flax seed	Kiwi	Red onion
Cayenne pepper	Grapefruit	Pecan	Tomato
Cilantro	Green leaf lettuce	Pinto bean	
Corn	Jalapeño	Pistachio	

Day 3

Almond	Blackberry	Green beans	Yellow bell
Apple	Brown rice	Green onion	pepper
Beets	Butter leaf lettuce	Pumpkin seed	Yellow squash

Day 4

Banana	Chicken	Oats	Yam
Brazil nut	Curry	Poppy seed	Yellow onion
Cashew	Fig	Snow peas	
Cauliflower	Green bell pepper	Spinach	

Day 5

Amaranth	Coconut	Jicama	Red bell pepper
Artichoke	Green cabbage	Macadamia	Red leaf lettuce
Blueberry	Green onion	Peach	Sesame
Carrots	Hazelnut	Potato	

Simple and Quick Five-Day Rotation Menu

Day 1

Breakfast	*Lunch*	*Dinner*	*Snack*
Cracked wheat cereal with either	Grilled goat cheese whole wheat sandwich	Whole wheat pasta with Basil	Pinenuts Walnuts Sunflower seeds
Walnuts	Cucumber	Feta cheese	Plum
Sunflower seeds	Zucchini	Mushrooms	Pear
or Pinenuts	Mushrooms	Garlic	Zucchini
Goat milk	Pear or plum	Zucchini	Cucumber
Pear	**or**	Romaine lettuce	Wheat crackers
or	Trail mix with	salad with	
Whole wheat bread toast with	Walnut Pinenuts Sunflower	Feta cheese dressing	
Sunflower butter or	seeds	**or**	
Goat cheese	Cucumber	Whole wheat pasta with	
Pear or plum	Zucchini	Basil	
or	Pear or plum	Zucchini	
Whole wheat bagel with	**or**	Mushrooms	
Goat cheese	Wheat crackers with	**or**	
Walnuts	Sunflower seed	Pasta salad with	
Pear or plum	butter	Zucchini	
	Cucumber	Cucumber	
	Zucchini	Garlic	
	Pear or plum	Oil dressing	
		or	
		Tabouli salad with	
		Zucchini	
		Cucumber	
		Garlic	
		Oil dressing	

Day 2

Breakfast
Corn cereal
Coconut milk
Grapefruit
or
Corn muffin or
   cornbread
Grapefruit
or
Corn muffin or
   tortilla with
   pistachio
   butter
Grapefruit
or
Corn tortilla with
   Avocado
Kiwi

Lunch
Taco or tortilla
   with
   Pinto beans
   Avocado
   Green leaf
      lettuce
   Tomato
   Red onion
   Jalapeño
   Cayenne
      pepper
or
Taco salad with
   Cilantro
   Pinto beans
   Avocado
   Green leaf
      lettuce
   Tomato
   Red onion
   Jalapeño
   Cayenne
      pepper
or
Corn chips with
   salsa
   pinto bean dip
   or Guacamole

Dinner
Polenta with
   Tomato sauce
Green leaf lettuce
   salad with
   Tomato
   Red onion
Kiwi
or
Corn pasta with
   Tomato sauce
Green leaf lettuce
   salad with
   Tomato
   Red onion
or
Taco with
   Pinto beans
   Avocado
   Green leaf
      lettuce
   Tomato
   Red onion
   Jalapeño
   Cayenne
      pepper

Snack
Pecans
Pistachio
Corn chips
Tomato
Avocado
Kiwi
Grapefruit

Day 3

Breakfast

Rice pancakes
  with
  Blackberry
  jam melt
Blackberries or
  Apple
or
Cream of rice
  cereal with
  Almonds
  Apple
  Rice milk or
  Amazaki
Baked apple
or
Rice cakes with
  Almond butter
  Blackberry
  jam
  Blackberries or
  Apple
or
Puffed rice cereal
  with
  Rice milk or
  Amazaki
  Almonds
  Blackberries or
  Apple

Lunch

Rice cakes with
  Almond butter
  Blackberry
  jam
Pumpkin seeds
Apple
Yellow bell
  pepper
Green beans
or
Trail mix with
  Almonds
  Pumpkin
  seeds
  Apple
Yellow bell
  pepper
Green beans
or
Rice cakes
Butter leaf lettuce
  salad with
  Green onion
  Yellow bell
  pepper
  Beets
  Green beans
Almonds or
  Pumpkin
  seeds

Dinner

Brown rice pasta
  with
  Yellow squash
  Yellow bell
  pepper
  Green onion
Steamed green
  beans
Butter leaf lettuce
  salad with
  Beet greens
Applesauce or
  Baked apple
or
Brown rice with
  green onions
Yellow squash
Green beans
Beet greens
Beets
Applesauce or
  Baked apple

Snack

Almonds
Apple
Pumpkin seeds
Blackberries
Rice cakes
Yellow bell
  pepper
Green beans
Beets

Day 4

Breakfast	*Lunch*	*Dinner*	*Snack*
Oatmeal with	Oatmeal muffin	Chicken with	Oat muffin
Cashew milk	Spinach salad	Curry powder	Fig
Cashews	with	Cashews	Banana
Fig or Banana	Snow peas	Yellow onion	Cashews
Cinnamon	Yellow onion	Green bell	Brazil nuts
or	Green bell	pepper	Snow peas
Oatmeal crepes	pepper	Spinach salad	Cauliflower
with	Cauliflower	with	Green bell pepper
Banana	Poppy seed	Poppy seed	
Cashew	dressing	dressing	
Fig or Banana	**or**	Steamed	
or	Trail mix with	Cauliflower	
Oatmeal banana	Brazil nuts	with	
muffin	Cashews	Snow peas	
Cashew butter	Fig or Banana	**or**	
Fig or Banana	Snow peas	Baked yam	
or	Cauliflower	Steamed spinach	
Oat granola with	**or**	Cauliflower	
Cashew milk	Baked yam	Snow peas	
Fig or Banana	Spinach salad	Green bell pepper	
	with	Fig	
	Poppy seed		
	dressing		
	Steamed or		
	stir fried		
	Spinach		
	Snow peas		
	Cauliflower		
	Green bell		
	pepper		

Day 5

Breakfast	Lunch	Dinner	Snack
Amaranth blueberry pancakes with Blueberry jam melt	Trail mix with Hazelnuts Macadamia Coconut Blueberries	Baked potato Steamed Artichokes with Sesame butter or Mayonnaise	Peach Blueberries Macadamia Hazelnuts Sesame seeds
Blueberries or Peach	Tahini dip with Jicama Carrot Red bell pepper	Red leaf lettuce salad with Shallot Red bell pepper Jicama Carrot	Red bell pepper Jicama Carrot Cold artichoke
or			
Amaranth cereal with Coconut milk Hazelnuts	Blueberries or Peach		
Peach	**or**		
or	Amaranth muffin	Amaranth salad with Shallot Red bell pepper Jicama Carrots Hazelnut or Macadamia Peach	
Cottage fries with Shallot Red bell pepper	Green cabbage salad with Shallot Red bell pepper Jicama Carrot Peach		
Peach Hazelnuts			

And you thought a five-day rotation diet is going to be boring, limited, and dull. The combinations can be delightful to the eye and delicious to the palate. Variations are only limited by your imagination. Enjoy, explore, and have fun!

PART III

Food and Recipes

Now for the fun! The following section contains recipes for different levels of cooking skills and degrees of health. This is not a Candida cookbook, but the principles will apply to most, if not all, allergy and immune based problems. If you do not have allergies and are simply looking for good recipes that taste great and are healthy, then enjoy! If you have Candida, do not use the recipes with a safe sweetener and check before using a fruit juice sweetener. If any type of sweetener is out, then these recipes are to be filed away for the day when you can eat them.

Most of the recipes are low fat and some are nonfat. Most of the recipes in the dessert and baked goods chapters contain fats or oils and can be converted to other nonfat methods of cooking you may already know.

Substitution is the foundation for allergy free eating. With substitution you can exchange one food for another in a recipe without altering the results. A major frustration for those with allergies is "What can I eat? I can no longer have my favorites! What CAN I cook? It is going to be boring and tasteless! If I can't have _____, what can I have?" For those who do not have allergies, but are trying to implement a healthier lifestyle, substitution is the answer. If you are attempting to avoid wheat, other grains can be substituted for the wheat in recipes without using combinations of several grains. Your favorite muffin or pancake recipe could use spelt, kamut, or brown rice flour instead of wheat. To support those with Candida and other immune disorders, allergies, and for those seeking to avoid foods that can create major health problems, the following recipes are free of yeast, cow's milk dairy, and sugar. As it is appropriate, each recipe will list the substitutes that are available for the various possibilities. These will include different foods (like vegetables or legumes), grains, sweeteners, dairy, egg replacers, and spices. Trust your own creativity and explore new foods and new ideas. Try using substitution with your favorite recipe. The following recipes will provide many opportunities.

Explore, enjoy, and bon appetit!

CHAPTER 13

Grains—The Staff of Life

GRAINS HAVE BEEN THE mainstay in diets for thousands of years. When whole grains are used, they provide the complex carbohydrates our bodies require for energy. Leaving them whole also supplies the bran for fiber and germ for a concentration of vitamins and minerals. Grains are naturally low in fat and versatile.

Most of us have eaten only a few major grains like rice, wheat, or corn. However, there is a whole new realm of other grains to explore. The world does not have to end when an allergy to wheat, corn, or another grain is diagnosed. You do not have to give up pasta! Wonderful new products are available on the market, including yeast-free bagels using alternative grains. See the chart at the end of this chapter and Sources on page 459. Make it an adventure as you try the common and exotic other grains.

Whole grains are the foundation to a good diet, providing you are not carbohydrate intolerant. When the grains are left whole and unrefined, the bran and fiber, the germ, the amino acids, and the vitamins and minerals remain intact. Refining destroys the integrity of the product.

In discussing the grains below, only the whole grains will be listed. The only exception will be white rice, which is mentioned to include all the forms of rice.

Grains

Amaranth	Kamut	Rice	Teff
Barley	Millet	Rye	Triticale
Buckwheat	Oats	Soy	Wheat
Corn	Quinoa	Spelt	Wild Rice

Each grain is different and has its own unique taste and character-istics. The following information below will help you become acquainted with the different grains. There is nothing mysterious or difficult in mak-ing the transition from one grain to another, only some of the names are a bit odd. Enjoy the adventure!

Amaranth

Amaranth is a seed known as the ancient grain of the Aztecs. It has the highest protein content of the grains and when cooked is very low gluten. Although its texture when cooked is pudding-like, its taste is strong and nutty. The whole grain is best used as different forms of cereal and in casseroles. The flour works well in cookies, pasta, breads, and other baked goods. It is frequently mixed with other whole grain flours.

Barley

Barley is one of the original cultivated grains and is well known in the Middle East. Recently, it has made a renaissance with its claim to help lower cholesterol, as well as with the high chlorophyll content contained in barley greens. It has an earthy, nutty taste with a smooth texture and is easy to digest. Barley can be used like rice, is especially good in soups, makes a great cereal (much like oatmeal), and even works well in sal-ads. The flour also is interesting. Barley/spinach pasta is a wonderful new addition to your pasta repertoire. It makes wonderful pancakes when mixed with buckwheat. Although more moist than wheat and with a smoother texture, barley muffins are an interesting alternative.

Buckwheat

Buckwheat is a hearty grain from central Europe and Russia. It is not a wheat nor is it in the grass family. Those allergic to wheat can usually tolerate buckwheat. It is also low in gluten and can be easily tolerated by those with Candida. Buckwheat is high in protein, calcium, and bioflavonoids. It has a strong and earthy taste. Buckwheat is best known for buckwheat groats or kasha. Groats are great in pilafs, salads, and as a replacement for rice. The flour is smooth and elastic. Pure buckwheat pasta is creamy, light, and easy to digest.

Corn

Delicious tender ears of corn are a wonderful summer treat; there is nothing like picking your own fresh corn. Fresh corn is a vegetable and as the corn dries it increases in starch and becomes a grain. Depending upon your area of the country, corn is not normally thought of as a grain. Corn originally grew in a variety of colors; today we have yellow, white, and blue corn. Cornmeal is used to make polenta, cornbread, and corn muffins, or cooked as a cereal and there are many forms of corn flakes. The flour is made into a pure corn pasta available in different shapes, tortillas, and, everyone's favorite, corn chips.

Kamut

This ancient grain from Egypt is related to modern durum wheat but is slightly grayish in color. It has recently become more available, with more protein than regular bread wheat and a nice nutty flavor. Kamut is found in pastas, pancake mixes, cereals, bagels, and sprouted breads.

Millet

Millet is a staple part of the diet used by the long-living Hunzas in the Himalayas. Millet is not acid in the body and well tolerated by those with Candida. Its tiny yellow beads have a nice nutty taste. When looking for a substitute for rice, do not overlook millet. It makes a great hot breakfast cereal, and combines well in loaves, casseroles, and stuffing. The flour can be used to make good biscuits or pancakes.

Oats

When we think of oats, the picture is of a steaming bowl of hot oatmeal swimming in butter, milk, and brown sugar. We can still have the warm bowl of oatmeal, but we may have to change what we put on it. Whole oats retain the beneficial bran (oat bran also helps lower cholesterol) and germ. Rolled oats are steamed and rolled flat, while steel cut oats are the whole oats sliced into small pieces. Oats can be used as a cereal or kneaded into loaves for bread. The sweet flavor transfers beautifully to the flour and pastas, which are usually mixed with another grain.

Quinoa

This Peruvian seed grain is high in protein and calcium. Its pale, small beads have a mild nutty flavor. It is excellent served as a stuffing, in cold vegetable salads (like tabouli), and casseroles. Use it as you would rice or millet. The pasta is usually found mixed with another grain, like corn or wheat. Quinoa cooks quickly.

Rice

Rice originated in India, Southeast Asia, and China about 4000 BC. and is still a mainstay in these places. This second-most-produced grain in the world is a staple food for more than one half of the world's population. Whole grain rice is an excellent source of B vitamins. It has a mild flavor and can be used well in combination with other foods and all other grains. There are many different varieties of rice, each with its own unique quality. Japonia is purple when cooked and usually mixed with other rices. Rice lends itself very nicely to many dishes, including pilafs, casseroles, stuffings, salads, and desserts.

Pure rice pasta maintains its firmness when cooked and its mild flavor is adaptable to different sauces. Rice flour is slightly course in texture with a flat taste which is great for blending with other flavors. There are rice cakes, crackers, and snacks. See the Cooking Rice chart on the next page for varieties and cooking times.

Rye

Rye originated in Central Asia and is popular today in Central Europe. Rye bread is a great alternative to wheat, whether it is regular, sourdough, or a yeast free variety. Working with rye flour to make your own bread is a challenge but well worth it. Rye has a unique, strong, sweet taste. There are wonderful yeast-free rye crackers, breads, and cereals available.

Soy

Soy is not a grain, it is a legume, but because of the prevalent use of soy flour in making pasta and baked goods, it is listed here. For more information on soy, see page 147.

Spelt

Like Kamut, spelt is related to wheat. It has been grown commercially in Europe for thousands of years and recently has been introduced into

Cooking Rice

Type	Amount	Water	Time	Comment
Brown Basmati	1 cup	2 cups	35 minutes	light and flavorful
Brown long grain	1 cup	2 cups	40 minutes	semi-dry, nutty
Brown medium	1 cup	2 cups	45 minutes	sticky and moist
Brown short	1 cup	2 cups	35 minutes	sticky and moist
Japonia (short)	1 cup	2 cups	40 minutes	rich black color
Sweet rice	1 cup	2 cups	35 minutes	sticky, glutinous
Wehani	1 cup	2¼ cups	60 minutes	russet color, strong flavor
White Basmati	1 cup	2 cups	20 minutes	mild and flavorful
White long grain	1 cup	2 cups	15 minutes	semi-dry, light
White short	1 cup	2 cups	15 minutes	moist and light

the United States. It is not a hybrid, like wheat, and can be grown without fertilizers, pesticides, and insecticides. Spelt is higher in protein and lower in gluten than common wheat, and has lots of vitamins and minerals. The taste is rich and nutty and it is easily digested, and well-tolerated by those allergic to wheat. The most popular product, and the easiest to obtain, is spelt pasta. It is also available in whole grain and flour forms, cereals, bread, and bagels. Spelt substitutes beautifully in any recipe in which you would use wheat.

Teff
Well-known in the Middle East, teff has the tiniest seeds of all the whole grains. Teff is a bread grain high in calcium and other minerals. It is sweet in flavor and makes a good cereal, casserole, or salad. The flour is mild and adapts or blends well in most dishes.

Triticale
Triticale is a grain which was developed in the 1960s and is a cross between wheat and rye. This grain is high in lysine (an amino acid) and has good, solid, protein value. The taste is stronger than wheat and milder than rye. It is available in whole grain berries, flakes (rolled), and flour.

The uses for triticale are similar to wheat. Like bulgur wheat, it is great for stuffing or salads and mixes well with rice. If you are allergic to either wheat or rye, then you will need to avoid this grain.

Wheat
Wheat is the most common grain produced throughout the world and most of it is cultivated in the United States. It has been around for thousands of years. When wheat was removed from King Tutankamon's tomb in Egypt after almost 3,500 years of storage, it was still good. Wheat even precedes King Tut and goes back to Neolithic times. Whole wheat is a good source of the B complex vitamins, vitamin E, and minerals. Wheat is used in many dishes and there is a tremendous variety of products on the market. Be sure that you are getting whole wheat, whether it is cereal, flour, or bread. The label should read 100 percent stone ground whole wheat, especially in breads, otherwise the manufacturer can legally say whole wheat because white flour is wheat. They neglect to inform you that the whole wheat has been stripped of its nutrients and then been enriched artificially with synthetic vitamins and minerals, usually in the form of malted barley. Malted barley is both a sugar and a yeast and white flour acts very much like sugar in the bloodstream.

Different Types of Wheat

Whole wheat pastry flour is a finely ground wheat flour and is excellent for baking cakes, pies, and other foods where you want a finer texture.

Regular whole wheat flour is the choice for making bread, quick bread, muffins, or pancakes.

Bulgur wheat is a precooked cracked wheat. It has been steamed, parched, and then cracked. Bulgur wheat is quick to prepare and is wonderful in casseroles, pilafs, salads (tabouli), stuffings, and other dishes.

Whole wheat berries, usually the hard, red winter wheat, are normally ground into flour for bread or cracked for cereal. The wheat berries can also be sprouted or grown for wheat grass.

Cracked wheat is the whole berry is broken into smaller pieces. It has a texture similar to bulgur wheat when cooked and makes a great hot cereal.

Couscous is made from refined durum wheat by steaming, drying, and cracking. It is another quick cooking form of wheat. Upon cooking, it becomes fluffy and can be used in puddings, salads, and with vegetable combinations. This is refined and has less nutritional value.

Durum wheat is a hard spring wheat and produced as a refined or nonrefined flour. Durum pasta available in health food stores is generally a whole grain pasta. Couscous is usually make from refined durum wheat.

Semolina wheat is a granular, milled product made from durum wheat. It is used for very fine pasta and is even more refined than white flour.

Cooking Wheat

Type	Amount	Water	Time	Comment
Wheat berries	1 cup	3½ cups	60 minutes	pour into boiling water and stir often
Cracked wheat	1 cup	3 cups	35 minutes	pour into boiling water and stir often
Bulgur wheat	1 cup	2 cups	30 minutes	pour boiling water over it and let stand 30 minutes
Couscous	1 cup	3 cups	15 minutes	add to boiling water, cook 1 minute, allow to sit for 15 minutes

Wild rice

Wild rice is harvested from the wild and is not a rice. It comes from the seed of an aquatic grass. The North American Indians were the first to cultivate wild rice. It is very high in protein and has a strong, earthy, but also nutty taste. Usually it is mixed with other rice, and also does well in salads, pilafs, and soups.

There is no real mystery to the preparation of the grains. All you need is a little confidence and information. One cup of dry grain (to be cooked) will feed 2 to 3 people, depending upon appetite. For most grains, ⅓ cup of grain to 1 cup of water, is enough for a single serving. Check with the chart below for any variations.

Cooking Grains

(see rice and wheat chart for varieties and cooking times)

Grain	Amount	Water	Cooking Time
Amaranth	1 cup	1½ cups	20 minutes
Barley	1 cup	3 cups	45 minutes
Buckwheat groats	1 cup	2 cups	15 minutes
Corn (polenta)	1 cup	4 cups	25 minutes
Millet	1 cup	3 cups	35 to 40 minutes
Oats (whole)	1 cup	2 cups	45 to 60 minutes
Quinoa	1 cup	2 cups	15 minutes
Teff	½ cup	2 cups	15 to 20 minutes
Triticale	1 cup	3½ cups	60 minutes
Wheat (cracked)	1 cup	3 cups	40 minutes
Wild Rice	1 cup	3 cups	40 minutes

Be sure to check the package or box if you have anything other than the basic whole grain forms (whole barley, cracked wheat, millet) for cooking instructions. It will be slightly different for each grain.

Packaged grains, especially cream of rye, rice, buckwheat, or other cereals have been processed to some degree. Liz has had clients that were sensitive to that small amount of processing. The whole grain was fine for them, but the processing was not. Most of the packaging are of the whole grains themselves, the flours, or flakes (like oatmeal).

❦ Cereal Toppings

What do you do without the butter, milk, and brown sugar? Here is an opportunity to be creative and to explore new tastes. Read through this section with a happy and adventurous heart.

Alternative cereal toppings

Liquid	Sweet	Liquid & Sweet
Coconut milk	Blackstrap molasses	Amazaki
Goat milk	Date sugar	Apple juice (unfiltered)
Nut milk	Honey	Apricot juice
Rice milk	Honey and blackstrap	Berry juice
Soy milk	molasses	Peach juice
	Maple syrup	Pear juice
		Pineapple juice

Amazaki is a creamy, rice-based liquid. It is both sweet and moist, and available in plain, almond, apricot, and carob.

If you can have sweeteners, and you are not allergic to either one, honey and blackstrap molasses mixed together in the right proportion tastes very much like brown sugar. For cereal, use 1 teaspoon honey and slight ⅛ teaspoon blackstrap.

Depending upon allergy restrictions, try adding cinnamon, nutmeg, chopped nuts, whole or chopped seeds, or dried fruit: raisins, currants, apples, apricots, prunes, and others.

Forms of Grains

The following chart shows the various forms in which different grains are available. The forms are pure and yeast free. If there is a question mark after a product, it means the product is mixed with another grain. Check the labels carefully before purchasing. Buckwheat pasta is found both as a pure pasta and one mixed with wheat. Often they are lumped together in the same area in the store. See Sources on page 459 for product names and distributors for these items.

Forms of Grains

Amaranth

Cereals
Cookies?
Flour
Pasta?
Whole

Barley

Bits of barley cereal
Cereal (flakes)
Flour
Spinach pasta
Sprouts
Whole

Buckwheat

Cream of
Flour
Groats (kasha)
Pasta
Sprouts

Corn

Chips
Cornmeal
Flour
Pasta
Polenta
Tortillas

Kamut

Bagels
Cereal
Flour

Pasta
Sprouts

Millet

Cereal
Flour

Oats

Cereal
Flour
Pasta?

Quinoa

Cakes
Flour
Pasta?

Rice

Cakes
Crackers
Cream of
Flour
Pasta
Snacks

Rye

Bread
Crackers
Cream of
Flour
Rye flakes

Soy

Crackers

Flour
Pasta

Spelt

Bagel
Bread
Cereal
Flour
Pasta

Teff

Cereal
Flour
Whole

Triticale

Flour
Whole

Wheat

Bread
Bulgur
Cereal
Crackers
Cream of
Flours
Pasta
Sprouts

Wild Rice

Whole

🦋 Dry Roasting Grains

Grains have a richer, fuller flavor when roasted. This process opens the grain and will also shorten cooking time. Several grains can be done at once by this method. Set aside some time once a month to do this and store the grain in glass jars. Grains can be roasted in the oven or on the stove top. Larger quantities of grains (three to five cups) are better roasted in the oven. For oven roasting, rinse and drain the grain and spread it on a cookie sheet. Place in an oven preheated to 300 degrees F. Stir the grain every 10 minutes until the moisture has evaporated and the aroma and color are more intense. Each grain will take a different time, from 20 to 40 minutes. For roasting on top of the stove, use a heavy-bottomed skillet and place on medium heat. When the skillet is hot, put the grain in the pan. Using a wooden spoon, turn the grain so the kernels are uniformly roasted. This will take about 15 minutes, depending upon the grain. Although this step is not necessary to enjoy any grain, it enhances the flavor.

For additional information on grains, check the references on page 469 for further reading. Recipes for the use of grains are given in the baked goods, desserts, salads, and vegetarian entrees chapters.

CHAPTER 14

Nuts and Seeds

OST OF US AVOID nuts and seeds mainly because we do not understand them and their importance in good nutrition. They are high in calories, mostly from their fat content. But, nuts and seeds do contain essential fatty acids, are a good source of vitamins and minerals, and are high in protein. For instance, pumpkin seeds are noted to be very beneficial, especially for men. They can kill the parasite responsible for problems associated with the prostate gland. Pumpkin seeds are also included in the formulas for fighting Candida. Flax seed is an excellent intestinal cleanser, providing fiber and bulk. Flax seed oil is a wonderful source of omega 3 fatty acids which helps to reduce blood cholesterol. Nuts and seeds are a fun food, a crunchy snack. They are very filling and high in energy. There are many varieties available, and the only nuts that are interrelated in a food family are walnuts and pecans. The other nuts are in separate food families, which is good news for those with allergies. However, because of their association with fun, nuts can be psychologically addictive for some people.

Nuts are the seeds of certain plants, mainly trees. Seeds are the seeds of various members of the plant family. Nuts and seeds are versatile and delectable. There is an abundant variety with multiple choices available. They both can be enjoyed raw, roasted, cooked, sprouted, or in the forms of flour or butters. However, when talking about nuts and seeds, we are referring to them in the raw form, not the roasted, salted, oiled variety we are accustomed to. They are delicious with everything from soup to dessert.

The nut and seed butters make a wonderful replacement for peanut butter. The butters are often well tolerated by those who cannot eat the whole nut or seed. The whole nut or seed is high in fiber and can be rough on a delicate digestive system. There are many delicious commercial varieties available at your local health food store.

Nut or seed milk provides a wonderful alternative to dairy for use on cereal, in soups, dressings, sauces, dips, and for baking. Included in this chapter are recipes for basic nut and seed milk. See page 148 for more information.

Nuts or seeds will store quite well in their shells providing they are not cracked or otherwise damaged. Because of their high oil content, nuts and seeds can be oxidized easily and become rancid. Raw, shelled nuts or seeds should be stored in an airtight container in the refrigerator or other cool location. They will also freeze well.

For those who have Candida or are highly sensitive to molds, nuts and seeds can be a potential problem. This can be resolved by placing a thin layer of the nuts or seeds on a baking sheet and roasting in an oven at 300 degrees F for 5 minutes. It will slightly alter their nutritional value.

The following charts will help make you aware of the delicious variety of nuts and seeds that available.

Nuts and Seeds

Nuts	Nut Butters	Nut Dairy
Almond	Almond	Almondrella cheeses
Brazil	Cashew	Nut milk
Cashew	Hazelnut (filbert)	
Chestnut	Macadamia	
Coconut	Pistachio	
Hazelnut (filbert)		
Macadamia		
Pecan		
Pinenut		
Pistachio		
Walnut		
Water Chestnut		

Seeds for Snacking	**Seeds for Sprouting**	**Herb Seeds**
Flax	Alfalfa	Anise
Poppy	Fenugreek	Caraway
Pumpkin	Radish	Celery
Sesame	Red clover	Coriander
Sunflower	Sunflower	Cumin
		Dill
	Seed Butters	Fenugreek
	Sesame (tahini)	
	Sunflower	

See page 303 for sprouting directions.

From the preceeding lists, one can see that there is a wide variety of nuts and seeds. On a five-day rotation plan one can have two nuts and one seed per day, depending upon allergy restrictions.

Nuts and seeds are very high in calories and packed with nutrition, so a little goes a long way. If you are trying to loose weight, or are restricting calories for one reason or another, then the following guidelines will be helpful: 10 to 20 nuts per day (depending upon their size), and ⅛ to ¼ cup of seeds per day; and 1 to 2 tablespoons per day of the butters. The nuts or seeds may be eaten raw or used to dress up a vegetable or cereal. If you use nut milk or have a nut loaf, then you will have had your allotment for the day.

Nuts and Seeds Recipes

Nut Cream

Makes 1 cup

    1 cup nuts
    1 cup water

Blanch the nuts in boiling water for 2 to 3 minutes. Drain the nuts and reserve the water. In a blender, coarsely grind the nuts. Add the water and blend until smooth. Refrigerate in a covered container or use immediately.

Nut Milk

Makes 3 cups

    1 cup nuts
    2½ cups water

Grind the nuts to a powder in a blender or food processor. Gradually add the water to desired consistency. For variation, vanilla or almond extract/flavoring may be added.

Sesame Seed Milk

Makes 2 cups

    ½ cup sesame seeds
    2 cups water

Blend well together in a blender. For variation two dates may be added for a little sweetness.

Sunflower Seed Milk

Makes 2½ cups

    1 cup sunflower seeds
    2 cups water

Grind the sunflower seeds to a powder in a blender or food processor. Gradually add the water to the desired consistency. For variation, vanilla extract/flavoring, honey, or dates may be added.

Nuts and seeds are used in recipes throughout *Allergy Free Eating*. Check the different recipe chapters for delightful, fun, and delicious ideas.

CHAPTER 15

Baked Goods

MAJOR PORTION OF DAILY life and eating habits are centered around the use of grains, especially in the form of muffins, pancakes, quick breads, waffles, crepes, and biscuits. These foods are familiar, comforting, and frequently begin the day. When it comes to making the transition from a white flour or limited grain diet, there is a profound sense of deprivation and being overwhelmed. Recipes and sources are limited with regard to the substitution with other grains and are often confusing; added to this is the problem of needing to eliminate dairy, eggs, or other items.

The following recipes taste good and some are absolutely delicious. We have provided substitutions and lots of variety for allergy concerns. However, some of the recipes will have more sweetener in them and will not be suitable for those with Candida or severe dietary restrictions. These are a wonderful alternative for a continuation of a healthy lifestyle. Most of the recipes are adaptable for those with Candida.

Alternative grains means alternative tastes, and what one person thinks tastes good the other may not. When using alternative grains, do not expect a puffy, three-inch or super-sweet muffin. But you will find the results more dense and rich, have different textures, be hearty, and have unique, delightful, and delicious flavors. They will fulfill your need for a warm muffin or a stack of pancakes at breakfast.

Considering that this is one of the most difficult areas of transition, our advice is to simply go for it! You will be pleased by the results. If it doesn't turn out the way you are used to, alter the ingredients to suit your individual taste (like more sweetener, nuts, or liquid). Following are some guidelines to assist you in achieving baked goods which you will be happy with. It will be a challenge, but by keeping open to experimentation and new taste sensations, you will find success.

🦋 *The secret* to working with the whole grains is to sift together all the dry ingredients two to three times and thoroughly beat together the wet ingredients. The sifting of the dry ingredients adds lightness, fluffiness, and even distribution of all the dry ingredients. Applying these techniques will lead to a quality baked good. The beating together of the wet ingredients whips air and lightness into the mixture while evenly dispersing the ingredients. Depending upon the recipe, alternating adding the wet and dry ingredients together will also contribute to the quality of the final product.

🦋 Troubleshooting

If you are you consistently having a problem with your baked goods, make sure that:

The baking powder is fresh.
The flour(s) are sifted adequately two to three times.
The wet ingredients are thoroughly beaten together with a hand mixer or egg beater.
The oven is preheated to the proper temperature and not too hot or too cold.
The correct amount of liquid is used.
Eggs or Egg Replacer or binder (page 140) are used, according to the grain in the recipe.

Based on our cooking experience with various flours, we discovered that barley, teff, amaranth, quinoa, and buckwheat require a little more liquid added to the recipe than the other flours. The whole grain flours absorb liquid quickly. For the best results, combine the flour mixture and the egg mixture efficiently and bake or cook them immediately. With grains other than wheat, baking time is usually five to ten minutes longer and require a lower temperature.

Baked goods require the use of butter or oil for cooking, texture, and taste. In keeping with the desire for lower fat consumption, concentrated fruit (like applesauce, pureed prunes, pears, and peaches) may be substituted for the fat in the recipe. As appropriate, substitute one cup of pureed fruit for one cup of fat. The following will be helpful if using substitutions with grains to determine which flour will work well with an egg replacer or actually need an egg.

Which Grains Need Egg or Egg Replacer or Binder?

Needs Egg	**Egg or Egg Replacer or binder** (page 140)
Barley flour	Amaranth flour
Oat flour	Buckwheat flour
Soy flour	Corn flour
	Millet flour
	Quinoa flour
	Rice flour
	Spelt flour
	Teff flour
	Wheat flour

❦ Important Guidelines

The following guidelines are a result of our winter days together baking and tasting muffins by the dozen.

NOTE: When using just water or juice in a recipe, DO NOT use baking soda as it will alter the taste of the product. Baking soda works great with milk products. Because baking powder often contains allergic or questionable ingredients, baking soda or other rising agents may be necessary. A substitute for baking powder is ¼ teaspoon baking soda and 1 teaspoon lemon juice. For other ideas see page 139.

Combination Suggestions

Amaranth

All nuts
Applesauce
Banana
Cardamom
Cinnamon
Cloves
Corn
Date sugar
Grape juice concentrate
Honey
Spelt
Vegetable glycerin
Wheat

Barley

All milks
All nuts
Apple
Banana
Cardamom
Cinnamon
Date sugar
Grape juice concentrate
Honey
Nutmeg
Pineapple
Rice syrup
Vegetable glycerin
Water

Brown Rice

All milks
All nuts

All seeds
Apple
Apricot
Banana
Blueberry
Cardamom
Cinnamon
Date sugar
Grape juice concentrate
Honey
Nutmeg
Orange
Pineapple
Rice syrup
Vanilla
Vegetable glycerin

Corn

All milks
All nuts
All seeds
All sweeteners
Apple
Blueberry
Orange
Pineapple
Vanilla
Water

Millet

All milks
Almond
Apple
Apricot
Banana

Cinnamon
Date sugar
Grape juice concentrate
Hazelnut
Honey
Orange
Rice syrup
Sunflower seeds
Vanilla
Vegetable glycerin

Oats

All milks
All nuts
All seeds
Apple
Apricot
Banana
Blueberry
Cardamom
Cinnamon
Date sugar
Grape juice concentrate
Honey
Nutmeg
Oat bran
Orange
Pineapple
Rice syrup
Vanilla
Vegetable glycerin

Quinoa

Applesauce
Banana

Combination Suggestions *continued*

Cardamom	Vanilla	All seeds
Cinnamon	Vegetable glycerin	All sweeteners
Cloves		Cardamom
Date sugar	**Spelt**	Cinnamon
Grape juice concentrate	All fruits	Nutmeg
Honey	All milks	Vanilla
Nut or rice milks	All nuts	
Other grains	All seeds	**Wheat**
Vegetable glycerin	All sweeteners	All fruits
	Cardamom	All milks
Soy	Cinnamon	All nuts
All nuts	Cloves	All seeds
All seeds	Ginger	All sweeteners
Apple	Nutmeg	Cardamom
Banana	Vanilla	Cinnamon
Date sugar	Water	Clove
Grape juice concentrate		Ginger
Honey	**Teff**	Nutmeg
Pineapple	All fruits	Vanilla
Rice or soy milk	All milks	Water
Rice syrup	All nuts	

🦋 Tasty Tidbits

One of the problems confronting those with Candida and other allergies is a sensitivity to yeast. Common extracts which can add a lot of flavor, contain alcohol, which contains yeast. A tasty solution is at hand!

Vanilla
Take a 2-inch section of vanilla bean and boil it in 2 to 3 tablespoons of water in a very small pan for 5 minutes. Let cool. Remove the bean and use the liquid in the recipe. For a stronger flavor, let the bean remain in the liquid overnight. For 1 teaspoon of extract, use 2 teaspoon of vanilla liquid or to taste.

Lemon

Replace 1 teaspoon of lemon extract with l teaspoon fresh lemon juice and 1 teaspoon of grated lemon rind.

Orange

Replace 1 teaspoon of orange extract with l teaspoon fresh orange juice and 1 teaspoon of grated orange rind.

Mint

Place 5 fresh mint leaves in 3 tablespoons of water and boil for 5 minutes. Cool and strain. Or use a mint tea bag in ⅓ cup of boiling water and let steep until the desired flavor is reached.

Almond

Place an almond tea bag in ⅓ cup of boiling water and let steep until the desired flavor is reached. For 1 teaspoon of extract, use 2 teaspoons of almond liquid or to taste.

❦ Muffins

Basic Muffins

Makes 12 muffins

- 2 cups whole wheat pastry flour
- 2 teaspoons baking powder
- ½ teaspoon cinnamon (optional)
- 1 cup water
- 1 egg
- 2 tablespoons honey
- ¼ cup melted butter or margarine

SUBSTITUTIONS

Whole wheat pastry flour: 2 cups spelt, barley, or kamut flour

Water: 1 cup nut, rice, goat, or soy milk

Honey: 2 tablespoons rice syrup; 3 tablespoons date sugar; 2 tablespoons barley malt

Butter: ¼ cup olive or canola oil plus ¼ teaspoon sea salt

Preheat oven to 400 degrees F and butter muffin pans. In a mixing bowl, combine the flour, baking powder, and cinnamon and sift together 2 to 3 times. In another bowl, beat together the water, egg, honey, and butter with an egg beater. Combine the flour mixture and the egg mixture, blending until just moistened. Fill the muffin pans to ¾ full and bake for 20 to 25 minutes.

VARIATIONS

Add ½ cup chopped nuts or seeds to the dry ingredients after sifting.

Increase the sweetener by 1 tablespoon and add 1 cup grated apple, blueberries, crushed pineapple, dates, or berries. Or replace the liquid and sweetener with 1 cup of juice and add 1 cup of the same fruit. One teaspoon cinnamon (sifted with the dry ingredients) with apple or dates is an excellent complement. Fold in the fruit last.

Amazing Amaranth Muffins

Makes 12 muffins

- 2 cups amaranth flour
- 2 teaspoons baking powder
- 1 teaspoon cinnamon
- 2 tablespoons water
- 1 egg
- 3 tablespoons grape juice concentrate
- ¼ cup melted butter or margarine
- 1 cup mashed banana
- ½ cup chopped nuts

SUBSTITUTIONS

Amaranth flour: 2 cups quinoa flour

Cinnamon: ¼ teaspoon clove or nutmeg

Egg: 1 teaspoon Egg Replacer or binder (page 140)

Grape juice concentrate: 3 tablespoons honey; 2 tablespoons vegetable glycerin

Butter: ¼ cup olive or canola oil plus ¼ teaspoon sea salt

Banana: 1 cup applesauce

Preheat oven to 400 degrees F and butter muffin pans. In a mixing bowl, combine the flour, baking powder, and cinnamon and sift together 2 to 3 times. In another bowl, beat together the water, egg, grape juice concentrate, and butter with an egg beater. Combine the flour mixture and egg mixture, blending until just moistened, and fold in the bananas and nuts. Fill the muffin pans to ¾ full and bake for 25 to 30 minutes.

Bountiful Brown Rice Muffins

Makes 12 muffins

- 2 cups brown rice flour
- 2 teaspoons baking powder
- 1 teaspoon cinnamon
- 1 egg
- ¼ cup melted butter or margarine
- 1 cup pineapple juice
- ½ cup crushed, well-drained pineapple
- ½ cup nuts or sunflower seeds (optional)

SUBSTITUTIONS

Cinnamon: 1 teaspoon cardamom
Egg: 1 teaspoon Egg Replacer or binder (page 140)
Butter: ¼ cup olive or canola oil plus ¼ teaspoon sea salt
Pineapple juice: 1 cup orange, apple or blueberry juice
Pineapple: ½ cup blueberries or grated apple

Preheat oven to 400 degrees F and butter muffin pans. In a mixing bowl, combine the flour, baking powder, and cinnamon and sift together 2 to 3 times. In another bowl, beat together the egg, butter, and pineapple juice with an egg beater. Combine the flour mixture and the egg mixture, blending until just moistened, and fold in the pineapple and nuts. Fill the muffin pans to ¾ full and bake for 25 to 30 minutes.

VARIATION

Replace the fruit juice and fruit with 1 cup of rice milk and 2 tablespoons rice syrup.

Colorful Corn Muffins

Makes 12 muffins

1¼ cups yellow or blue corn flour
1 cup cornmeal
2 teaspoons baking powder
1 teaspoon baking soda
¼ teaspoon sea salt
1 egg
¾ cup soy milk
¼ cup olive or canola oil
    juice of ½ orange
    ¼ cup honey
2 teaspoons grated orange rind
½ teaspoon vanilla extract

SUBSTITUTIONS
Soy milk: ¾ cup goat or rice milk, or water
Honey: ⅓ cup rice syrup or 1 tablespoon vegetable glycerin
Vanilla extract: 1 teaspoon vanilla liquid (page 205)

Preheat oven to 400 degrees F and butter muffin pans. In a mixing bowl, combine the flour, cornmeal, baking powder, baking soda, and salt and sift together 2 to 3 times. In another bowl, beat together the egg, soy milk, olive oil, orange juice, honey, orange rind, and vanilla extract with an egg beater. Combine the flour mixture and the egg mixture, blending until just moistened. Fill the muffin pans to ⅓ full and bake for 20 minutes.

Marvelous Millet Muffins

Makes 12 muffins

2 cups millet flour
2 teaspoons baking powder
1 egg
1 cup plus 3 tablespoons rice milk
¼ cup melted butter or margarine
2 tablespoons rice syrup
½ cup chopped almonds

Egg: 1 teaspoon Egg Replacer or binder (page 140)
Rice milk: 1 cup plus 3 tablespoons goat, soy, or nut milk
Butter: ¼ cup olive or canola oil plus ¼ teaspoon sea salt
Almond: ½ cup chopped hazelnut or sunflower seeds

Preheat oven to 400 degrees F and butter muffin pans. In a mixing bowl, combine the flour and baking powder and sift together 2 to 3 times. In another bowl, beat together the egg, rice milk, butter, and rice syrup with an egg beater. Combine the flour mixture and the egg mixture, blending until just moistened, and fold in the almonds. Fill the muffin pans to ¾ full and bake for 25 to 30 minutes. Don't worry if the mixture appears too liquid; it bakes beautifully.

VARIATION
Replace the rice milk and syrup with 1 cup orange, apple, or apricot juice and 1 cup chopped or grated fruit. If using orange juice, add 2 teaspoons grated orange rind. If using apricot or apple juice, add 4 tablespoons melted and cooled apricot or apple sugarless jam.

Old Fashioned Oat Muffins
Makes 12 muffins

> 1½ cups oat flour
> ½ cup oat bran
> ¼ cup date sugar
> 2 teaspoons baking powder
> ½ teaspoon cinnamon
> 1 egg
> ¼ cup melted butter or margarine
> 1 cup nut milk
> ½ cup chopped nuts

SUBSTITUTIONS
Cinnamon: ½ teaspoon cardamom
Butter: ¼ cup olive or canola oil plus ¼ teaspoon sea salt
Date sugar: 2 tablespoons grape juice concentrate or maple syrup
Nut milk: 1 cup rice or goat milk

Preheat oven to 400 degrees F and butter muffin pans. In a mixing bowl, combine the flour, oat bran, baking powder, and cinnamon and sift together 2 to 3 times. In another bowl, beat together the egg, butter, and date sugar with an egg beater. Alternately add the flour mixture and the nut milk to the egg mixture, blending until just moistened, and fold in the nuts. Fill the muffin pans ¾ full and bake for 25 minutes.

VARIATION
Replace the milk with 1 cup apple, apricot, or peach juice or 1 cup mashed banana or applesauce. When using the juice, fold in one cup of the same fruit just before putting the batter into the muffin pan.

Satisfying Soy Muffins
Makes 12 muffins

- 2 cups soy flour
- 2 teaspoons baking powder
- 1 egg
- 1 cup soy milk
- 2 tablespoons honey
- ¼ cup melted butter or margarine

SUBSTITUTIONS
Soy milk: 1 cup rice or goat milk
Honey: 2 tablespoons grape juice concentrate or maple syrup
Butter: ¼ cup olive or canola oil plus ¼ teaspoon sea salt

Preheat oven to 350 degrees F and butter muffin pans. In a mixing bowl, combine the flour and baking powder and sift together 2 to 3 times. In another bowl, beat together the egg, soy milk, honey, and butter with an egg beater. Combine the flour mixture and the egg mixture, blending until just moistened. Fill the muffin pans to ¾ full and bake for 30 minutes.

VARIATIONS
Add ½ cup chopped nuts of choice. DO NOT add nut milk or water— the results are bland and flat tasting. Optional: ½ teaspoon of vanilla extract or 1 teaspoon of vanilla liquid.

Add 1 cup grated apple or crushed pineapple. Fruit juice will not work.

Replace the liquid with 1 cup mashed banana. Add 2 to 3 tablespoons or more of milk for desired consistency.

Teff Muffins

Makes 12 muffins

- 1¾ cup teff flour
- 2 teaspoons baking powder
- ½ teaspoon cinnamon (optional)
- 1 egg
- 1 cup plus 3 tablespoons rice milk
- 2 tablespoons rice syrup
- ¼ cup melted butter or margarine
- ½ cup chopped nuts or seeds

SUBSTITUTIONS
Egg: 1 teaspoon Egg Replacer or binder (page 140)
Rice milk: 1 cup plus 3 tablespoons soy, goat, or nut milk
Rice syrup: 2 tablespoons barley malt
Butter: ¼ cup olive or canola oil plus ¼ teaspoon sea salt

Preheat oven to 400 degrees F and butter muffin pans. In a mixing bowl, combine the flour, baking powder, and cinnamon and sift together 2 to 3 times. In another bowl, beat together the egg, rice milk, rice syrup, and butter with an egg beater. Combine the flour mixture and the egg mixture, blending until just moistened, and fold in nuts. Fill the muffin pans to ¾ full and bake for 25 minutes.

VARIATION
Add 1 cup of any fruit.

Marge's Mixed Muffins

Makes 12 muffins

- ⅓ cup millet flour
- ⅓ cup brown rice flour

⅓ cup quinoa flour
2 teaspoons baking powder
¼ teaspoon baking soda
½ teaspoon cinnamon (optional)
2 eggs
½ cup rice milk
1 tablespoon honey
¼ cup melted butter or margarine
1 cup blueberries (optional)

SUBSTITUTIONS
Egg: 2 teaspoons Egg Replacer or binder (page 140)
Honey: 1 tablespoon rice syrup or 1 teaspoon vegetable glycerin
Butter: ¼ cup olive or canola oil plus ¼ teaspoon sea salt

Preheat oven to 350 degrees F and butter muffin pans. In a mixing bowl, combine the flours, baking powder, baking soda, and cinnamon and sift together 2 to 3 times. In another bowl, beat together the eggs, rice milk, honey, and butter with an egg beater. Combine the flour mixture and the egg mixture, blending until just moistened, and fold in blueberries. Fill the muffin pans to ⅔ full and bake for 15 to 20 minutes. These muffins are delicious, but are not low in fat.

🦋 Pancakes, Waffles, and Crepes

Liz's Basic Pancakes

Serves 3

1 tablespoon olive or canola oil for frying
1 cup whole wheat flour
1 teaspoon baking powder
1 egg
2 tablespoons honey (optional)
2 tablespoons olive or canola oil
½ teaspoon vanilla extract (optional)
1 cup water

SUBSTITUTIONS
Whole wheat flour: spelt, kamut, brown rice, barley, or oat flour
Egg: 1 teaspoon Egg Replacer or binder (page 140) or baking powder
Water: 1 cup goat, rice, soy, or nut milk (use rice milk when using rice
    flour)
Vanilla extract: 1 teaspoon vanilla or lemon liquid (page 205)

Heat oil in griddle or frying pan over medium-high heat. In a mixing
bowl, combine the flour and baking powder and sift together 2 to 3
times. In another bowl, beat together the egg, honey, oil, and vanilla
extract with an egg beater. Alternately blend the flour and water into the
egg mixture. Add enough water to maintain a pourable and fairly thin
consistency. As the grain sits, it will absorb liquid and thicken; adding
more water as needed will not alter the pancake. Drop the batter by large
spoonfuls on to the hot griddle and brown pancakes on both sides. Serve
at once or keep pancakes warm in a 200 degree F oven.

VARIATION
Fold in ¼ cup ground nuts or seeds.
    Increase the sweetener by 1 tablespoon and add ½ cup blueberries.

Barley Buckwheat Pancakes
Serves 3

     1   tablespoon olive or canola oil for frying
     ½   cup barley flour
     ½   cup buckwheat flour
     1   teaspoon baking powder
     1   egg
     2   tablespoons honey (optional)
     2   tablespoons olive or canola oil
     ½   teaspoon vanilla extract (optional)
     1   cup water

SUBSTITUTIONS
Egg: 1 teaspoon Egg Replacer or binder (page 140) or baking powder
Water: 1 cup goat, rice, soy, or nut milk
Vanilla extract: 1 teaspoon vanilla or lemon liquid (page 205)

Heat oil in griddle or frying pan over medium-high heat. In a mixing bowl, combine the flours and baking powder and sift together 2 to 3 times. In another bowl, beat together the egg, honey, oil, and vanilla extract with an egg beater. Alternately blend the flour and water into the egg mixture. Buckwheat will absorb water so more will be needed to maintain consistency. Drop the batter by large spoonfuls on to the hot griddle and brown pancakes on both sides. Serve at once or keep pancakes warm in a 200 degree F oven.

My Grandma's Waffles

Serves 4

- 2 cups whole wheat pastry flour
- 4 teaspoons baking powder
- 3 eggs
- 4 tablespoons olive or canola oil
- 1 teaspoon vanilla extract
- 1½ cups water

SUBSTITUTIONS

Whole wheat pastry flour: 2 cups brown rice, spelt, kamut, or oat flour
Vanilla extract: 2 teaspoons vanilla liquid (page 205)
Water: 1½ cups rice, soy, or goat milk

Heat the waffle iron. In a mixing bowl, combine the flours and baking powder and sift together 2 to 3 times. Separate the eggs and beat the egg whites with a hand mixer until stiff peaks form. In another bowl, beat together the yolks, oil, and vanilla extract with an egg beater. Alternately add the flour and milk to the egg mixture, beating until smooth and well blended. Fold in the beaten egg whites. Depending upon your waffle iron, lightly butter the cooking surface.

Cover the grid of the waffle iron about ⅔ with the batter and cook for about 4 minutes or until done. Either serve at once or keep waffles warm in a 200 degree F oven. When buying a waffle iron, look for one that cooks quickly at a high temperature. This will produce a light, fluffy, and delectable waffle.

Pancake and Waffle Toppings

Maple syrup
Heated honey/rice syrup
Melted sugarless jam
Chopped nuts
Chopped fruit
Pureed fruit
Goat or soy yogurt

Joanna's Basic Crepes

Serves 4 (16 crepes)

1   cup whole wheat pastry flour
2   large eggs
1   cup rice milk
¼   teaspoon sea salt
1   tablespoon olive or canola oil

SUBSTITUTIONS

Whole wheat pastry flour: 1 cup brown rice, barley, oat, spelt, kamut, or millet flour
Egg: 3 teaspoons Egg Replacer or binder (page 140)
Rice milk: 1 cup goat milk

In a blender, combine all the ingredients and blend until smooth. Let mixture sit for one hour. The mixture should be thin and pour easily. If not, add up to ½ cup of additional rice milk. Lightly oil a skillet or crepe pan and place over high heat. Pour a small amount of batter into the pan and swirl it until it barely covers the bottom of the pan. Cook for 2 to 3 minutes checking the underside of the crepe for a light brown color. Quickly turn and cook the other side to the same light brown (1 to 2 minutes). Either serve at once or keep crepes warm in a 200 degree F oven.

Crepes can be used for breakfast, as a lunch or dinner entree, or even as a dessert. Traditionally, crepes are filled with 2 tablespoons of filling, rolled, and served with a sauce. For entree ideas, see page 318. For breakfast crepes try:

Crushed or chopped strawberries topped with melted, sugarless strawberry jam, sprinkled with slivered almonds.

Blueberries or other berries topped with melted, sugarless blueberry jam.

Crushed or chopped peaches, nectarines, kiwi, or apricot topped with goat or soy yogurt and pieces of fruit or coarsely ground nuts. Sprinkle with cinnamon.

❧ Biscuits

Basic Biscuits

Makes 24 biscuits

- 2 cups spelt flour
- 2 teaspoons baking powder
- ¼ teaspoon sea salt
- 4 to 6 tablespoons butter or margarine
- ¾ cup goat milk

SUBSTITUTIONS

Spelt flour: 2 cups whole wheat pastry flour, millet, kamut, or brown rice flour

Goat milk: ¾ cup soy or rice milk

Preheat oven to 450 degrees F. In a mixing bowl, combine the flour, baking powder, and salt and sift together 2 to 3 times. With two knives or pastry blender, quickly cut the butter into the flour mixture until it is the consistency of oatmeal. Make a well in the center of the mixture. Pour in the milk and stir with a fork until blended. It will be a slightly sticky dough. Knead briefly on a floured surface. Roll out into a sheet from ½ to 1 inch thick. Cut the dough with a floured biscuit cutter, glass, or knife into rounds. Place on a lightly oiled cookie sheet and bake for 12 to 15 minutes.

VARIATIONS

Herb Biscuits

Add ½ cup minced parsley, basil, or chive or 1½ tablespoons tarragon or 2 tablespoons dill to flour mixture before adding the milk.

Seed Biscuits
Add 2 teaspoons of celery seed, cumin seed, poppy seed, caraway seed, or anise to flour mixture before adding the milk.

Vegetable Biscuits

Makes 18 biscuits

- 1 cup millet flour
- 2 teaspoons baking powder
- ¼ teaspoon nutmeg
- ¼ teaspoon sea salt
- 6 tablespoons butter or margarine
- 6 tablespoons rice milk
- 1 cup cooked and mashed sweet potato
  sesame seeds or poppy seeds (optional)

SUBSTITUTIONS
Millet flour: 1 cup whole wheat pastry, spelt, or brown rice flour
Rice milk: 6 tablespoons soy or goat milk
Sweet potato: 1 cup cooked and mashed butternut squash, yam, or
   pumpkin
Nutmeg: ½ teaspoon cinnamon

Preheat oven to 450 degrees F. In a mixing bowl, combine the flour, baking powder, nutmeg, and salt and sift together 2 to 3 times. With two knives or pastry blender, quickly cut the butter into the flour mixture until it is the consistency of oatmeal. Make a well in the center of the mixture. Add the milk and sweet potato and stir with a fork until blended. Knead briefly on a floured surface. Roll out into a sheet from ½ to 1 inch thick. Cut the dough with a floured biscuit cutter, glass, or knife into rounds. Sprinkle surface of biscuits with sesame seeds. Place on a lightly oiled cookie sheet and bake for 12 to 15 minutes.

🦋 Dumplings

Basic Flour Dumplings

Serves 4

> 1 cup sifted whole wheat pastry flour
> 2 teaspoons baking powder
> ¼ teaspoon sea salt
> ¼ cup chopped parsley
> ¼ cup minced chives (optional)
> 1 egg
> ⅓ cup soy milk
> 2 tablespoons butter or margarine

SUBSTITUTIONS

Whole wheat pastry flour: 1 cup spelt, rice, kamut, or millet flour
Chives: ¼ cup chopped fresh basil or 1 tablespoon tarragon or dill
Egg: 1 teaspoon Egg Replacer or binder (page 140)
Soy milk: ⅓ cup goat, rice, or nut milk

In a mixing bowl, combine the flour, baking powder, and salt and sift together 2 to 3 times. With two knives or pastry blender, quickly cut the butter into the flour mixture until it is the consistency of oatmeal. Stir in the chopped herbs. In another bowl, beat together the egg, milk, and butter with an egg beater. Add ¾ of the egg mixture to the flour mixture, stirring with a fork to make a stiff dough. Do not over mix. Add the rest of the liquid, if needed. Drop the batter by spoonfuls into heated vegetable stock, soup, or stew and cover. Simmer for 5 minutes, remove lid and turn dumplings, then replace lid and simmer for another 5 minutes.

VARIATION

The dumplings may be made without butter. Add the egg mixture to the dry ingredients and proceed.

Potato Dumplings

Serves 4

     4 large potatoes
  1½ cups rice flour
     ½ teaspoon sea salt
     1 egg
     2 tablespoons parsley (optional)

SUBSTITUTIONS

Rice flour: 1½ cups whole wheat pastry, spelt, oat, kamut, millet, ama-
    ranth, or barley flour
Egg: 1 teaspoon Egg Replacer or binder (page 140)

Peel, coarsely chop, and boil the potatoes in salted water until tender.
Drain the potatoes and work them through a ricer. When cool, transfer potatoes to a mixing bowl and beat in the flour, salt, egg, and parsley. Work the mixture into a dough with your hands, adding more flour
if the dough is too moist. Shape into golf ball size dumplings. Drop them
into a large kettle of boiling, salted water and boil for 15 minutes. Serve
with a gravy or sauce.

❦ Flatbreads and Crackers

Kate's Barley Flatbread

Makes 12 flatbreads

     ½ cup sesame seeds
     1 cup barley flour
     1 teaspoon sesame oil
     ¼ cup minced onion (optional)
     ½ teaspoon sea salt
     ¼ cup cold water
         sesame seed and sea salt for topping

SUBSTITUTIONS

Barley flour: 1 cup spelt or kamut flour; 1½ cups rye flour
Sesame oil: 1 teaspoon olive or canola oil

Topping: caraway seed and sea salt for rye; cumin, flax, or sesame and sea salt for spelt or kamut

Preheat oven to 400 degrees F. In a blender or grinder, grind the sesame seeds to make ½ cup flour. In a mixing bowl, combine sesame seed flour and barley flour and sift together 2 to 3 times. Add the oil, onion, and salt and mix well. Make a well in the center of the mixture and slowly pour in the water, stirring with a fork until well blended and mixture leaves the sides of the bowl. Break the mixture into four balls and roll them on a floured board. Cut in large, even circles like a cereal bowl. Sprinkle 1 teaspoon sesame seeds and ¼ teaspoon sea salt on each round and press lightly with rolling pin. Transfer to a baking sheet and bake for 15 minutes.

Joanna's Poppy Seed Crackers

Makes 24 crackers

- 1½ cups millet flour
- 2½ teaspoons baking powder
- ¼ teaspoon sea salt
- ¼ teaspoon baking soda
- 4 tablespoons butter or margarine
- ¾ cup rice milk
- ½ cup poppy seeds
- 2 tablespoons dry parsley (optional)

SUBSTITUTIONS

Millet: 1½ cup spelt, oat, whole wheat, kamut, amaranth, or quinoa flour
Rice milk: ¾ cup goat milk or water

Preheat oven to 400 degrees F. In a mixing bowl, combine millet, baking powder, baking soda, and salt and sift together 2 to 3 times. With two knives or pastry blender, quickly cut the butter into the flour mixture until it is the consistency of oatmeal. Stir in poppy seeds and make a well in the center of the mixture. Pour in the milk and stir with a fork until well blended and mixture leaves the sides of the bowl. Knead briefly on a floured surface. Roll out into a sheet from ¼-inch thick. Sprinkle lightly with salt and additional poppy seeds. Cut into 3-inch squares and transfer to a baking sheet. Bake 12 to 15 minutes.

🦋 Quick breads

Banana Bread

Makes 1 loaf

> 3 large, ripe bananas
> 2 cups sifted whole wheat pastry flour
> 3 teaspoons baking powder
> 1 teaspoon cinnamon
> ½ cup butter or margarine
> ⅓ cup honey plus enough blackstrap molasses to make ½ cup
> 2 eggs
> 1 teaspoon vanilla extract
> ½ cup chopped nuts

SUBSTITUTIONS

Whole wheat pastry flour: 2 cups barley, spelt, kamut, brown rice, or quinoa flour

Cinnamon: 1 teaspoon cardamom

Honey: ⅔ cup date sugar, ¾ cup grape or apple juice concentrate, or ¾ cup rice syrup

Eggs: 2 teaspoons Egg Replacer or binder (page 140)

Vanilla extract: 2 teaspoons vanilla liquid (page 205)

Preheat oven to 350 degrees F. Mash bananas and set aside. In a mixing bowl, combine flour, baking powder, and cinnamon and sift together 2 to 3 times. In another bowl, cream the honey and butter until light. Beat in the eggs and vanilla and stir in the mashed banana. Add the flour to the creamed mixture, blending well. Depending on the flour, add water if needed. Fold in the nuts and pour mixture into a lightly oiled loaf pan. Bake for one hour.

Corn Bread

Makes 6 servings

- 1 cup corn flour
- 1 cup cornmeal
- 4 teaspoons baking powder
- 2 eggs
- 1 cup water
- ¼ cup melted butter or margarine
- 2 tablespoons honey
- 1 teaspoon blackstrap molasses

SUBSTITUTIONS

Corn flour: 1 cup spelt, amaranth, whole wheat pastry, kamut, or millet flour

Water: 1 cup rice, soy, or goat milk

Honey: 3 tablespoons rice syrup or 2 tablespoons grape/rice granular concentrate

Preheat oven to 425 degrees F. In a mixing bowl, combine the flour, cornmeal, and baking powder and sift together 2 to 3 times. In another bowl, beat together the eggs, water, honey, molasses, and butter with an egg beater. Add the flour mixture and water and blend until smooth. Pour mixture into a buttered 9 x 9 x 2 pan and bake for 25 minutes. Serve warm.

Oat Bread

Makes 1 loaf

- 1¾ cups oat flour
- 4 teaspoons baking powder
- ¼ teaspoon sea salt
- ¼ teaspoon ginger
- ¼ teaspoon nutmeg
- ½ teaspoon cinnamon
- ¼ cup oat bran
- 1 cup oatmeal

2 eggs
1 cup goat milk
⅓ cup oil
⅓ cup honey and enough blackstrap molasses to make ½ cup
½ cup chopped nuts (optional)

SUBSTITUTIONS
Goat milk: 1 cup rice or soy milk
Honey: ½ cup date sugar; ⅓ cup maple syrup

Preheat oven to 350 degrees F. In a mixing bowl, combine the flour, baking powder, salt, ginger, nutmeg, and cinnamon and sift together 2 to 3 times. Stir in the oat bran and oatmeal. In another bowl, beat together the eggs, milk, oil, and honey with an egg beater. Make a well in the flour mixture and add the egg and milk mixture and blend until just moistened. Fold in the nuts. Butter a large loaf pan, line bottom with wax paper and grease the paper. Pour batter into the loaf pan and bake for 45 to 50 minutes. Store covered for 24 hours. Slice and serve.

Date Nut Loaf

Makes 1 loaf

2 cups chopped dates
1 cup chopped walnuts
1 cup boiling water
2 cups of sifted whole wheat pastry flour
1 teaspoon baking soda
1 teaspoon baking powder
1 teaspoon cinnamon (optional)
¼ cup butter or margarine
½ cup date sugar
1 egg
1 teaspoon vanilla extract (optional)
   5 tablespoons cold water

SUBSTITUTIONS
Walnuts: 1 cup pecans, hazelnuts, or Brazil nuts
Whole wheat pastry flour: 2 cups brown rice, soy, spelt, kamut, or millet
   flour

Date sugar: ¼ cup honey plus blackstrap molasses to make ⅓ cup; ½ cup rice syrup or barley malt

Vanilla extract: 2 teaspoons vanilla liquid (page 205)

Preheat oven to 350 degrees F. In a medium bowl, combine the dates, nuts, and boiling water. Set aside. In a mixing bowl, combine the flour, baking soda, baking powder, and cinnamon and sift together 2 to 3 times. In another bowl, cream the butter and date sugar. Add the egg and vanilla and beat thoroughly. Alternately add the flour mixture and date and nut mixture to the egg mixture and blend well. Stir in the water and butter a large loaf pan. Pour batter into the loaf pan and bake for 45 to 50 minutes or until done.

NOTE: If using soy flour, preheat oven to 300 degrees F and bake for 1 hour or until done.

Apple Loaf

Makes 1 loaf

  2 cups whole wheat pastry flour
1½ teaspoons baking powder
  1 teaspoon cinnamon
  ¼ cup butter or margarine
  ¼ cup honey and enough blackstrap molasses to make ⅓ cup
  2 eggs
  1 cup grated apple
  ¼ cup chopped nuts (optional)
    water

SUBSTITUTIONS

Whole wheat pastry flour: 2 cups spelt, brown rice, amaranth, millet kamut, or barley flour

Cinnamon: 1 teaspoon cardamom; ½ teaspoon nutmeg and ¼ teaspoon clove

Honey: ½ cup apple juice concentrate, rice syrup, or date sugar

Egg: 2 teaspoons Egg Replacer or binder (page 140)

Preheat oven to 350 degrees F. In a mixing bowl, combine the flour, baking powder, and cinnamon and sift together 2 to 3 times. In another bowl, cream the butter and honey. Add the eggs and beat thoroughly. Add the apple and the flour mixture and blend well. Fold in the nuts and enough water, if necessary, to make a thick but moist batter. Butter a large loaf pan and spoon in batter. Bake for 60 to 70 minutes or until done.

Liz's Pumpkin Bread

Makes 1 loaf

    2 cups spelt flour
    1 teaspoon baking soda
    ½ teaspoon nutmeg
    ½ teaspoon cinnamon
    ¼ teaspoon ginger
    ¼ teaspoon sea salt
    1 cup cooked pumpkin
    ½ cup olive or canola oil
    2 eggs
    ⅓ cup honey plus enough blackstrap molasses to make ½ cup
    ½ cup chopped walnuts
    1 cup raisins (optional)
    ¼ cup water

SUBSTITUTIONS

Spelt flour: 2 cups whole wheat pastry, brown rice, millet, or kamut flour; 1½ cups oat flour and ½ cup oat bran
Cinnamon: ½ teaspoon cardamom
Pumpkin: 1 cup cooked sweet potato, yam, or squash
Egg: 2 teaspoons Egg Replacer or binder (page 140)
Honey: ½ cup date sugar, rice syrup, or maple syrup
Walnuts: ½ cup almonds, pecans, or hazelnuts
Raisins: 1 cup currants

Preheat oven to 350 degrees F. In a mixing bowl, combine the flour, baking soda, nutmeg, and cinnamon and sift together 2 to 3 times. In another bowl, combine the pumpkin, oil, eggs, and honey and beat well. Mix in the flour mixture until well blended. Fold in the walnuts and stir in water. Add more water, if necessary, to make a thick but very moist batter. Grease a large loaf pan and spoon in batter. Bake for 65 to 70 minutes or until done.

Zucchini Bread

Makes 1 loaf

- 1¼ cups of whole wheat pastry flour
- 1 teaspoon baking powder
- ½ teaspoon baking soda
- ½ teaspoon nutmeg
- ½ teaspoon cinnamon
- ½ cup butter or margarine
- ¼ cup honey plus 1 tablespoons blackstrap molasses
- 1 cup grated zucchini
- 2 eggs
- ½ teaspoon lemon extract
- ½ cups raisins or currants (optional)

SUBSTITUTIONS

Whole wheat pastry flour: 1¼ cup spelt, brown rice, millet, amaranth, or quinoa flour
Honey: ⅓ cup rice syrup, barley malt, apple juice concentrate
Zucchini: 1 cup grated carrot
Egg: 2 teaspoons Egg Replacer or binder (page 140)
Lemon extract: 1 teaspoon lemon juice

Preheat oven to 350 degrees F. In a mixing bowl, combine the flour, baking powder, baking soda, nutmeg, and cinnamon and sift together 2 to 3 times. In another bowl, cream the butter and honey until light and smooth. Add the eggs and lemon extract and beat well. Add the zucchini and flour mixture and mix until well blended. Fold in the raisins. If necessary, add water to make a thick but very moist batter. Grease a large loaf pan and spoon in batter. Bake for 1 hour or until done.

Citrus Tea Bread

Makes 1 loaf

- 3 medium oranges, peeled and cut into narrow strips
- 2 cups water
- 1 cup honey
- 2¾ cups whole wheat pastry flour

  4 teaspoons baking powder
  ¾ teaspoon sea salt
  1 cup almond or hazelnut milk
  ½ teaspoon almond extract
  ½ cup chopped almond

SUBSTITUTIONS

Orange: 4 lemons, 5 tangerines, or 3 tangelos

Honey: 1¼ cup rice syrup, grape or apple juice concentrate, or 1 cup
    maple syrup

Whole wheat pastry flour: 2¾ cups spelt, millet, kamut, or brown rice
    flour; 2¼ cups oat flour and ½ cup oat bran

Almond milk: 1 cup hazelnut milk

Almonds: ½ cup chopped hazelnuts (nuts should match the milk)

In a medium saucepan, combine orange strips and water. Simmer over
medium heat for 30 to 45 minutes, or until peels are tender and only ¼
cup of water remains. Add the honey, bring to boil and cook until syrup
thickens. Preheat oven to 325 degrees F. In a mixing bowl, combine the
flour, baking powder, and salt and sift together 2 to 3 times. To the flour
mixture, gradually add the milk, almond extract, and warm orange strips
and syrup and beat well. Stir in the chopped nuts. Butter a large loaf
pan, line bottom with wax paper and grease the paper. Spoon batter into
the loaf pan and bake for 1 hour or until done and let cool before serving.

CHAPTER 16

Nurturing and Delicious Soups

he soups presented here are wonderful as part of a meal, great for lunch, or a meal in itself with a salad and whole grain cracker, muffin, or roll. They are especially nurturing and satisfying on a cold day. Frequently, directions are given for sautéing some of the vegetables in a little oil. It improves the flavor, but the step can be omitted.

An excellent and economical poultry stock can be made from the leftover carcass or parts of chicken, turkey, or game hens. In the process of preparing the stock, you will find that quite a bit of meat will be left. It can be added to the soup, used for a poultry/rice casserole, or be combined with a sauce to serve over pasta and grains. Be generous with the water when you are preparing the stock. You may have three meals out of that chicken instead of merely one!

Soup Stocks

Quick Herb Stock

Makes 4 cups

- 2 quarts cold water
- 1 medium onion, thinly sliced
- ¼ cup chopped fresh parsley
- 2 tablespoons dried thyme
- 1 tablespoon dried oregano
- 1 tablespoon black pepper
- 4 bay leaves
- 1 teaspoon sea salt

SUBSTITUTIONS
Onion: 1 large leek, thinly sliced; 3 minced shallots; 1 bunch chopped green onions
Thyme: 2 tablespoons dried marjoram or rosemary

In a soup pot, combine all ingredients and bring to a boil. Simmer until the liquid is reduced by half. Pass through a fine strainer and let cool. Transfer to a covered container and refrigerate or freeze until ready to use.

Vegetable Stock

Makes 4 quarts

- 2 tablespoons olive or canola oil
- 3 sliced onions
- 3 cloves minced garlic
- 5 chopped carrots
- 4 stalks chopped celery plus leaves
- 6 quarts water
- 2 bay leaves
- 1 teaspoon thyme
- 1 teaspoon oregano

SUBSTITUTIONS
Onion: 3 large leeks, thinly sliced; 8 minced shallots
Thyme: 1 teaspoon dried marjoram or rosemary

In a soup pot, heat the oil and sauté the onions, garlic, carrots, and celery until tender. Add the water, bay leaves, thyme, and oregano and bring to a boil. Reduce heat to simmer and cook covered for 30 minutes. Pass through a fine strainer and let cool. Transfer to a covered container and refrigerate or freeze until ready to use.

Poultry Stock

Makes 1½ quarts

- 1 or more poultry carcass (or fresh cut or whole) plus the giblets and neck
- 2 quarts water

  2 stalks chopped celery plus leaves
  1 chopped onion
  1 chopped carrot
  ½ cup chopped fresh parsley
  1 teaspoon thyme
  1 teaspoon sage
    sea salt and black pepper

SUBSTITUTIONS
Onion: 2 sliced leeks; 3 minced shallots
Thyme: 1 teaspoon marjoram or rosemary

In a soup pot, combine all ingredients and bring to a boil. Simmer 2 to 4 hours. Let sit to cool, strain out the bones, and reserve the meat. Leave in the vegetables depending on the use of the stock. Transfer to a covered container and refrigerate or freeze until ready to use.

✤ Barley Soups

Liz's Barley Soup

Serves 4

  2 tablespoons olive or canola oil
  1 sliced large onion
  2 medium chopped carrots
  2 stalks chopped celery plus leaves
  2 cups chopped tomatoes
  1 cup whole barley
  ⅓ cup chopped fresh parsley
    sea salt and black pepper
  4 cups water
    cayenne pepper

SUBSTITUTIONS
Onion: 2 sliced leeks; 3 minced shallots
Carrot: 1 cup chopped jicama
In a soup pot, heat the oil and sauté the onion, carrot, and celery in the oil for about 10 minutes. Add the tomatoes, barley, parsley, a little

salt and pepper, and water. Bring to a boil and correct the seasonings with salt and cayenne pepper. Simmer for 1 hour, adding more water if necessary. and serve hot. Barley will grow and absorb liquid.

Barley Cabbage Soup

Serves 6

    2 tablespoons olive or canola oil
    1 medium sliced onion
    2 medium sliced carrots
    2 stalks chopped celery plus the leaves
    1 cup whole barley
    6 cups water
  ¼ cup chopped fresh parsley
    2 cups shredded green cabbage
      sea salt and black pepper

SUBSTITUTIONS
Carrot: 1 large diced red bell pepper or jicama
Celery: 1½ cups chopped celery root
Barley: 1 cup kasha, whole wheat berries, or spelt berries
Water: 6 cups Quick Herb Stock (page 229)
Green cabbage: 2 cups shredded red, Napa, Chinese, or Savoy cabbage

In a soup pot, heat the oil and sauté the onion, carrot, and celery in the oil for about 10 minutes. Add the barley, broth, parsley, salt and pepper. Bring to a boil, then reduce heat and simmer for 2 hours. Add the cabbage and more water if necessary, and salt and pepper. Cook for 30 minutes and serve hot.

Barley Mushroom Soup

Serves 6

    2 tablespoons olive or canola oil
    1 large sliced onion
    2 chopped carrots
    1 stalk chopped celery plus leaves
    1 cup sliced mushrooms
    2 peeled, chopped potatoes

8 cups Quick Herb Stock (page 229)
1 cup whole barley
¼ cup chopped fresh parsley
½ teaspoon celery seed
1 teaspoon thyme
1 cup chopped green beans
  sea salt and black pepper

SUBSTITUTIONS
Onion: 2 sliced leeks; ¾ cup minced shallots
Carrots: 1 cup chopped jicama
Celery: ½ cup chopped celery root
Quick Herb Stock: 8 cups water
Barley: 1 cup kasha
Celery seed: ½ teaspoon dill seed
Green beans: 1 cup peas
Thyme: 1 teaspoon rosemary

In a soup pot, heat the oil and sauté the onion, carrot, and celery in the oil for about 10 minutes. Add the sliced mushrooms and potatoes and sauté briefly. Add the stock, barley, parsley, celery seed, and thyme. Bring to a boil and simmer for about 2 hours. Add the green beans, salt and pepper and cook for 30 minutes. Serve hot.

Barley Pea Soup

Serves 4

1 tablespoon olive or canola oil
1 cup chopped onion
5 cups water
½ cup whole barley
1 cup split peas
½ teaspoon thyme
  sea salt and black pepper

SUBSTITUTIONS
Onion: ½ cup minced shallots; 4 cloves minced garlic
Barley: ½ cup millet or triticale
Thyme: ½ teaspoon basil

In a soup pot, heat the oil and sauté the onion for 3 to 5 minutes or until transparent. Add the water, barley, split peas, and thyme and bring to a boil. Reduce heat and let simmer for 1½ to 2 hours. Add salt and pepper and serve.

🦋 Legume Soups

Basic Split Pea Soup

Serves 6

- 8 cups of water
- 2 cups split peas
- 2 large ham hocks (optional)
  sea salt and black pepper
- 1 large chopped carrot
- 1 large chopped onion
- 2 large stalks chopped celery plus leaves
- 2 diced potatoes
- ½ cup chopped fresh parsley
- 1 cup goat milk (optional)

SUBSTITUTIONS
Ham hocks: ½ cup kombu
Onion: ¾ cup minced shallots; 2 sliced leeks
Goat milk: 1 cup soy or rice milk

In a large soup pot, combine the water, split peas, ham, and salt and pepper and bring to a boil (watch because it will boil over easily). Add the carrot, onion, celery, potatoes, and parsley and simmer for 2 hours. Remove the ham, discarding the rind, chop into serving pieces. The soup can be presented three ways: 1. Add the chopped ham and serve as a chunky soup. 2. Puree the soup in a blender, add the chopped ham and serve. 3. Milk may be added to either for a richer soup.

NOTES: Carrot, potato, celery, or parsley may be omitted from the soup without much effect on the flavor.

A good substitute for the ham hocks is kombu, or seaweed. It provides similar salt flavoring and is rich in vitamins. Use any dry seaweed, break into pieces, and add in place of the ham hocks.

Curried Split Pea Soup

Serves 4

- 4 cups water
- 1 cup yellow split peas
- 1 medium chopped onion
  sea salt and black pepper
- 2 teaspoons curry powder
- 1 cup rice milk

SUBSTITUTIONS
Onion: ½ cup minced shallots; 1 sliced leek
Rice milk: 1 cup goat or soy milk

In a large soup pot, combine the water, split peas, onion, and salt and pepper. Bring to a boil, then reduce heat and simmer for 45 minutes. In a blender, puree the mixture along with the curry powder and milk. Reheat and serve. For a thinner soup, add an additional cup of rice milk or water.

Curried Lentil Soup

Serves 6

- 1 tablespoon olive or canola oil
- 1 medium chopped onion
- 1 chopped carrot
- 6 cups water
- 2 cups lentils
- 1 bay leaf
- 2 teaspoons curry powder
  sea salt and black pepper

SUBSTITUTIONS
Onion: ½ cup minced shallots; 1 sliced leek; 4 cloves minced garlic
Carrot: ½ cup chopped red bell pepper; 1 chopped celery stalk

In a soup pot, heat the oil and sauté the onion and carrot for 3 to 5 minutes or until onion is transparent. Add the lentils, water, and bay leaf. Bring to a boil, then reduce heat and simmer for 1 hour. In a blender, puree the mixture along with the curry powder and salt and pepper. Reheat and serve. For a thinner soup, add an additional cup of water.

Luscious Lentil Soup

Serves 4

- ¼ cup olive or canola oil
- 2 large sliced onions
- 1 chopped carrot
- 3 cups water
- 1 cup lentils
- 2 chopped tomatoes
- ¼ cup unfiltered apple juice
- ⅓ cup chopped fresh parsley
- ¼ teaspoon thyme
- ¼ teaspoon marjoram
  sea salt and black pepper

SUBSTITUTIONS
Onion: 2 sliced leeks; 1 cup minced shallots
Carrot: 1 diced red bell pepper; 1 cup chopped jicama
Apple juice: ¼ cup unfiltered pear juice

In a soup pot, heat the oil and sauté the onion and carrot for 3 to 5 minutes or until onion is transparent. Add the water, lentils, tomatoes, apple juice, parsley, thyme, marjoram, and salt and pepper. Bring to a boil and simmer for 1 to 2 hours. Serve hot.

White Bean and Ham Soup

Serves 6

- 8 cups water
- 1 pound Navy beans
- 2 ham hocks (optional)
- 2 stalks chopped celery plus leaves

    1 chopped carrot
    1 chopped onion
        sea salt and black pepper

SUBSTITUTIONS

Navy beans: 1 pound small lima or small northern beans

Ham hocks: 1 teaspoon thyme, 1 teaspoon allspice, and ½ teaspoon sea
    salt

Carrot: ½ cup chopped red bell pepper or jicama

Onion: ½ cup shallots or 5 cloves minced garlic

In a soup pot, combine all the ingredients and bring to a boil. Reduce
heat and simmer for 2 to 3 hours. If using the ham, remove from the
soup. Discard the rind, chop the ham and return it to the soup. Serve
hot.

🦋 Vegetable Soups

Corn Chowder

Serves 4

    2 teaspoons olive or canola oil
  1½ cups chopped green onions
    1 sliced red bell pepper
    3 tablespoons corn flour
    4 cups goat milk
  2½ cups fresh corn niblets
    2 teaspoons dill
        sea salt and black pepper

SUBSTITUTIONS

Green onion: 1 cup chopped onion; ¾ cup minced shallots

Corn flour: 3 tablespoons whole wheat, amaranth, barley, buckwheat,
    kamut, millet, oat, rice, rye, spelt, quinoa, or teff flour

Goat milk: 4 cups soy or rice milk

In a soup pot, heat the oil and sauté the onions and bell pepper for 3 to
5 minutes. Reduce heat and add flour, stirring for several minutes. Add

the milk slowly, stirring constantly. Add the corn, dill, and salt and pepper and cook for 15 minutes. Adjust the seasonings if necessary. Serve hot.

Tomato Vegetable Soup

Serves 4

> 2 tablespoons olive or canola oil
> 1 chopped onion
> 2 chopped carrots
> 2 chopped celery stalks plus leaves
> 1⅓ cups chopped okra
> 2 chopped tomatoes
> 3 bay leaves
> ¾ teaspoon thyme
> 2 tablespoons chopped fresh basil
> 4 cups tomato juice
> 1 cup water
> sea salt and black pepper

SUBSTITUTIONS

Onion: 1 cup chopped green onion; ½ cup minced shallots; 4 cloves minced garlic
Carrots: 1 cup chopped jicama
Celery: 1 cup diced red or green bell peppers
Okra: 1⅓ cups chopped summer squash or zucchini
Thyme: ¾ teaspoon rosemary

In a soup pot, heat the oil and sauté the onion, carrot, and celery for 3 to 5 minutes or until onion is transparent. Add the okra, tomatoes, bay leaves, thyme, and basil and sauté for several more minutes. Add the tomato juice, water, and salt and pepper and simmer for 15 to 20 minutes. Serve hot.

Carrot and Ginger Soup

Serves 4

> 1-inch ginger root
> 12 chopped carrots

> 2 cups unfiltered apple juice
> sea salt and black pepper

SUBSTITUTION
Apple juice: 2 cups orange juice

Peel and grate the ginger root. In a soup pot, combine the ginger, carrots, and apple juice and cook for 10 minutes or until carrots are tender. In a blender, puree the mixture with more apple juice if necessary and add salt and pepper. Reheat and serve hot.

Curried Squash Soup

Serves 4

> 2 butternut squash
> 2 tablespoons butter or margarine
> 1 cup chopped onion
> 2 cups unfiltered apple juice
> 2 teaspoons curry powder
> 1 teaspoon dill
> sea salt and black pepper

SUBSTITUTIONS
Butternut squash: 2 acorn squash
Onions: ½ cup minced shallots; 1 cup chopped green onion
Apple juice: 2 cups pear, apricot, or cranberry juice

Preheat oven to 350 degrees F. Cut the squash in half and place cut side down on a cookie sheet. Bake for 45 minutes. Scoop the squash from the shell and set aside. In a frying pan, melt the butter and sauté the onions for 5 minutes or until they are browned. In a blender, combine the squash, onions, apple juice, curry powder, and dill and puree. Add the salt and pepper and additional curry powder if desired. In a soup pot, reheat the mixture slowly over low heat. Serve hot.

Potato Leek Soup

Serves 4

> 2 tablespoons butter or margarine
> 2 large chopped leeks

4 cups water
4 large peeled, diced potatoes
⅓ cup chopped fresh parsley
2 teaspoons dill (optional)
     sea salt and black pepper

SUBSTITUTIONS
Leeks: 1 large chopped onion
Dill: 1 teaspoon celery seed

In a soup pot, melt the butter and sauté the leeks for 5 minutes or until tender. Add the water, potatoes, parsley, dill, and salt and pepper and cook until the potatoes have fallen apart. If desired, puree all or half of the soup. Reheat, adjust seasonings, and serve garnished with chopped parsley.

Pasta and Vegetable Soup

Serves 6

2 tablespoons butter or margarine
3 peeled, diced potatoes
3 chopped zucchini
2 cups peeled, chopped tomatoes
2 quarts Vegetable Stock (page 230)
1 cup chopped green beans
2 cups small whole grain pasta
1 tablespoon basil
     sea salt and black pepper
½ cup grated soy or goat cheese (optional)

SUBSTITUTIONS
Zucchini: 3 chopped summer squash or carrots; 1 cup sliced okra
Green beans: 1 cup sugar snap peas

In a soup pot, melt the butter and sauté the potatoes, zucchini, and tomatoes for 10 minutes or until tender. Pour in half the stock and salt and pepper, and cook for 15 to 20 minutes. Add the rest of the stock and bring to a boil. When the stock is boiling, add the pasta, then reduce heat and simmer until pasta is cooked al dente. Serve hot with cheese if desired.

Celery Root and Chicken Stock Soup

Serves 6

 2 quarts Poultry (chicken) Stock (page 230)
 1 large peeled, chopped celery root
 1 bunch chopped leeks
   sea salt and black pepper
 1 cup grated soy or goat Parmesan cheese (optional)

In a soup pot, combine the stock, celery root, leeks, and any meat from the bone, if desired. Bring to a boil, then reduce heat and simmer for 1 hour. Correct the seasoning with salt and pepper. Serve hot with cheese if desired.

Gazpacho

Serves 4

 4 cups tomato juice
 2 cups diced tomatoes
 1 cup chopped green onion
 1 cup chopped cucumber
 ¼ cup chopped fresh parsley
   juice of one lemon
 1 tablespoon basil
   sea salt and black pepper
   cucumber slices and minced green onion for garnish

In a blender, combine all the ingredients and blend until smooth. Transfer to a covered container and refrigerate for about 3 hours or until chilled. Garnish with cucumber slices and green onion and serve cold.

Coconut Curry Vegetable Soup

Serves 6

 2 tablespoons butter or margarine
 4 cloves minced garlic
 3 large peeled, diced potatoes
 2 large chopped carrots
 3 cups Vegetable Stock (page 230)

   1 teaspoon cumin seed
   1 tablespoon anise seed
   1 teaspoon whole cloves
   2 teaspoons curry powder
      sea salt and black pepper
   4 cups Coconut Milk (page 149)
   2 cups chopped zucchini
   2 bunches chopped spinach

SUBSTITUTIONS

Garlic: 1 chopped onion; 1 cup chopped green onion
Carrots: 1 large chopped red bell pepper
Vegetable Stock: 3 cups water
Coconut milk: 4 cups rice or soy milk
Zucchini: 2 cups chopped summer squash
Spinach: 2 bunches chopped chard or beet greens

In a soup pot, melt the butter and sauté the garlic for 3 minutes. Add
the potatoes and carrots and sauté for 2 minutes. Add the vegetable
stock, cumin, anise, cloves, curry powder, and salt and pepper, and cook
for 10 minutes on medium heat. Add the coconut milk and the squash.
Cook until the vegetables are tender. Just before serving add the chopped
spinach. Serve hot.

🦋 Cream Soups

Traditional Cream Soup

Serves 6

   ¼ cup butter or margarine
   ½ cup rice flour
   2 quarts Poultry Stock (page 230)
   1 chopped onion
   1 stalk chopped celery
   2 sprigs chopped fresh parsley
      sea salt
   1 cup cream

SUBSTITUTIONS
Rice flour: ½ cup teff, oat, whole wheat pastry, spelt, or millet flour
Onion: 2 chopped leeks; 3 minced shallots
Celery: ½ cup chopped chard stems
Cream: 1 cup goat, rice, or soy milk

In a soup pot, melt the butter and stir in the flour, cooking until the mixture turns golden brown. Add the stock, stirring constantly until the mixture is smooth. Add the onion, celery, parsley, and salt. Reduce heat and simmer for 30 minutes. Strain the stock, removing the stock vegetables. Add soup vegetable of choice (pureed or whole) and simmer for 15 to 30 minutes. Stir in the cream, correct seasonings, and serve hot.

VARIATION: Quick Cream

Add 1 cup rice milk directly to 2 quarts of vegetable or poultry stock. This base is not thick and creamy, but has the taste of a cream base. If you wish to thicken the milk, heat the milk and add one teaspoon of arrowroot and stir until thickened. Adjust the amount of arrowroot to your desired consistency.

Ideas for Cream Soups

Here are several suggestions for cream soups. The vegetables are combined with 1 recipe of Traditional Cream Soup. Spices may be added to increase the flavors.

Spinach

Steam 1 pound of spinach until tender. In a blender, combine spinach with ½ cup of the soup and puree until smooth. Add 1 teaspoon nutmeg, combine spinach mixture with remaining soup and reheat. Serve hot.

Celery

Steam 1½ cups chopped celery stalk or celery root until tender. In a blender, combine celery with ½ cup of the soup and puree. Combine celery mixture with remaining soup and reheat. Serve hot.

Tomato

Add 6 large chopped tomatoes or 4 cups of tomato puree and 1 clove minced garlic to soup. Cook for 1 hour. In a blender, puree until smooth. Reheat and serve hot.

Green Beans

Add 1½ cups chopped green beans to soup and simmer for 15 minutes or until beans are tender. In a blender, puree until smooth. Reheat and serve hot.

Broccoli

Add 2 cups chopped broccoli to soup and simmer for 15 minutes or until broccoli is tender. In a blender, puree until smooth. Reheat and serve hot.

Mushroom

In a frying pan, melt 2 tablespoons butter or margarine and sauté 2 cups chopped mushrooms until tender. In a blender, combine mushrooms with ½ cup of the soup and puree until smooth. Combine mushroom mixture with remaining soup and reheat. Serve hot.

Cauliflower

Add 2 cups chopped cauliflower to soup and simmer 15 minutes or until cauliflower is tender. In a blender, puree until smooth. Reheat and serve hot.

Asparagus

Steam 2 cups chopped asparagus until tender. In a blender, combine asparagus with ½ cup of the soup and puree until smooth. Combine asparagus mixture with remaining soup and reheat. Serve hot.

Squash (summer or winter variety)

Steam 2 cups of chopped squash until tender. In a blender, combine squash with ½ cup of the soup and puree until smooth. Combine squash mixture with remaining soup and reheat. Serve hot.

Beet Borscht

Serves 6

        1   large bunch beets
        1   tablespoon olive or canola oil
        1   cup chopped onion
        1   teaspoon caraway seeds
        6   cups Vegetable Stock (page 230)
    ½   cup tomato puree (optional)
        2   sliced carrots
        1   tablespoon fresh dill (1½ teaspoons dried)
            sea salt and black pepper
    ½   head chopped green cabbage
            juice of 1 lemon

SUBSTITUTIONS
Onion: 1 cup chopped green onions; 2 chopped leeks
Vegetable Stock: 6 cups water
Green cabbage: ½ head red, Savoy, Napa, or Chinese cabbage

In a saucepan, place the unpeeled beets with enough water to cover them. Bring to a boil and then simmer for about 45 minutes or until tender. Drain, peel, and chop the beets. In a soup pot, heat the oil and sauté the onion and caraway seeds for 3 to 5 minutes or until onions are transparent. Add the beets, vegetable stock, tomato puree, carrots, and dill. Add salt and pepper and simmer for 20 minutes. Add the cabbage and the lemon and cook for 15 minutes. Adjust the seasonings, garnish with dill, and serve either hot or cold.

✤ Poultry Soup

Chicken or Turkey Soup

Serves 6

        8   cups Poultry Stock (page 230)
    ½   cup barley
        1   large chopped onion

2 sliced carrots
2 stalks chopped celery plus leaves
½ cup chopped fresh parsley
1 teaspoon thyme
½ teaspoon sage
   sea salt and black pepper
1 cup shredded poultry meat
2 cups uncooked spelt pasta
1 cup peas

SUBSTITUTIONS

Barley: ½ cup quinoa, kasha, wheat berries, or spelt berries
Onion: ¾ cup minced shallot; 3 chopped leeks
Carrot: 1 cup chopped jicama
Celery: 1 cup chopped celery root
Spelt pasta: 2 cups amaranth, barley, corn, kamut, rice, buckwheat, or
    wheat pasta; ½ cup rice
Peas: 1 cup chopped summer squash or green beans; 1 cup snow peas

In a soup pot, bring the stock to a boil and add the barley, onion, carrots, celery, parsley, thyme, and sage and salt and pepper. Let simmer
for one to two hours. Add the meat, pasta, and peas and cook for another
20 minutes or until pasta and peas are done. Serve hot.

CHAPTER 17

Colorful and Creative Salads

A SALAD CAN BE A side dish or a complete meal and range from elegant to hearty. The choices and combinations are endless, determined only by your taste buds and imagination. Here are some recipes to spark your creativity. Some dressings will be listed with the recipes; see page 407 for additional dressings.

The following recipes call for 1 cup of greens per person and accompany a meal. Make adjustments according to your individual needs. For those that are rotating or are allergic to some of the various ingredients, do not hesitate to substitute. If the lettuce is added last and no dressing is applied, the salad will keep until serving time. Toss with the dressing at the last minute.

For different flavors, textures, colors, and adventures, expand your horizons with one or more of the following interesting greens that are available. It will delight your eye and liven up the salad bowl. Try growing a few in your garden. To add additional delight to the salad, explore the wide variety of oils and vinegars. For ideas and lists see page 407.

Exotic and Delicious Greens

Arugula	Miner's lettuce
Curly dock	Mustard greens
Dandelion greens	Purslane
Escarole	Radicchio
Lamb's-quarters	Wild sorrel

Other nutritious additions for your salad are: sunflower seeds, sprouts of all kinds, sesame seeds, nuts (especially pinenuts and almonds), flax seeds, nasturtium leaves and flowers, pomegranate seeds, kale, beet greens, turnip greens, collard greens.

Green Salad

Serves 1

For a simple green salad, place a cup of washed and dried torn butter, romaine, or red leaf lettuce on a chilled plate. Serve with 2 tablespoons of your favorite dressing and fresh cracked black pepper.

Butter Lettuce Salad

Serves 4

    4 cups torn butter lettuce
    1 grated carrot
    1 chopped green onion
    3 large sliced mushrooms
       cracked black pepper
    ½ cup Lemonette Dressing (page 413) or your favorite oil and
       vinegar

Wash and dry the lettuce. In a salad bowl, combine the carrot, green onion, and mushrooms. Add the butter lettuce leaves and mix well. Add pepper and a sprinkle of the herb used in the dressing. Toss with dressing and serve.

Winter Surprise Salad

Serves 4

    4 cups torn green leaf lettuce
    1 thinly sliced cooked beet
    ½ cup chopped jicama
    1 tablespoon chopped chives
       sea salt or kelp and cracked black pepper
    ½ cup Close-to-Thousand Island Dressing (page 411)

SUBSTITUTIONS
Dressing: ½ cup Almost Ranch Dressing (page 412)

Wash and dry the lettuce. In a salad bowl, combine lettuce, beet, and jicama. Just before serving, add chives and salt and pepper. Toss with dressing and serve.

Early Spring Surprise Salad

Serves 4

> 4 cups torn spinach
> ½ cup sliced mushrooms
> ½ cup sliced red onion
> 1 grated egg (optional)
> sea salt or kelp and cracked black pepper
> ½ cup Poppy Seed Dressing (page 415)

Wash the spinach thoroughly. Break off and discard the stems. Place spinach on a kitchen towel or paper towel to dry and let crisp in the refrigerator for a 30 minutes to 1 hour (can be prepared up to a day ahead of time). In a salad bowl, combine the mushrooms and onions. Add the spinach, egg, and salt and pepper. Toss with dressing and serve.

Summer Wonder

Serves 4

> 4 cups torn red leaf lettuce
> ½ sliced green bell pepper
> 1 small sliced zucchini
> 3 sliced radishes
> ¼ cup chopped shallot
> sea salt or kelp and cracked black pepper
> ½ cup Creamy Basil Dressing (page 418)

Wash and dry the lettuce. In a salad bowl, combine the bell pepper, zucchini, radishes, and shallot. Add the torn lettuce and salt and pepper. Toss with dressing and serve.

Liz's Cabbage Salad

Serves 4

> 3 cups green cabbage
> 1 grated carrot

   1 stalk chopped celery
   2 tablespoons minced yellow onion
      sea salt or kelp and cracked black pepper
   2 tablespoons Eggless "REAL" Mayonnaise (page 408)

SUBSTITUTIONS
Green cabbage: 3 cups Napa or Chinese cabbage
Carrot: ½ cup chopped jicama or red bell pepper
Onion: 2 tablespoons chopped green onion

Wash, dry, and shred the cabbage. In a salad bowl, combine the cabbage, carrot, celery, onion, and salt and pepper. Toss with mayonnaise and serve.

VARIATION
For a low fat dressing, combine 2 teaspoons of olive or canola oil and 2 to 3 teaspoons of lemon or lime juice or vinegar. Add salt and pepper and cayenne pepper to taste and mix well. Cumin or caraway seed can also be added for extra flavor.

Cool Green Salad

Serves 4

   2 cups watercress
  ½ peeled, sliced cucumber
   1 cup snow peas
      sea salt or kelp and cracked black pepper
  ½ cup Cucumber Dressing (page 419)

Wash and dry the watercress. Break off and discard the large stems. In a salad bowl, combine the cucumber and snow peas. Add the watercress and salt and pepper. Toss with dressing and serve.

Summer Color Salad

Serves 4

   4 cups torn romaine lettuce
   1 clove garlic
  ½ cup chopped tomato or whole cherry tomatoes
  ½ cup cauliflower

½ cup chopped green beans
sea salt or kelp and cracked black pepper
½ cup Practically It "Blue Cheese" Dressing (page 412)

SUBSTITUTION
Dressing: ½ cup Zesty Tomato Dressing (page 00)
Green beans: ½ cup sugar snap peas

Wash and dry the lettuce. Peel the garlic and cut in half. In a salad bowl, rub the garlic around the inside. Add the tomato, cauliflower, green beans, lettuce, and salt and pepper. Toss with dressing and serve.

Fall Fun Salad

Serves 4

4 cups Napa cabbage
½ red bell pepper
1 cup sliced jicama
2 tablespoons chopped leek
sea salt or kelp and cracked black pepper
½ cup Sesame Seed Dressing (page 414)

Wash, dry, and shred the cabbage. In a salad bowl, combine the bell pepper, jicama, and leek. Add the cabbage and salt and pepper. Toss with dressing and serve.

Delve into Endive Salad

Serves 4

1 large endive
½ sliced avocado
½ cup chopped walnuts
sea salt or kelp and cracked black pepper
½ cup Lemon Thyme Dressing (page 413)

Cut the base off the endive, separate the leaves, and wash and dry. Arrange leaves on individual serving plates, about 3 leaves per plate. Divide the avocado slices equally and place on top of the leaves with walnuts. Lightly salt and pepper. Drizzle with dressing and serve.

❧ Vegetable Salads

Cauliflower Salad

Serves 4

   3 cups cauliflower flowerettes
  ½ cup julienned red bell pepper
  1 small sliced zucchini
  2 chopped green onions

Dressing:
  ½ cup Lemonette Dressing (page 413)
  ¼ teaspoon marjoram

SUBSTITUTIONS

Red bell pepper: ½ cup chopped tomato; ½ cup sliced radishes
Zucchini: 1 small sliced summer squash

In a small bowl, combine the dressing ingredients and mix well. In a
salad bowl, combine dressing with all the salad ingredients. Refrigerate
for 30 minutes before serving or until chilled to let the flavors marry.

Chilled Broccoli Salad

Serves 4

  1 bunch broccoli
  1 cup halved cherry tomatoes
  ½ cup minced shallots
  2 tablespoons chives
  2 tablespoons chopped fresh parsley
  ½ cup Lemonette Dressing (page 413)

SUBSTITUTIONS

Shallots: ½ cup chopped green onion
Chives: 1 tablespoon minced shallots; 1 tablespoon chopped green onion
Parsley: 2 tablespoons chopped fresh cilantro

Clean and chop the broccoli into bite-size pieces, discarding the lower
tough part of the stem. In a salad bowl, combine the ingredients and
serve.

Crunch Surprise Salad

Serves 4

    1 sliced jicama
    ¾ cup petit peas
    ½ cup cashews
    2 chopped green onions
    ½ cup Cashew Mayonnaise (page 409)

SUBSTITUTIONS
Green onions: 2 tablespoons chopped chives
Jicama: 2 sliced carrots

In a salad bowl, combine the ingredients and serve.

Oriental Slaw

Serves 4

    ½ head shredded green cabbage
    ½ thinly sliced jicama
    1 large peeled, seeded, sectioned orange
    ½ chopped green bell pepper
    ¼ medium sliced red onion
    ⅛ cup chopped fresh cilantro
    ¼ cup pinenuts
Dressing:
    2 tablespoons olive, canola, or safflower oil
    1 tablespoon honey
  1½ tablespoons rice vinegar
    ½ tablespoon sesame oil (optional)
    ¼ teaspoon dry mustard
        sea salt or kelp

SUBSTITUTIONS
Cabbage: ½ head shredded Napa or Chinese cabbage
Jicama: 2 thinly sliced carrots
Orange: 2 tangerines; 1 large mandarin orange
Pinenuts: ¼ cup peanuts or sunflower seeds

Red onion: ¼ chopped yellow onion; 1 minced shallot; 2 chopped green
   onions
Honey: 1 tablespoon concentrated grape juice or rice syrup
Rice vinegar: 1½ tablespoons lemon juice
Sea salt: 1 teaspoon soy sauce

In a small bowl, combine the dressing ingredients and mix well. In a
salad bowl, combine the cabbage, jicama, orange, bell pepper, onion,
cilantro, and pinenuts. Add dressing and toss. Cover and refrigerate for
3 hours or until chilled.

Summer Garden Salad

Serves 4

    1 large sliced zucchini
    1 sliced yellow squash
    1 sliced carrot
    1 cup snow peas
    1 chopped red bell pepper
    ½ cup chopped walnuts
Dressing:
    1 tablespoons apple juice
    2 teaspoons minced fresh ginger (1½ teaspoons powdered
       ginger)
    ¼ teaspoons cayenne pepper
    2 tablespoons walnut oil
    ½ cup rice vinegar

SUBSTITUTIONS
Carrot: ½ cup sliced jicama
Snow peas: 1 cup sugar snap peas
Walnuts: ½ cup chopped pecans or hazelnuts
Walnut oil: 2 tablespoons olive or peanut oil
Vinegar: ½ cup lemon juice

In a small bowl, combine the dressing ingredients and mix well. The
salad can be presented in two ways. 1. Slice the vegetables, leaving the
snow peas whole. In a salad bowl, toss the vegetables with dressing and

walnuts and serve. 2. Cut the vegetables into 2½ inch lengths and arrange on a serving platter in a pinwheel or circular pattern. Drizzle the dressing over the salad, garnish with walnuts, and serve.

Celery Italiano

Serves 4

> 2 chopped tomatoes
> 4 medium celery stalks cut into ½-inch pieces
> 1 tablespoon fresh basil (2 teaspoons dried basil)
> ¼ cup grated soy or goat Parmesan cheese
>   cracked black pepper

Dressing:
> ½ cup Lemonette dressing (page 413)
> ¼ teaspoon basil

In a small bowl, combine the dressing ingredients and mix well. In a salad bowl, combine the tomatoes, celery, basil, and pepper. Toss with dressing and add cheese. Cover and refrigerate for one hour or until chilled. Serve on lettuce leaves on a chilled plate.

Humble Cucumber Salad

Serve 4

> 1 peeled, sliced cucumber
> 1 tablespoon chives
>   sea salt or kelp and cracked black pepper

On a serving dish, arrange the cucumber. Sprinkle with salt and pepper and chives and serve.

VARIATIONS

In a salad bowl, combine the cucumber and ½ sliced red onion. Sprinkle with salt and black pepper and ½ teaspoon tarragon or dill. Pour ¼ cup vinegar over the vegetables and add enough water to cover. Cover and refrigerate overnight for the flavors to marry.

Add 1 sliced tomato to the above.

Substitute ½ cup Zesty Mint Dressing for the vinegar and water. Chill as above and serve with chopped mint leaves for garnish.

Add 2 tablespoons goat yogurt or soy sour cream.

Kohlrabi Salad

Serve 4

2 cups peeled, shredded kohlrabi
½ cup sliced radish

Dressing:

3 tablespoons Eggless "REAL" Mayonnaise (page 408)
2 tablespoons lemon juice
¼ teaspoon paprika
½ teaspoon dry mustard

In a small bowl, combine the dressing ingredients and mix well. In a salad bowl, combine the kohlrabi and radishes. Add the dressing and toss and serve. Garnish servings with paprika.

Ultimate Purple Passion Salad

Serves 4

1 eggplant
3 cloves minced garlic
⅓ cup chopped fresh parsley
1 medium chopped tomato
½ small minced yellow onion
½ teaspoon marjoram
½ teaspoon oregano
juice of ½ lemon
2 tablespoons olive or canola oil
sea salt or kelp and cracked black pepper

SUBSTITUTION

Onion: 2 tablespoons minced shallots

Preheat oven to 350 degrees F. Place eggplant on baking sheet and bake for 45 minutes. Let cool, then peel and chop. In a salad bowl, combine the eggplant with remaining ingredients and toss and serve.

For added flavor, grill the eggplant on a barbecue, under a broiler, or over a gas flame until the skin is charred. Then bake as above.

Spring Delight Salad

Serves 4

> 2 cups chopped asparagus
> juice of ½ lemon
> ½ teaspoon rosemary
> cracked black pepper

In a vegetable steamer, lightly steam asparagus for 5 to 10 minutes or until cooked al dente. Rinse the asparagus under cold water to cool and stop the cooking process. In a serving dish, place the asparagus and sprinkle with lemon juice and rosemary. Refrigerate for ½ hour or until chilled. Arrange on a bed of red leaf lettuce or beet greens and garnish with a thin strip of pimento, red bell pepper, or sprinkle with paprika. Serve with cracked black pepper.

Rouge et Vert Salad

Serves 4

> 1 cup cooked sliced beets
> ½ cup cooked green beans
> ¼ cup sliced mushrooms
> ¼ cup chopped green onion
> ¼ teaspoon dill

Dressing:

> ½ cup Almost Ranch Dressing (page 412)
> ¼ teaspoon dill
> chopped green onion for garnish

SUBSTITUTION

Almost Ranch Dressing: ½ cup Lemonette Dressing
Green onion: ⅓ cup chopped chives

In a salad bowl, combine the beets, beans, mushrooms, green onion, and dill. Toss with dressing and serve on a bed of lettuce. Garnish with green onion.

Hearts of Green Salad

Serves 4

16 artichoke hearts (frozen and defrosted or water-packed)
¼ cup chopped green bell pepper
½ cup chopped celery
 2 cloves minced garlic
½ teaspoon oregano
½ cup Lemonette Dressing (page 413)
    cracked black pepper

In a salad bowl, combine all the ingredients. Cover and refrigerate overnight to let the flavors marry. Serve on a bed of endive spears and garnish with cracked black pepper.

Root Surprise Salad

Serves 4

 1 medium peeled, trimmed, cubed celery root
 2 tablespoons chopped green onion
 2 tablespoons chopped fresh parsley
¼ cup chopped walnuts (optional)

Dressing:
1½ tablespoons lemon juice
     sea salt or kelp and cracked black pepper
 1 tablespoon dry mustard
½ teaspoon tarragon
 3 tablespoons olive or canola oil
 3 tablespoons soy sour cream

SUBSTITUTIONS
Celery root: 1 medium peeled, trimmed, cubed parsley root
Green onion: 3 tablespoons chopped chives
Walnuts: ¼ cup chopped almonds or hazelnuts
Tarragon: ½ teaspoon dill or marjoram
Sour cream: 3 tablespoons goat ricotta cheese

In a small bowl, combine the lemon juice, salt and pepper, mustard, and tarragon. Gradually whisk in the oil and then the sour cream. In a salad bowl, combine the celery root with dressing and toss until thoroughly until well coated. Cover and refrigerate for overnight for the flavors to marry. Before serving, add the parsley, green onion, and walnuts. Toss and serve on a bed of radicchio or red leaf lettuce. Garnish with parsley.

Hearty Winter Salad with Raspberry Vinaigrette

Serves 4

> 4 cups shredded red cabbage
> 1 large grated carrot
> 1 grated turnip
> 1 small chopped leek
> caraway seeds

Dressing:

> 2 tablespoons walnut oil
> 2 tablespoons raspberry vinegar
> ¼ teaspoon caraway seed
> sea salt or kelp and cracked black pepper

SUBSTITUTION

Raspberry vinegar: 2 tablespoons lemon juice

In a small bowl, combine the dressing ingredients and mix well. In a salad bowl, combine cabbage, carrot, turnip, and leek and sprinkle with caraway seeds. Toss with dressing and serve.

Rays of the Sun Salad

Serves 4

> 1 cup alfalfa or red clover sprouts
> 1 large carrot, thinly sliced lengthwise
> 1 cup jicama, thinly sliced lengthwise
> ¼ cup sunflower seeds
> ¼ cup sunflower sprouts

Dressing:

> 2 minced shallots
> ½ teaspoons paprika
> ¼ cup lemon juice
> sea salt or kelp and cracked black pepper

In a blender, combine the shallots, paprika, lemon juice, and salt and pepper. Blend until smooth. On a individual plates, arrange the sprouts in a thin layer. Alternate carrot and jicama on sprouts in an overlapping circle to form spokes. Sprinkle with sunflower seeds and sprouts. Pour ¼ of dressing over each salad. Garnish with paprika and pepper and serve.

Orange Surprise Salad
Serves 4

    1   medium halved, seeded spaghetti squash
    1   large peeled, sectioned orange
    1   cup walnuts
    1   medium diced red bell pepper
    ½   cup currants (optional)
        2-inch piece peeled, thinly sliced fresh ginger
Dressing:
    2   tablespoons cornstarch
    4   tablespoons warm water
    1   cup orange juice
    2   cloves minced garlic
    2   tablespoons lemon juice
    ¼   teaspoon thyme
    ¼   teaspoon oregano
    1   teaspoon chopped fresh parsley

SUBSTITUTIONS
Walnuts: 1 cup toasted hazelnuts, pinenuts, or almonds
Red bell pepper: 1 medium diced green bell pepper; ½ cup diced celery
Ginger: ½ teaspoon nutmeg
Cornstarch: 2 tablespoons arrowroot

Preheat the oven to 350 degrees F. Place the squash in shallow baking dish, cut side down with about ½ inch of water to cover the bottom of the dish. Cook for 1 hour or until tender. Cool and remove the pulp. While the squash is baking, place the walnuts on a baking sheet in a thin layer and bake for 15 minutes. Set aside and let cool. In a small bowl, combine the cornstarch and water. Mix well and set aside. In another bowl, combine orange juice, garlic, lemon juice, thyme, oregano, and parsley. Blend in the cornstarch mixture and mix well. In a small bowl, combine the currants, ½ cup walnuts, ginger, and squash. In a serving dish, spread the squash mixture and arrange the orange sections and bell pepper on top. Pour dressing over the salad and garnish with the remaining nuts.

Old-Fashion Favorites

Liz's Potato Salad

Serves 4

> 2 pounds russet or white rose potatoes
> 1 medium chopped red onion
> 2 stalks chopped celery
> ¼ cup chopped fresh parsley
> 2 large diced dill pickles (regular or nonvinegar/yeast-free variety)
> 3 hard boiled eggs, diced or wedged (optional)

Dressing:

> 1 cup Eggless "REAL" Mayonnaise (page 408)
> 2 teaspoons onion powder
> ½ teaspoons paprika
> ¼ cup lemon juice
> sea salt or kelp and cracked black pepper

Wash and boil or bake potatoes until barely fork tender. Let cool, peel, cut into bite-size pieces, and place in a salad bowl. Add the onion, celery, parsley, pickles, and eggs. In a small bowl, combine the dressing ingredients and mix well. Add dressing to potatoes and mix well. Cover and refrigerate overnight for the flavors to marry.

VARIATION

For a low fat dressing, combine 1 cup goat yogurt (or nonfat cow's milk yogurt if tolerated), 3 teaspoons of lemon or lime juice, and salt and pepper. Paprika, basil, dill, onion powder, and garlic powder can be added for extra flavor. Mix well and use in place of mayonnaise.

Joanna's Potato Salad

Serves 4

2 pounds red potatoes
½ cup chopped green onions
¼ cup chopped celery
¼ cup chopped red bell pepper
1 tablespoon dill
   red bell pepper rings for garnish

Dressing:
1 cup Eggless "REAL" Mayonnaise (page 408)
1 teaspoon Dijon mustard or dry mustard
1 tablespoon dill
   sea salt or kelp and cracked black pepper

Wash and boil or bake potatoes until barely fork tender. Let cool, peel, cut into quarters or slices., and place in a salad bowl. Add the onion, celery, parsley, and dill. In a small bowl, combine the dressing ingredients and mix well. Add dressing to potatoes and mix well. Cover and refrigerate overnight for the flavors to marry.

Traditional Macaroni Salad

Serves 4

4 cups whole grain macaroni
2 stalks chopped celery
1 small chopped yellow onion
3 hard-boiled eggs (optional)
½ cup chopped or sliced olives (optional)
1 4-ounce jar pimento (¼ cup fresh)

Dressing:
1 cup Eggless "REAL" Mayonnaise (page 408)
2 teaspoons onion powder
½ teaspoon paprika
¼ cup lemon juice
   sea salt or kelp and cracked black pepper

In a large pot, bring 2 quarts of water and a little salt to a boil. Add macaroni and cook for 10 to 15 minutes or until al dente. Drain and set aside. In a small bowl, combine the dressing ingredients and mix well. Mix well. In a salad bowl, combine macaroni, celery, and onion. Add dressing and mix well. Garnish with eggs, paprika, and olives and serve.

VARIATIONS

Many interesting or necessary substitutes can be added to macaroni salad: sliced radishes, grated or chopped carrot, green or red bell pepper, diced green onions, minced garlic, red onion, jicama, fresh chopped parsley, chopped zucchini, snow peas, cherry tomatoes, and herbs like basil, marjoram, or dill. Dry mustard or catsup can be added to the dressing for a different taste.

🦋 Bean Salads

Beans with a Heart Salad

Serves 4

>   2 cups cooked Great Northern beans
>   1 jar drained, water-packed artichoke hearts
>   1 cup sliced celery •
>   ½ cup sliced red onion
>   1 teaspoon thyme
> Dressing:
>   ½ cup Lemonette Dressing (page 413)
>   ¼ teaspoon Dijon or dry mustard

SUBSTITUTIONS

Great Northern beans: 2 cups cooked kidney, pinto, or Anasazi beans
Celery: 1 cup sliced jicama
Red onion: ½ cup chopped green onion; 2 minced shallots; 2 cloves minced garlic
Thyme: 1 teaspoon oregano or marjoram

In a small bowl, combine the dressing ingredients and mix well. In a serving dish, combine the beans, artichoke hearts, celery, onion, and thyme. Add dressing and mix well. Cover and refrigerate for at least 2 hours or until chilled.

Three Bean Salad

Serves 4

    1 cup cooked kidney beans or 1 can drained (reserve liquid)
    1 cup cooked garbanzo beans or 1 can drained (reserve liquid)
    1 cup cooked green beans
    ½ sliced medium red onion
    2 cloves minced garlic
    ¼ cup chopped fresh parsley
       sea salt or kelp and cracked black pepper
Dressing:
    ¼ cup Lemonette Dressing (page 413)
    ¼ cup reserved liquid from beans
    ¼ teaspoon oregano

SUBSTITUTIONS
Kidney beans: 1 cup cooked red, pinto, or pink beans
Green beans: 1 cup cooked wax beans
Red onion: ½ sliced yellow onion; ½ cup chopped green onion

In a salad bowl, combine all the ingredients. In a small bowl, combine
the dressing ingredients and mix well. Add the dressing with enough
liquid from the beans to cover vegetables. Cover and refrigerate overnight
to let the flavors marry. Serve using a slotted spoon on a bed of lettuce.

Black Bean Salad

Serves 4

    2 cups cooked black beans
    ½ cup chopped yellow onion
    ½ cup cooked corn (optional)
    ½ cup chopped red bell pepper
    ¼ cup chopped fresh cilantro
Dressing:
    ½ cup Lemonette Dressing (page 413)
    1 clove minced garlic
    1 pinch cayenne pepper (optional)
       sea salt or kelp and cracked black pepper

SUBSTITUTIONS
Yellow onion: ½ cup chopped red onion or green onion; 3 minced shallots
Red bell pepper: ½ cup chopped green bell pepper; 1 chopped dried red
    chili pepper; 1 chopped jalapeño
Garlic: 1 tablespoon minced onion

In a small bowl, combine the dressing ingredients and mix well. In a
salad bowl, combine the beans, onions, corn, bell pepper, and cilantro.
Add dressing to salad, mix well, and refrigerate for 2 hours or until
chilled. Serve on a bed of butter or green leaf lettuce.

Ceci Salad

Serves 4

    1 cup uncooked couscous
    1 cup cooked garbanzo beans (or 1 drained 8-ounce can)
    4 chopped green onions
    1 cup chopped red bell pepper
    ½ cup peeled, seeded, chopped cucumber
    ½ cup diced black olives (optional)
    ½ cup Zesty Mint Dressing (page 415)
       Fresh mint leaves for garnish

SUBSTITUTIONS
Couscous: 1 cup uncooked quinoa, amaranth, or teff
Green onions: ½ cup chopped white or yellow onions
Red bell pepper: 1 cup chopped green pepper; ½ cup sliced radishes; 1
    large sliced carrot

In a large pot, bring 1¾ cups of water to a boil. In a salad bowl, place
couscous and pour boiling water on top. Let stand for 5 minutes and
then fluff with a fork. (If using one of the other grains, see page 192 for
cooking instructions.) Add the beans, onions, bell pepper, cucumber,
and olives to the couscous. Toss with dressing and refrigerate for 2 hours
or until chilled. Serve on romaine lettuce and garnish with mint.

🦋 Grain and Pasta Salads

Simple Supper Salad

Serves 4

    10   ounces pasta, in any shape except spaghetti, linguini, or lasagna
     2   chopped, tomatoes
    ½   cup small chopped yellow onion
    ½   cup snow peas
    ¼   cup chopped fresh parsley
    ½   teaspoon fresh basil (1 teaspoon dried basil)
         sea salt and cracked black pepper
    ½   cup Lemonette Dressing (page 413)

SUBSTITUTIONS

Yellow onion: ½ cup chopped green onion
Snow peas: ½ cup sugar snap peas
Basil: ½ teaspoon marjoram or oregano

In a large pot, bring 2 quarts of water with a little salt to a boil and add pasta. Cook for about 10 minutes or until al dente. Drain and cool. In a salad bowl, combine the pasta, tomatoes, onion, peas, parsley, basil, and salt and pepper. Toss with dressing and serve.

Pepper Pasta Salad

Serves 4

     8   ounces pasta
    1½ cups chopped, cooked broccoli
    ⅓   cup chopped red onion
    ¼   cup chopped red bell pepper
    ¼   cup chopped green bell pepper
    ¼   cup chopped yellow bell pepper
    ¼   cup chopped purple bell pepper
    ½   cup Almost Ranch Dressing (page 412)

SUBSTITUTION

Red onion: ⅓ cup chopped yellow or white onion
Dressing: ½ cup Lemonette Dressing (page 413)

In a large pot, bring 2 quarts of water with a little salt to a boil and add the pasta. Cook for about 10 minutes or until al dente. Drain and cool. In a salad bowl, combine the pasta, broccoli, onion, and bell peppers. Toss with dressing and serve.

Hot Pasta Salad

Serves 4

    8   ounces pasta
    2   diced zucchini
    1   small chopped yellow onion
    ½   cup chopped celery
    1   4-ounce can diced green chili
    ¼   cup sliced olives (optional)
    2   tablespoons chopped fresh cilantro
Dressing:
    ¼   cup of olive or canola oil
    ⅓   cup lime juice
    ¼   cup chopped fresh cilantro
    1½ teaspoons chili powder
    ½   teaspoon onion powder
        sea salt or kelp and cracked black pepper

SUBSTITUTIONS
Zucchini: 2 diced patty or yellow squash
Onion: 2 cloves minced garlic
Cilantro: 2 tablespoons chopped fresh parsley
Onion powder: ½ teaspoon garlic powder

In a small bowl, combine the dressing ingredients and mix well. In a large pot, bring 2 quarts of water with a little salt to a boil and add the pasta. Cook for about 10 minutes or until al dente. Drain and cool. In a salad bowl, combine the pasta, zucchini, onion, celery, chili, and olives. Toss with dressing and refrigerate overnight for the flavors to marry. Garnish with cilantro and serve.

Chinese Pasta Salad

Serves 4

    8 ounces buckwheat noodles
    ½ cup snow peas
    ½ cup sliced water chestnuts
    ¼ cup sliced mushrooms
    2 chopped green onions
    ½ chopped red bell pepper
    2 tablespoons toasted sesame seeds
       sea salt or kelp and cracked black pepper

Dressing:
    2 tablespoons toasted sesame oil
    2 tablespoons rice vinegar
    ¼ teaspoon onion powder
    ¼ teaspoon grated fresh ginger root (½ teaspoon powdered ginger)

SUBSTITUTION

Buckwheat noodles: 8 ounces rice noodles
Rice vinegar: 2 tablespoons lemon juice

In a small bowl, combine the dressing ingredients and mix well. In a large pot, bring 2 quarts of water with a little salt to a boil and add the noodles. Cook for about 15 minutes or until al dente. Drain and cool. In a salad bowl, combine the noodles, snow peas, water chestnuts, mushrooms, green onion, bell pepper, and salt and pepper. Toss with dressing, garnish with sesame seeds, and serve.

Wild Salad

Serves 4

    ⅓ cup wild rice
    ½ cup long grain rice
    1 cup cooked corn niblets
    1 chopped red bell pepper
    1 cup cooked, chopped green beans
    2 tablespoons chopped fresh parsley

Dressing:
- 6 tablespoons olive or canola oil
- 3 tablespoons lemon juice
- 2 tablespoons chopped chives
- 1 teaspoons Dijon or dry mustard
- 1 pinch ground mace

SUBSTITUTIONS
Corn: 1 cup steamed chopped carrots
Red bell pepper: 1 chopped green or yellow bell pepper
Green beans: 1 cup cooked snow peas, sugar snap peas, or peas
Chives: 2 tablespoons chopped chives

In a saucepan, bring 1 cup of water and a little salt to a boil and add the wild rice. Cook for about 30 to 40 minutes or until the water is evaporated. In another saucepan, bring 1 cup of water and a little salt to a boil and add the long grain rice. Cook for about 20 to 30 minutes or until the water is evaporated. In a small bowl, combine the dressing ingredients and mix well. In a salad bowl, combine the rices, corn, bell pepper, and beans. Toss with dressing, salt and pepper, garnish with the parsley, and serve.

Traditional Tabouli

Serves 4

- 1 cup bulgur
- ¾ cup chopped tomatoes
- ½ cup peeled, seeded, chopped cucumber
- 1 cup chopped green onions
- 1½ cups chopped fresh parsley
- ½ cup chopped fresh mint or cilantro

Dressing:
- ⅓ cup lemon juice
- ¼ cup olive or canola oil
  sea salt or kelp and cracked black pepper

SUBSTITUTIONS
Bulgur: 1 cup rice, millet, teff, or quinoa
Tomatoes: ½ cup chopped red bell pepper

Green onions: 2 cloves minced garlic
Mint: ½ cup chopped fresh cilantro
Lemon juice: ¼ cup lime or grapefruit juice

In a salad bowl, place the bulgur and pour boiling water on top. Let stand for 45 minutes until water is absorb. Drain any excess water. (If using one of the other grains, see page 192 for cooking instructions.) In a small bowl, combine the dressing ingredients and mix well. Add tomatoes, cucumber, green onion, parsley, and mint to bulgur and mix well. Toss with dressing and refrigerate for 1 hour or until chilled. Serve on romaine lettuce and garnish with mint.

VARIATIONS
The following additions can provide interest and varieties, or substitutes, to traditional tabouli: ½ cup crumbled feta cheese, 1 cup cooked garbanzo beans, ½ cup chopped summer squash, 1 cup diced poultry, ½ cup nuts or seeds, ⅓ cup grated carrot, ⅓ cup sliced radishes, ½ cup chopped red, green, yellow, or purple bell pepper, ½ cup jicama diced, ½ cup celery, ¼ cup grated beet.

Unberry Salad
Serves 4

    1 cup wheat berries
    ½ cup grated carrot (optional)
    ½ cup chopped green onions
    ½ cup chopped fresh parsley
    2 teaspoons fresh dill
       sea salt or kelp and cracked black pepper
Dressing:
    ½ cup Lemonette Dressing (page 413)
    ½ teaspoon dill

SUBSTITUTIONS
Wheat berries: 1 cup rye, buckwheat, spelt, or kasha
Carrot: ½ cup chopped red bell pepper; ¼ cup grated beet
Dill: 2 teaspoons fresh basil
Dill: ½ teaspoon basil

lorf Salad

lopes Knox gelatin
 unfiltered apple juice
oons honey (optional)
 diced red apple
chopped celery
chopped walnuts
 of cinnamon

ONS
: 2 tablespoons gelatin powder; 4 tablespoons agar; 1 table-
w-methoxyl pectin
aspoons concentrated grape juice or rice syrup
up chopped almonds, pecans, or hazelnuts

n, pour 1 cup of the juice and honey and sprinkle the gelatin
op. When gelatin is softened (about 3 to 5 minutes), heat
 high heat until dissolved. In a bowl or mold, combine gelatin
th remaining juice and refrigerate for 30 minutes or until
gins to thicken. Fold in the apple, celery, walnuts, and cin-
 chill until firm. To unmold, dip the mold in hot water quickly
es and then invert on a serving dish.

it Avocado Salad

velope Knox gelatin
p unsweetened grapefruit juice
blespoons honey
rge peeled, sectioned grapefruit
up diced avocado
up diced celery
iced pimento stuffed green olives (optional)

In a large bowl, soak the berries overnight in enough water to cover. In a large pot, bring 3½ cups of water to a boil. Drain wheat berries and add to boiling water. Cook for about 1 hour or until tender and most of the water is absorbed. Drain if necessary. (If using another grain, soak it overnight, and then cook according to directions on page 192). In a small bowl, combine the dressing ingredients and mix well. In a salad bowl, combine wheat berries, carrot, green onions, parsley, dill, and salt and pepper. Toss with dressing and serve garnished with parsley and green onions.

Middle East Salad

Serves 4

> 1½ cups cooked brown rice
> 1 cup cooked yellow or brown lentils
> 1 large thinly sliced carrot
> ⅓ cup chopped green onions

Dressing:
> 1 tablespoon olive or canola oil
> 2½ tablespoons lime or lemon juice
> 1 teaspoon curry powder
> 1 clove minced garlic
> sea salt or kelp and cracked black pepper

SUBSTITUTIONS
Carrot: 1 large stalk sliced celery; ½ cup peas; ½ cup chopped jicama; ½ cup chopped kohlrabi
Green onion: 1 chopped leek; ⅓ cup chopped yellow or red onion; 2 minced shallots; 2 cloves minced garlic
Curry powder: 1 teaspoon Dijon or dry mustard
Garlic: 1 tablespoon minced green onion

In a small bowl, combine the dressing ingredients and mix well. In a salad bowl, combine rice, lentils, carrot, and green onion. Toss with dressing and serve on a bed of romaine or red leaf lettuce.

Peruvian Salad

Serves 4

    2 cups cooked quinoa
    ½ cup chopped carrot
    ½ cup sunflower seeds
    ⅓ cup chopped fresh parsley
    2 cloves minced garlic
    ½ cup Lemon Thyme Dressing (page 413)

SUBSTITUTIONS

Quinoa: 2 cups cooked amaranth, teff, millet, or buckwheat groats
Garlic: ⅓ cup chopped onion

In a salad bowl, combine all the ingredients. Mix well and refrigerate for ½ hour or until chilled. Serve on a chilled plate on a bed of purslane or romaine lettuce.

VARIATIONS

Many interesting or necessary substitutes can be added to Peruvian salad: 1 wedged tomato, ½ cup chopped red or green bell pepper, ½ cup chopped or thinly sliced zucchini, ½ cup chopped nuts, ¼ cup sliced mushrooms, ½ cup chopped cucumber, ½ cup chopped celery, ¼ cup sliced olives.

❧ Gelatin Salads

Most of us have grown up with Jell-O salads and their fruity, fun taste. However, the commercial types are loaded with sugar, chemicals, or both. There are delicious alternatives. Kids will love the new taste treat and even prefer it to the old standbys. Gelatin (1 tablespoon), methoxyl (½ tablespoon), or agar (2 tablespoons) will jell 1¾ cups of juice. Try variations according to your taste preferences.

Gelatin is derived from animal sources (bones, tissues, skin, tendons, and ligaments of fish and mammals), methoxyl is a type of pectin from citrus, and agar comes from sea vegetables.

Basic Fruit Gelatin Salad

    1 envelope Knox gelatin
    1¾ cup unsweetened fruit j
    1 cup of fruit

SUBSTITUTION

Knox gelatin: 1 tablespoon gelati
    spoon low-methoxyl pectin

In a saucepan, pour ½ cup of the
on top. When gelatin is softened
over high heat until dissolved. In a
ture with remaining juice and ref
ture begins to thicken. Fold in the
dip the mold in hot water quickl
serving dish.

Fruit Com

Pineapple juice with banana and
Orange juice with mandarin oran
Raspberry or boysenberry juice w
Black cherry juice with apple and
Lemonade with raspberries or pea
Grape juice with grapes
Peach juice with peaches and bana
Pear juice with pears and nuts
Papaya juice with pear, peach, or gr
Pureed strawberries with strawberri

Apple Wal

Serves 6

    2 enve
    3½ cups
    2 teas
    1½ cups
    ¼ cup
    ¼ cup
        das

SUBSTITUTI

Knox gelati
    spoon l
Honey: 2 te
Walnut: ¼

In a saucep
evenly on
quickly ove
mixture w
mixture be
namon and
several tim

Grapefru

Serves 4

    1 er
    1¾ cu
    2 ta
    1 la
    ¾ cu
    ¼ c
    ⅛ s

SUBSTITUTIONS

Knox gelatin: 1 tablespoon gelatin powder; 2 tablespoons agar; ½ tablespoon low-methoxyl pectin

Honey: 2 tablespoons grape juice concentrate or rice syrup

In a saucepan, pour ½ cup of the juice and honey and sprinkle the gelatin
evenly on top. When gelatin is softened (about 3 to 5 minutes), heat
quickly over high heat until dissolved. In a bowl or mold, combine gelatin
mixture with remaining juice and refrigerate for 30 minutes or until
mixture begins to thicken. Fold in the grapefruit, avocado, celery, and
olives and chill until firm. To unmold, dip the mold in hot water quickly
several times and then invert on a serving dish. This salad is delicious
with poultry.

Dash of Spice Salad

Serves 4

2½ cups black cherry juice
 1 tablespoon honey (optional)
 3 tablespoons agar
 1 teaspoon grated orange peel
 1 stick cinnamon
 1 tablespoon lemon juice

SUBSTITUTION

Honey: 1 tablespoon grape juice concentrate or rice syrup

Agar: 1½ tablespoons gelatin

Orange peel: 1 teaspoon grated tangerine or tangelo peel

In a saucepan, pour ½ cup of the juice and honey and sprinkle the agar
evenly on top. Set aside and let sit for 30 minutes. In another saucepan,
combine ½ cup of the juice and cinnamon stick and heat until warm.
Set aside and let sit for 30 minutes. In a bowl or mold, combine the
remaining juice and orange peel. Heat agar mixture quickly under high
heat and dissolve agar. Combine the agar with the cinnamon and juice
mixture in the mold with the lemon juice and chill until firm. To unmold,
dip the mold in hot water quickly several times and then invert on a
serving dish.

Classic Tomato Salad

Serves 4

1¾ cup tomato juice
½ teaspoon grated fresh horseradish
¼ teaspoon paprika
1 teaspoon lemon juice
½ tablespoon low-methoxyl pectin
½ tablespoon calcium water solution
½ cup small, deveined shrimp
¼ cup finely chopped celery
1½ tablespoons minced green onion

SUBSTITUTIONS

Shrimp: ½ cup crab
Green onion: 1½ tablespoons minced yellow or white onion
Celery: ¼ cup chopped green bell pepper
Paprika: ¼ teaspoon tarragon
Lemon juice: 1 teaspoon lime juice
Low-methoxyl pectin: 1 tablespoon gelatin (follow Basic Fruit Gelatin
    Salad directions)

In a saucepan, combine the tomato juice, horseradish, paprika, and
lemon juice and heat to boiling. In a blender, combine tomato juice mixture and pectin and blend for 1 minute. Add the calcium solution and
process for 10 seconds. In a bowl or mold, combine the shrimp, celery,
and green onion and pour in juice mixture. Refrigerate for 1 hour or
until firm. To unmold, dip the mold in hot water quickly several times
and then invert on a serving dish. Serve on a bed of watercress.

VARIATIONS

Replace tomato juice with: 1¾ cup Very Veggie tomato juice; 1¾ cup
tomato juice with ¼ cup diced green bell pepper, ¼ cup diced celery, 1
tablespoon diced onion; 1¾ cup tomato juice with ½ chopped cucumber and 2 teaspoons minced chives; 1¾ cup tomato juice with ¼ cup
diced avocado, 1 tablespoon diced onion, 1 teaspoon chopped fresh
parsley, dash of cayenne pepper.

CHAPTER 18

Don't Forget the Vegetables

VEGETABLES ARE RICH IN vitamins (A, Bs, C), minerals (calcium, magnesium, iron, and potassium), and fiber. They are low in calories and fat free. The diversity of colors, textures, and flavors delight both the eye and the palate. This chapter contains a list of odd and uncommon vegetables to give you broader choices and a chart showing the calcium distribution in vegetables. This will answer the question, if I give up dairy, where will I get my calcium? Vegetables provide an abundant resource for minerals.

Fresh vegetables are much better than canned and frozen. There is no mystery in their preparation; it takes only a little more time. And the experience of selecting fresh vegetables from your garden, local produce stand, or market can be rewarding and stimulating.

If you have been tested sensitive to food grade vegetable petroleum, beeswax, or lactase resin base wax and resin, be extra careful about choosing your produce. Organic is always best. Below is a list of commercially grown vegetables that may contain one or more of these additives.

Vegetables That May Contain Additives

Avocado	Sugar cane
Bell pepper	Squash
Chili pepper	Sweet potato
Cucumber	Tomato
Eggplant	Turnip
Parsnip	Yucca
Rutabaga	

Explore the New and Different World of Vegetables

Bok choy
An Oriental vegetable with a thick stalk like celery and dark green leaves. The flavor is mild and delicious in stir fry.

Brocoflower
A new cross between cauliflower and broccoli, with a sweet milder flavor and yellow green in color.

Broccoli-rabe
Another broccoli and cauliflower combination except the flowerettes have a stronger flavor.

Celery root
A hardy winter vegetable with a mild celery flavor and a cream colored flesh. It is great in soups or grated raw for salads.

Chinese cabbage
A delicate, crinkly leafed cabbage with a mild flavor. Use as you would any other cabbage.

Jicama
This root vegetable is frequently used in Mexican cuisine. Peel the light brown skin to reveal a crunchy, white, mild-flavored flesh.

Kale
This nutrient treasure is over 2000 years old. It is a hardy winter vegetable from the cabbage family which is good steamed, braised, sautéed, and in soups.

Kohlrabi
A light green bulb with leaves growing out of it. Peel the outer skin and enjoy the delicate flavor, which is similar to broccoli with a pinch of turnip.

Okra
Okra is usually found in Southern cooking and is very good for the stomach. The flavor is unique and excellent in soups, casseroles, and chowders.

Potatoes
Yellow firs, Yukon gold, and purple potatoes each have their unique taste and color.

Savoy cabbage
This cabbage has pale green, crumpled leaves with a light flavor.

🦋 Greens

Greens or tops are frequently the most nutritious part of the vegetable and often are discarded or neglected. They can be eaten raw, braised, sautéed, and added to soups and stews.

Greens	
Beet greens	Kale
Broccoli stems	Leek
Celery leaves	Mustard greens
Chives	Red or green chard
Collards	Spinach
Dandelion greens	Turnip greens

Forgotten Oldies

Acorn squash	Shallot
Banana squash	Snow pea
Fava bean	Spaghetti squash
Hubbard squash	Sugar snap pea
Italian bean	Turnip
Parsnip	Wax bean
Rutabaga	

Nondairy Sources of Calcium

Food	Calcium (mgs.)	Calories
1 cup cooked Bok choy	300	25
1 cup cooked collards	300	60
1 cup cooked spinach	300	60
1 cup cooked kale	300	60
2 cups cooked broccoli	300	80
1 cup Chinese cabbage	100	9
1 leek	100	76
1 cup okra	100	38
1 cup parsley	125	26
1 cup parsnips	100	102
1 cup rutabaga	100	64
1 cup turnip greens	105	15
2½ tablespoons blackstrap molasses	300	110

Compared to	Calcium (mgs.)	Calories
12 ounces ice cream	300	450-1000
2 cups low fat cottage cheese	300	410
3½ ounces sardines	300	200
5 ounces canned salmon	300	235
1 cup whole cow's milk	300	150

🦋 How to Steam

Most vegetables in the following recipes are steamed. Steaming preserves the nutrients, retains the color, and controls the quality of flavor. In a pot, place about 1 inch of water and add a steamer basket. Prepare the vegetable by washing, peeling tough skin, discarding decayed parts, chopping, and slicing as appropriate. Put the vegetable in the basket and bring the water to a boil. When boiling, turn down to a simmer. Cover and cook for required length of time. Herbs, nuts, or seeds, or vegetable combinations that complement each other can be added. Vegetables lightly steamed and served plain are also delicious.

🦋 Carrots

Mint Carrots

Serves 4

> 6 peeled, sliced carrots
> 1 tablespoon butter or margarine
> 1 tablespoon flour
> 2 tablespoons lemon juice
> 2 teaspoons honey (optional)
> 1 teaspoon grated lemon peel
> 1 tablespoon chopped mint leaves
>   sea salt and black pepper

SUBSTITUTIONS

Butter: 1 tablespoon olive or canola oil
Lemon juice: 2 tablespoons lime juice
Flour: 1 tablespoon arrowroot or cornstarch
Honey: 2 teaspoons rice syrup or apple or grape juice concentrate
Lemon peel: 1 teaspoon grated lime peel

In a pot, steam the carrots for 6 to 8 minutes or until tender. Reserve ⅓ cup of the carrot water. In a frying pan, melt the butter and stir in the flour. Cook until golden brown, stirring constantly. Add the lemon juice and carrot water and stir until well blended and slightly thick. Add the honey, lemon rind, mint leaves, and salt and pepper and stir well. Add the carrots, toss to glaze, and serve.

Cumin Carrots

Serves 4

> 6 peeled, sliced carrots
> 1 tablespoon butter or margarine
> ¼ teaspoon cumin
> 2 tablespoons chopped fresh parsley
>   sea salt and black pepper

In a pot, steam the carrots for 6 to 8 minutes or until tender. In a frying pan, melt the butter, add the carrots, cumin, parsley, and salt and pepper. Mix well and serve.

Replace the cumin with 4 tablespoons chopped onion, green onion, chives, or 2 tablespoons shallots. In a frying pan, melt the butter and sauté the onion and carrots until tender, yet crunchy. Add salt, pepper, and parsley and serve.

❦ Broccoli

Broccoli with Herbs

Serves 4

- 1 bunch broccoli
- 2 tablespoons butter or margarine
- 3 tablespoons lemon juice
- 1/4 teaspoon oregano
  - sea salt and black pepper

SUBSTITUTIONS
Broccoli: 1 bunch kohlrabi, brocoflower, or broccoli-rabe
Butter: 2 tablespoons olive or canola oil
Oregano: 1/4 teaspoon marjoram, tarragon, or thyme

Prepare the broccoli by cutting off about 1 inch of the tough end of the stalk. Trim any bruised or discolored spots. Chop into bite-size pieces, or cut lengthwise into smaller pieces. In a pot, steam the broccoli for 10 to 15 minutes or until tender, yet crunchy. In a small saucepan, melt the butter and add the lemon juice, oregano, and salt and pepper. Mix well and keep warm; sauce does not have to be over direct heat. (If you use oil instead of butter, add extra salt.) Pour sauce over the broccoli and serve.

VARIATIONS
Add sunflower seeds, cashews, pinenuts, or hazelnuts to sauce before
    serving.
    In the butter, sauté 2 cloves minced garlic.
    Garnish with chopped green onions or chives.
    Sprinkle 1/4 cup grated soy, goat, or Parmesan cheese over the hot
broccoli and serve.

🦋 Cauliflower

Hot Pickled Cauliflower

Serves 4

- 1 head cauliflower
- 2 tablespoons butter or margarine
- 2 tablespoons chopped red bell pepper
- 2 tablespoons chopped green bell pepper
- 3 tablespoons vinegar
- 1 teaspoon honey
  sea salt

SUBSTITUTIONS

Cauliflower: 1 head brocoflower or broccoli-rabe
Vinegar: 3 tablespoons lemon juice
Red bell pepper: 2 tablespoons chopped pimento
Honey: 1 tablespoon apple or grape juice concentrate, or rice syrup

Prepare the cauliflower by breaking into serving pieces. Trim any bruised or discolored spots. In a pot, steam the cauliflower for 10 to 15 minutes or until tender, yet crunchy. In a small saucepan, melt the butter and add the bell peppers, vinegar, honey, and salt. Cook over low heat for about 5 minutes. Pour over cauliflower and serve.

VARIATIONS

Follow recipe above. To the sauce, add one or more: 1 cup sautéed sliced mushrooms, seasoned with salt and black pepper; ½ cup sautéed sliced almonds or hazelnuts; ½ cup sliced, steamed carrots; ½ sliced, steamed celery; ¼ cup grated soy or goat cheese.

Serve with nut milk Basic Cream Sauce.

🦋 Spinach

Basic Spinach

Serves 4

- 1 bunch spinach
- 2 tablespoons butter or margarine

$\frac{1}{2}$ teaspoons nutmeg
  black pepper

SUBSTITUTIONS

Spinach: 1 bunch chard, beet greens, bok choy, kale, turnip greens, or
  mustard greens
Nutmeg: $\frac{1}{2}$ teaspoon cardamom

Thoroughly wash spinach under running water. Discard stems and any
wilted or discolored leaves and coarsely chop. (When preparing the chard
or kale, cut out the coarse stem in the center of the leaf. Discard or save
for use in place of celery.) In a pot, place the spinach with about $\frac{1}{2}$ inch
of water. Steam for 3 to 5 minutes to wilt the leaves, stirring occasionally. Drain the spinach. In a saucepan, melt the butter and add nutmeg
and pepper. Add the spinach and stir well. Serve hot. Spinach and other
greens, may also be braised by sautéing in oil or butter until wilted. Kale
is very good with a cream sauce and grated soy or goat cheese.

VARIATIONS

Follow recipe above. To the sauce, add one 1 cup sautéed sliced mushrooms and/or 1 tablespoon sautéed shallot or other onion.

In a blender, puree cooked spinach and add $\frac{1}{2}$ cup rice, soy, goat, or
nut milk and $\frac{1}{2}$ teaspoon nutmeg. Blend and return pan to heat.

🦋 Green Beans

Basic Green Beans

Serves 4

1 pound green or Italian beans
$\frac{1}{2}$ cup diced red bell pepper

SUBSTITUTION

Red bell pepper: $\frac{1}{2}$ cup diced yellow bell pepper or pimento

Prepare the green beans by cutting off the ends. Leave whole or cut into
1-inch pieces. In a pot, steam the beans and bell pepper for 10 to 15
minutes or until tender, yet crunchy. Serve hot.

VARIATIONS

Follow recipe above. Add one or more: 1 cup sautéed, sliced mushrooms and serve over the steamed green beans; steam ½ cup pearl onions with green beans; ¼ cup sautéed, sliced almonds; ¼ cup sesame or sunflower seeds sprinkled on top of steamed green beans.

❦ Asparagus

Basic Asparagus

Serves 4

- 1 pound asparagus
- 2 tablespoons butter or margarine
   juice of ½ lemon
- ¼ cup grated soy or goat cheese

Preheat oven to 375 degrees F. Prepare the asparagus by breaking off and discarding the tough stem. Wash and cut into 1 inch pieces or steam whole. In a pot, steam asparagus for 10 to 15 minutes or until tender, yet crunchy. In a buttered baking dish, arrange a layer of asparagus, dot with butter, sprinkle with lemon juice, and top with the cheese. Alternate the layers with as many as the dish will hold, ending with the butter, juice, and cheese. Bake for 10 minutes and serve.

VARIATIONS

Follow recipe above. In a frying pan, melt 2 tablespoons butter and sauté 1 tablespoon shallots and 2 teaspoons parsley. Toss with steamed asparagus and serve.

Steam asparagus with ½ cup snow peas or other peas and ¼ cup diced red bell pepper.

Sprinkle with 2 tablespoons toasted sesame seeds.

❦ Cabbage

Sautéed Cabbage

Serves 4

- 1 head Napa cabbage
- 2 tablespoons butter or margarine

½ cup chopped red onion
1 teaspoon caraway seeds
   sea salt and black pepper

SUBSTITUTIONS
Napa cabbage: 1 head red, green, Chinese, or Savoy cabbage or bok choy
Red onion: ½ cup chopped white or yellow onion; 1 chopped leek; ¼
   cup shallots
Caraway seed: 1 teaspoon celery seed or cumin
Butter: 2 tablespoons olive or canola oil

Prepare the cabbage by cutting out the hard core. Discard any wilted or discolored leaves. Shred the cabbage and set aside. In a frying pan, melt the butter and sauté the onion, caraway seeds, and cabbage until tender (different cabbages require different cooking times, from 6 to 15 minutes). Add salt and pepper and serve. Cabbage is delicious added to a soup, stew, or pot roast.

VARIATIONS
Add 3 cloves minced garlic and 1 teaspoon cumin seed and cook as directed above.

   Steam wedges of cabbage with onion, carrots, and caraway seed, cumin, or celery seed.

🦋 Peas

Perfect Peas

Serves 4

1 pound sugar snap peas
1 cup sliced mushrooms
1 tablespoon butter or margarine
   sea salt and black pepper

SUBSTITUTIONS
Sugar snap peas: 1 pound snow peas or shelled peas

Prepare sugar snap (or snow) peas, by pulling off the ends of the pods toward you and discard the string. (For shelled peas, open the pod with your fingers and scoop the peas into a container.) In a pot, steam the peas for about 5 minutes or until tender, yet crunchy. In a frying pan, melt the butter and sauté the mushrooms. Add the steamed peas, season with salt and pepper, and serve.

VARIATIONS

Follow recipe above. Add one or more: ½ cup boiling onions; add ¼ sliced water chestnuts and ½ teaspoon fresh ginger (or ¼ teaspoon dried ginger) and sauté for about 5 minutes; ¼ cup sliced almonds; 2 tablespoons toasted sesame seeds; 1 teaspoon thyme, mint, basil, or oregano.

Steam peas and carrots by cooking the carrots for about 5 minutes and then adding the peas.

𝕎 Squash

Summer Squash

Serves 4

    1   pound sliced or julienned zucchini
    1   tablespoons butter or margarine
    ½   chopped red onion
    ½   teaspoon cumin
        sea salt and black pepper

SUBSTITUTIONS

Zucchini: 1 pound sliced or julienned green, yellow, crook-neck, or patty squash
Butter: 1 tablespoon olive or canola oil
Red onion: ½ chopped yellow or white onion; 2 chopped green onions; 1 minced shallot

Wash the zucchini and chop off the ends. Cut into desired shapes. In a frying pan, melt the butter and sauté the onion, cumin, and salt and pepper for 3 to 5 minutes or until onion is transparent. Steam or sauté the zucchini for about 5 minutes or until tender. Combine with the onion mixture and serve.

VARIATIONS

Follow recipe above, omit the cumin and add 1 tomato chopped, 1 tablespoon fresh basil, and 2 cloves minced garlic.

Steam or sauté the squash with ½ cup chopped red bell pepper.
Steam or sauté the squash with 1 sliced carrot and ½ chopped onion.
Serve with ¼ cup grated parmesan, soy, or goat cheese.

Winter Squash

Serves 4

>   2 pounds acorn
> 1½ teaspoons nutmeg
>   1 tablespoon butter or margarine
>   sea salt and black pepper

SUBSTITUTIONS
Acorn squash: 2 pounds butternut, hubbard, or spaghetti squash
Nutmeg: 1½ teaspoons cinnamon, cardamom, or allspice

Preheat oven to 350 degrees F. Cut the squash in half and discard the
seeds. Place cut side down in a baking dish with a little water in the bottom. Bake for 1 hour, depending upon the size, or until done. Dot with
butter, sprinkle with nutmeg, salt and pepper, and serve. Squash can
also be steamed by cutting into 1-inch pieces or large wedges and steaming until tender.

VARIATIONS
To the above, add some drizzled honey or other sweetener and chopped
nuts.

To the almost-baked acorn squash, add salt and pepper, garlic or
onion powder, oregano or marjoram, 1 teaspoon butter for each squash
half, and grated soy or goat Parmesan cheese. Bake for an additional 10
minutes.

In a blender, puree the cooked, peeled squash. Strain and add enough
hazelnut or other milk to create desired consistency, season with nutmeg and top with chopped nuts.

Scoop out the cooked spaghetti squash. In a frying pan, melt 2 tablespoons of butter and sauté ½ chopped onion and ½ cup chopped green
bell pepper or zucchini for 5 minutes or until onion is transparent. Add
1 cup tomato sauce and ½ teaspoon oregano, marjoram, or basil. Toss
with the squash and serve.

🦋 Tomatoes

Baked Tomatoes

Serves 4

> 4 tomatoes
> 2 tablespoons cornmeal
> 1 clove minced garlic
> ¼ teaspoon oregano
>   sea salt and black pepper
> 1 tablespoon butter or margarine
> ¼ cup grated soy or goat cheese

SUBSTITUTIONS

Cornmeal: 2 tablespoons cooked rice, millet, kasha, bulgur, couscous, or quinoa; 2 tablespoons crushed rye, rice, or wheat crackers
Garlic: ¼ teaspoon garlic or onion powder; ½ minced shallot
Oregano: ¼ teaspoon basil, thyme, or marjoram
Butter: 1 tablespoon olive or canola oil

Preheat oven to 375 degrees F. Wash and core the tomatoes with a wide cut at the top, not cutting through the tomato. Scoop some of the pulp out, if desired. If the tomatoes are small, cut into large pieces and place in a baking dish. In a small bowl, combine the cornmeal, garlic, oregano, and salt and pepper. Fill tomatoes with cornmeal mixture. Dot with butter and top with grated cheese. Bake at 375 degrees for 15 to 20 minutes.

Stewed Tomatoes

Serves 4

> 1 pound tomatoes
> 1 small chopped onion
> ½ chopped green bell pepper
> ½ teaspoon oregano
> 1 teaspoon lemon juice (optional)
>   sea salt and black pepper

SUBSTITUTIONS

Onion: 1 minced shallot; 2 cloves minced garlic
Green bell pepper: ½ cup chopped celery or zucchini

Oregano: ½ teaspoon basil, marjoram, or parsley; ⅛ teaspoon cayenne powder

Wash, core, and chop the tomatoes. In a pot, combine all the ingredients, bring to a boil, and then simmer for 20 minutes.

❦ Eggplant

Eggplant Stew

Serves 4

- 1 tablespoon olive or canola oil
- 5 cloves minced garlic
- ½ cup chopped green bell pepper
- 1 teaspoon cumin
  sea salt and black pepper
- 1 peeled, chopped eggplant
- 2 chopped tomatoes
- ⅓ cup tomato juice
- 2 tablespoons chopped parsley
- ½ teaspoon paprika
- ¼ cup grated soy cheese for garnish (optional)

SUBSTITUTIONS
Garlic: 1 chopped onion, 2 minced shallots
Green bell pepper: ½ cup chopped red bell pepper or summer squash
Cumin: 1 teaspoon oregano or marjoram
Soy cheese: ¼ cup grate goat cheese; ¼ cup soy or goat yogurt

In a large pot, heat the oil and sauté the garlic for 2 to 3 minutes or until golden. Add the bell pepper, cumin, salt and pepper and stir well. Add the chopped eggplant, tomatoes, and juice. Cook until very soft. Garnish with parsley, paprika, and cheese and serve.

🦋 Beets

Basic Beets

Serves 4

    1 bunch beets (save the greens!)

Wash the beets and remove the greens. In a large pot, steam the beets for 30 minutes to 1 hour or until tender, yet crunchy. Remove beets, peel, and cut into desired shapes. Serve hot.

VARIATION
Preheat oven to 375 degrees F. Prepare beets as above and bake for 45 minutes to 1 hour.

    Prepare beets as above. In a frying pan, melt 2 tablespoons of butter and add ½ teaspoon dill or cumin. Pour over beets, garnish with chopped chives or green onions and serve.

Harvard Beets

Serves 4

    3 cups cooked beets (steamed or canned)
    1 cup water (or liquid from the can)
    3 tablespoons flour
  ⅓ cup vinegar
    1 tablespoon honey

SUBSTITUTIONS
Flour: 1 tablespoon arrowroot or cornstarch
Vinegar: ⅓ cup lemon juice
Honey: 1 tablespoon rice syrup or grape juice concentrate

In a saucepan, combine the beets and water on medium. Add the flour, vinegar, and honey and stir into the beets until well blended. Cook until sauce thickens and serve.

❦ Mushrooms

Stuffed Mushrooms

Serves 4

- 1 pound large mushrooms
- 3 tablespoons butter or margarine
- 2 tablespoons chopped shallot
- 1 tablespoon parsley
- 1 tablespoon tarragon
- 1 egg (optional)
- ½ cup crushed rye crackers
   sea salt and black pepper to taste

SUBSTITUTIONS

Shallot: 3 tablespoons chopped yellow or white onion; 2 tablespoons chopped chives

Tarragon: 1 tablespoon oregano, thyme, or marjoram

Rye crackers: ½ cup crushed rice or wheat crackers

Preheat oven to 375 degrees F. Wash and trim the mushrooms. Remove stems from caps and chop stems. In a frying pan, sauté the mushroom caps in 2 tablespoons butter until golden. Transfer caps to baking dish. In the remaining butter, sauté the stems and shallots. Add the tarragon, parsley, and salt and pepper. In a small bowl, combine the egg and crackers and add to mushroom/shallot mixture. Mix well. Fill each mushroom with the stuffing and bake (or broil) for a few minutes until browned and heated through. Serve hot.

VARIATIONS

Add one or more to the mushrooms, sautéed in a 1 tablespoon of butter: 1 minced clove garlic; 2 tablespoons minced onion; 1 tablespoon chopped parsley.

Garnish mushrooms with 2 tablespoons chopped chives, green onions, or minced red bell pepper.

🦋 Potatoes

Potatoes are filled with protein, vitamins, and minerals. They are versatile, delicious, and available in many different varieties: red, russet, Yukon gold, white rose, sweet, and yams. Potatoes can be steamed, boiled, baked, barbecued, and sautéed.

VARIATIONS

Steamed or boiled potatoes can be served with chopped parsley, chives, green onion, rosemary, dill, and cumin seed.

Boil small red potatoes and cut into serving size. In a frying pan, melt 1 tablespoon butter or margarine. Add the potatoes and 1 teaspoon parsley, ½ teaspoon rosemary, and sea salt and black pepper.

Preheat oven to 425 degrees F. Slice potatoes, sweet potatoes, or yams into French fry slices. Lightly oil a baking sheet with 2 tablespoons olive or canola oil. Arrange the fries in a single layer. Lightly salt the fries and bake in a hot oven for about 30 minutes. To brown them, broil for another 2 to 3 minutes. If desired, sprinkle with rosemary, thyme, or cumin.

In a frying pan, heat 2 tablespoons olive or canola oil and brown 1 cup grated potatoes per person. Cook until done and season with sea salt and black pepper. Add 2 tablespoons minced onion to oil if desired.

Baked potatoes can be topped with sautéed mushrooms, chopped green onions or chives, chopped parsley, Parmesan cheese, grated soy or goat cheese, salsa, cooked broccoli, or any herb.

In a frying pan, heat 1 tablespoon of olive or canola oil and brown 1 sliced potato, sweet potato, or yam per person. Season with salt and pepper or any herb.

Leftover Potatoes

In a frying pan, heat 2 tablespoons olive or canola oil and fry grated potatoes for delicious hash browns.

In a frying pan, heat 2 tablespoons olive or canola oil and stir fry chopped potatoes briefly with ¼ cup chopped onions and ¼ cup chopped red or green bell pepper. Add sea salt and black pepper and serve.

In a frying pan, melt 2 tablespoons of butter or margarine. Add ½ teaspoon curry powder, ¼ cup rice or other milk, and mix well. Add the chopped potatoes, sweet potatoes, or yams and heat through over low heat.

In a frying pan, melt 2 tablespoons of butter or margarine. Add 1 diced tomato, 1 clove minced garlic (or 1 tablespoon minced onion), and chopped potatoes. Season with salt and pepper. Garnish with salsa and 2 tablespoons chopped fresh cilantro (or parsley) or add 1 teaspoon chili powder or ⅛ teaspoon cayenne powder.

In a blender, puree the potatoes with a little liquid (cooking liquid, water, or any milk). For every cup of potatoes, add ½ cup cooked parsnips, turnip, or rutabaga and process. Garnish with paprika and serve hot.

Mashed Potatoes

Serves 4

- 4 medium potatoes
- 2 tablespoons butter or margarine
- ¼ cup rice milk
-    sea salt and black pepper

SUBSTITUTION
Rice milk: ¼ cup goat or soy milk

In a large pot, combine the potatoes with enough water to cover and a little salt. Cook covered for 20 to 40 minutes or until done. Drain and transfer to a bowl. With a potato masher, mash the potatoes with the butter (butter makes it taste richer and adds flavor; add only what you need). Add the salt and pepper to taste. Add the milk and mash and whip vigorously until you reach the desired consistency (thick or thinner, lumpy or very smooth). Adjust the salt and pepper and serve.

Scalloped Potatoes

Serves 4

- 4 thinly sliced potatoes
-    sea salt and black pepper
- 1 sliced yellow onion
- 2 tablespoons flour (optional)

¼ cup rice milk
2 tablespoons butter or margarine

SUBSTITUTIONS
Yellow onion: 1 sliced white onion; 3 sliced shallots; 1 large sliced leek
Rice milk: ¼ cup goat or soy milk

Preheat oven to 375 degrees F. Butter a casserole dish and arrange a layer of potato slices in the bottom of the dish. Season with the salt and pepper, cover with onion slices, and sprinkle layer with flour. For richer potatoes, dot each layer with butter. Continue until you reach the top of the dish. Pour enough milk to cover the layers. Bake for 30 to 45 minutes or until done. Serve hot.

VARIATION
Au Gratin Potatoes
Sprinkle ¼ cup grated soy or goat cheese on top of the onions on each layer. Top with the cheese and bake as above.

Traditional Holiday Sweet Potatoes

Serves 4

6 cooked, sliced sweet potatoes or yams
  sea salt and black pepper
⅓ cup honey and 1 tablespoon blackstrap molasses
1 teaspoon grated lemon peel
1½ tablespoons lemon juice
2 tablespoons butter or margarine
¼ teaspoon paprika

SUBSTITUTIONS
Honey: ¾ cup date sugar or ½ cup malted barley
Lemon peel: 1 teaspoon grated orange peel
Lemon juice: 1½ tablespoon orange juice

Preheat oven to 375 degrees F. Butter a 9 x 13 baking dish. Arrange the sliced sweet potatoes in a barely overlapping layer. Season with salt and pepper. Drizzle the honey and molasses mixture evenly over the potatoes. Sprinkle with the lemon peel and juice and dot with butter. Garnish with paprika. Bake for 20 minutes, basting frequently. Serve hot.

CHAPTER 19

Luscious Legumes

CCORDING TO THE BIBLE, Esau sold his inheritance for a bowl of lentils. Daniel impressed the King of Babylon with his good health and strength and his insistence on eating pulse, or legumes, instead of the king's heavy meats and drink. Legumes have been cultivated for many thousands of years. Archaeologists have dated remains of peas and lentils to about 5500 BC During the voyages to the Americas in the sixteenth century, legumes were consumed and valued for their rich source of protein and other nutrients.

Legumes are plants that have edible seeds within a pod. They are extremely versatile and their flavors, tastes, and textures provide an interesting addition to the diet. Their hearty character is a good substitute for regular protein foods, such as red meats and poultry. Since they are high in an incomplete protein (missing one or more of the essential amino acids), they should be combined with a grain, nut, seed, or goat dairy product to make a complete protein. A variety of foods is a major key to good nutrition.

Besides being high in protein, legumes are also an excellent source of iron, thiamine (B_1), riboflavin (B_2), and niacin (B_3), and contain other vitamins and minerals. When they are sprouted, their vitamin C content is high.

Preparation of legumes is relatively easy. The only problem is the time element. The cooking of legumes requires time. For this reason, people have a tendency to stay away from them. Legumes have become a forgotten food. In our search for the quick meal, our tastes have centered mainly on meat and potatoes. The time problem can be solved by planning ahead and applying some of following suggestions. Some of the recipes ask that you sauté some of the vegetables before adding to the dish. This improves the flavor, but this step can be eliminated.

Choose from this selection of delicious recipes or experiment with some of your old family favorites. Many of the beans are interchangeable in the recipes, which adapts well for those on a rotation diet. See Vegetarian Entrees for additional legume recipes.

Rediscover the Luscious Legume

Bean Varieties

Aduki
Anasazi
Black
Black-eyed peas
Fava
Garbanzo
Great Northern
Kidney
Lima
Mung
Navy
Pink
Pinto
Small red
Soybean

Other Legumes

Carob
Green and yellow split peas
Green beans
Peanut
Peas
Red and yellow lentils

For Sprouting

Aduki
Garbanzo

Lentil
Mung
Soybean

Vegetables

Fava
Green
Italian
Lima
String

Peas

Green
Snow
Sugar snap

Other

Bean chips
Bean pasta
Dried bean mixes for dips and
     other uses
Ice Bean (ice cream)

Bean Flours

Black bean
Garbanzo
Pinto bean
Soybean

If you do not know beans about beans, the following is a brief discussion about some of the lesser-known varieties.

Aduki
A small red bean which is rich in flavor and valued in macrobiotic cooking. This bean is good in soup and chili recipes and combines well with rice.

Anasazi
These beans were cultivated by the Anasazi Indians as early as 130 AD. Anasazi beans are one of the faster cooking beans. They are sweeter and mealier than most beans, and are great in Mexican foods. The bean is unusually tasty baked.

Black bean
The black bean is a small bean with a rich flavor. It is excellent in soups, salads, and stews and is a Mexican dietary staple.

Fava bean (broad bean)
It is a tan bean which resembles the lima bean but is stronger in taste. Fava beans can be used dry or fresh. Select the smaller, still-pale green beans for preparation as a fresh vegetable. The larger, dry beans can be used in legume recipes. Fava beans are rich in nitrogen and make a wonderful cover crop for your vegetable garden.

Garbanzo (chickpea)
This versatile, beige-colored, round bean is used in soups, salads, stews, and dips. It is known as the base bean for hummus. Hummus is a delicious and nutritious foundation for spreads, dips, and dressings.

Lima bean
The Lima bean is not well-known as a dry bean or as a fresh vegetable. Fresh, shelled, small green limas are delicious.

Mung bean

A mung bean is a small, round bean that is excellent for sprouting and popular in Chinese cooking. Bean thread noodles are translucent and are best in soups and salads.

Soybean

This sproutable bean originated in China. Soybeans are very high in protein and other nutrients, but are high in fat (35 percent). The dry bean can be prepared many ways, from flour to tofu. The bean itself can also be cooked as a bean for soups. The soybean is best known for its many available products.

🦋 Legume Information

Storage

Dry uncooked legumes should be stored in a dry cool location in a tightly covered container. Glass containers are preferred. They will keep for a very long time. Cooked legumes will not only store in the refrigerator for several days and but also freeze well, providing a nutritious, quick meal. This method provides excellent options for those on a rotation diet.

Soaking

Legumes do not necessarily have to be soaked. The purpose of soaking them is to shorten their cooking time. Cover the legumes with 1 to 2 inches of water and let soak overnight. Sometimes baking soda is added to the water to help to eliminate the gas problem associated with legumes; we feel that adding dulse to the cooking stage is a better and healthier alternative. To aid digestion, always drain and discard the soaking water.

Quick soaking

Cover the legumes with 1 to 2 inches of water. Bring to a boil. Turn off the heat and let sit for 1 hour.

🦋 Cooking Methods

There is no one right way to cook beans. There are several methods which work well. Choose the one that is the most adaptable to your needs and time considerations.

Top of the stove
After bringing the recipe's ingredients to a boil, let simmer for the required length of time. Stir occasionally.

Pressure cooker
The pressure cooker shortens the cooking time. Follow the directions in the recipe, adding one tablespoon of oil to prevent the beans from foaming, and cook for the allotted time. See the chart for cooking times.

Crock pot
The crock pot is an answer to time problems. Start it first thing in the morning and let it cook slowly all day. Assemble the same recipe ingredients and place them into the crock pot. You have two choices of cooking times, depending on how long you will be gone or when you want to have dinner. Five to six hours on high heat, or 10 to 12 hours on low heat.

Thermos
In the biggest thermos you can find, combine the beans with enough boiling water to cover them. The amounts will depend upon the size of the thermos.

Oven-baked
This method applies to certain types of legumes. Check recipes for ideas.

Fireplace
Pull out grandma's Dutch oven or cast iron pot. Gather wood and make a fire in your fireplace. Follow any of the recipes or choose one of your own favorites. While you are enjoying the fire and the aromas drifting through the air, do not forget to occasionally stir the beans.

Legume Cooking Chart

1 cup of dried legumes will yield 2 cups cooked

Legume	Water	Time	Soaked	Pressure Cooker Time	
				15 Pounds Pressure	10 Pounds Pressure
Aduki	3 cups	2 hours	1 hour	10 to 15 minutes	25 to 30 minutes
Anasazi	3 cups	2½ hours	1½ hours	10 minutes	20 minutes
Black	4 cups	1½ hours	1 hour	10 to 15 minutes	25 to 30 minutes
Black-eyed pea	3 cups	1 hour	no need	7 to 10 minutes	15 minutes
Fava	3 cups	3 hours	no need	10 to 15 minutes	25 to 30 minutes
Garbanzo	4 cups	3 hours	2½ hours	10 to 15 minutes	25 to 30 minutes
Great Northern	3 cups	2 hours	1½ hours	10 to 15 minutes	25 to 30 minutes
Kidney	3 cups	1½ hours	1½ hours	10 to 15 minutes	25 to 30 minutes
Lentils	3 cups	45 minutes	no need	7 to 10 minutes	15 minutes
Lima	3 cups	1¼ hours	no need	10 minutes	20 minutes
Mung	2½ cups	1½ hours	45 minutes	10 to 15 minutes	25 to 30 minutes
Navy	3 cups	2½ hours	1½ hours	10 minutes	20 minutes
Pink	3 cups	2½ hours	1½ hours	10 minutes	20 minutes
Pinto	3 cups	2½ hours	1½ hours	10 minutes	20 minutes
Small red	3 cups	3 hours	2½ hours	10 to 15 minutes	25 to 30 minutes
Split pea	4 cups	45 minutes	no need	7 to 10 minutes	15 minutes
Soybean	4 cups	3½ hours	no need	15 to 20 minutes	30 to 35 minutes

Cooking times vary depending whether you want the beans to be soft and mushy or crunchy. If the legumes have been stored for a long time, they will cook better if they are soaked. The actual cooking time will also be somewhat longer. The taste test is always best.

✿ Sprouting

Sprouting is a simple, easy, and inexpensive method to produce your own healthy food at home. Purchase a sprouting jar or make your own from a wide mouth jar and cheesecloth or a small screen. Place the legume (or grain or seed) that is to be sprouted into the jar to the depth of ½ inch. Cover with an inch of water and let sit overnight (12 hours for most; 18 hours for soybeans). Rinse and drain in the morning. Place the jar on its side in a cupboard or other area of the kitchen that does not receive much light and the temperature will remain fairly constant. Rinse and drain two to three times a day. Depending upon the size and type of legume that is being sprouted, it will require from three to five days for a mature sprout to appear. The length of the sprouts should be about 1 inch. Rinse and drain the sprouts well and they will keep in the refrigerator for three to five days. For those with Candida, always make sure that the sprouts are fresh. When in doubt, throw it out, as molds can grow quickly. Sprouting is fun and nutritious and children love to tend the mini-garden!

Black Bean Stew

Serves 4

1½	cups black beans
1	tablespoon olive or canola oil
1	medium diced onion
½	cup chopped red bell pepper
4	cups chopped tomatoes
½	minced jalapeño
	sea salt or kelp
½	bunch chopped fresh cilantro

SUBSTITUTIONS
Black beans: 1½ cups small red, pinto, or Anasazi beans
Onion: 2 minced shallots; 1 cup chopped green onion; 5 cloves minced
    garlic
Cilantro: ½ bunch chopped fresh parsley
Red bell pepper: ½ cup chopped green bell pepper; ½ cup chopped carrot

Rinse and soak beans for 6 hours or overnight. Drain and transfer to a
soup pot. Cover beans with an inch of water and bring to boil, skim-
ming the foam that rises. In a frying pan, heat the oil and sauté the onions
with the bell pepper for 3 to 5 minutes or until onion is transparent.
Add onions, bell pepper, tomatoes, jalapeño, and salt to the beans. Add
¾ of the cilantro. Reduce heat to simmer and stir occasionally for 1 hour.
Garnish with a strip of bell pepper and remaining cilantro when serving.

Curried Lentils

Serves 4

    1 cup dried lentils
       sea salt and black pepper
    1 tablespoon butter or margarine
    1 sliced onion
    ¼ cup diced celery
    1 tablespoon curry powder
    1 tablespoon flour
    ¼ cup unfiltered apple juice

SUBSTITUTIONS
Butter: 1 tablespoon olive or canola oil
Onion: 2 minced shallots
Celery: ¼ cup chopped red bell pepper or carrot
Apple juice: ¼ cup pear juice or rice milk

In a soup pot, cook lentils with salt and pepper and enough water to
cover for 30 minutes. Drain the lentils. In a frying pan, melt the butter
in skillet and sauté the onion and celery for 3 to 5 minutes or until onions
are transparent. Add the curry powder and ¼ cup water. Cover and simmer for 5 minutes. Mix flour with apple juice and stir into onion mixture. Add to lentils and simmer for 15 minutes.

Lentil Dal

Serves 4

1½	cups lentils
5	cups water
1	clove minced garlic
¼	teaspoon turmeric
1½	teaspoon cumin
2	teaspoon coriander
½	teaspoon sea salt or kelp
	black pepper

SUBSTITUTION
Lentils: 1½ cups yellow split pea or fava beans

In a soup pot, bring lentils and water to a boil. Add garlic, turmeric, cumin, coriander, salt, and pepper. Let simmer for 45 minutes, stirring occasionally so it does not stick. Stir with a whisk or wooden spoon briskly to form a puree, or place in a blender for a creamier consistency. There should be five cups of puree.

Dal, a traditional Indian dish, can be used in many ways, including as a side dish, a spread on flat bread, and a sauce on vegetables and lentil or nut loaf.

VARIATION
Spicy Dal
Follow recipe above. In a frying pan, heat 2 tablespoons olive or canola oil and sauté 4 cloves minced garlic, ½ teaspoon cumin, and 2 small dried crushed red peppers (or 1 tablespoon red pepper flakes) until garlic is brown. Stir into the dal and serve.

Almost-Old-Fashioned Baked Beans

Serves 4

2	cups dried navy beans
½	pound salt pork, cut in ½ (optional)
1	small chopped onion
½	teaspoon dry mustard

¼ cup blackstrap molasses

¼ cup honey

SUBSTITUTION

Navy beans: 2 cups dried small red, pink, small Great Northern, or black
 beans

Onion: 1 minced shallot

Honey: ¼ cup rice syrup or malted barley

Rinse and soak beans for 6 hours or overnight. Drain and transfer to a
large pot. Cover beans with an inch of water and bring to boil, then simmer for 1 hour. Drain and save the water. Preheat oven to 300 degrees
F. In a soup pot, place one piece of the salt pork. Add beans and remaining ingredients plus ½ cup of the bean water. Place the other piece of
salt pork on the top. Cover and bake for 5 hours. Add bean water if
needed. Uncover and bake for 1 hour.

Alternative cooking method: Use the crock pot on the low heat setting. Soak beans overnight, drain, and assemble the ingredients as directed
above. Add 1 cup of bean water, and bake at 275 degrees F setting for 8
hours. Uncover, transfer to a 300 degree F oven and bake for ½ hour.

Spicy Baked Beans

Serves 4

 2 cups navy beans
 1 tablespoon butter or margarine
 2 cups chopped onion
 3 cloves minced garlic
 1 chopped green bell pepper
 3 cups tomato juice
 4 tablespoons blackstrap molasses
 2 teaspoons thyme
   sea salt and black pepper

SUBSTITUTIONS

Navy beans: 2 cups pink, pinto, or small red beans

Butter: 1 tablespoon olive or canola oil

Onion: 1½ cups chopped shallots

Green bell pepper: 1 chopped chili pepper
Molasses: 5 tablespoons sorghum or malted barley
Thyme: 2 teaspoons marjoram or rosemary

In a large pot, cover the beans with water and cook covered for about 1 hour or until beans are barely tender. Drain the beans, reserving some of the liquid. Preheat oven to 275 degrees F. In a frying pan, melt the butter and sauté the onion, garlic, and bell pepper for 3 to 5 minutes or until onion is transparent. In a soup pot, combine the beans, onion mixture, tomato juice, molasses, and thyme, and salt and pepper. Cover and bake for 4 hours. Add more of the bean water if needed. Bake uncovered for another 30 minutes and serve.

Bean Cake

Serves 4

- 2 cups pinto beans
- 2 cloves minced garlic
- ¼ teaspoon crushed red pepper
- 1 teaspoon sea salt or kelp
- 2 tablespoons butter or margarine

SUBSTITUTIONS

Pinto beans: 2 cups dried lima, Great Northern, or navy beans
Red pepper: 1 minced chili pepper
Garlic: ¼ chopped onion; 1 tablespoon minced shallot
Butter: 2 tablespoons olive or canola oil

Rinse and soak beans for 6 hours or overnight. In a large pot, cover beans with water, bring to a boil, then reduce heat and simmer for 2 hours. Drain the beans. In a blender or food processor, combine the beans, garlic, red pepper, and salt and coarsely grind. Shape into small cakes. In a frying pan, melt the butter and sauté the cakes for 10 minutes or until golden brown. Four cups of canned beans may be substituted for the two cups of dried beans.

Basic Hummus

Serves 4

 1½ cups garbanzos
 ¼ cup tahini
 3 chopped green onions
 2 cloves minced garlic
 2 tablespoons lemon juice
 ¼ teaspoon cumin
 ¼ teaspoon coriander
 ¼ teaspoon paprika
 1 teaspoon sea salt or kelp

SUBSTITUTION
Lemon juice: 2 tablespoons lime or kumquat juice

Rinse and soak the beans for 6 hours or overnight. Drain beans and transfer to a large pot. Cover with water and cook covered for about 2 hours or until soft. Drain beans. In blender or food processor, combine the beans with the remaining ingredients and puree until smooth. Cover and refrigerate for least 1 hour or until chilled.

Fabulous Fava

Serves 4

 2½ cups fava beans
 2 chopped stalks celery plus leaves
 2 small chopped onions
 1 clove minced garlic
 4 sprigs chopped parsley
 4 whole cloves (optional)
 1 bay leaf
 ½ teaspoon sea salt
  fresh peppercorns
 3 tablespoons butter or margarine
 2 tablespoons flour
 ½ cup cashew Nut Cream (page 199)
 3 strips bacon (optional)

SUBSTITUTIONS
Fava beans: 2½ cups Great Northern or lima beans
Onions: 4 cloves minced garlic; 3 minced shallots
Parsley: 4 springs chopped cilantro
Butter: 3 tablespoons olive or canola oil
Nut Cream: ½ cup almond Nut Cream (page 199) or heavy cream

Rinse and soak the beans for 6 hours or overnight. Drain, transfer to a large pot, and cover with 1 inch of water. Add the onion, garlic, celery, parsley, cloves, bay leaf, salt, and pepper and bring to a boil. Simmer for 2 hours. Drain and reserve the liquid, discard the cloves and bay leaf. In a frying pan, melt the butter and stir in the flour. Gradually stir in 1½ cups of the reserved liquid and cook until the sauce is smooth and slightly thickened. Stir in the cream. Preheat oven to 350 degrees F. Place the beans in a buttered baking dish. Pour the sauce over the beans, arranging the strips of bacon on the top. Bake for 30 minutes and serve hot.

Alias Lima

Serves 4

- 2 cups lima beans
- 1 teaspoon sea salt or kelp
- 2 tablespoons butter or margarine
- 1 cup chopped onion
- 4 tablespoons chopped fresh parsley

SUBSTITUTIONS
Lima beans: 2 cups dried pinto, Great Northern, or navy beans
Onion: ¾ cup chopped shallot; 1 cup chopped green onion
Butter: 2 tablespoons olive or canola oil
Parsley: 4 tablespoons chopped fresh cilantro

In a large pot, combine the beans with the salt and cover with 1 inch of water. Cook for 1½ hours, stirring occasionally, and adding more water if needed. Drain and set aside. Preheat oven to 350 degrees F. In a frying pan, melt the butter and sauté the onion for 3 to 5 minutes or until transparent. In a blender, blend the beans until smooth or press the beans through a coarse sieve. Add all but 4 tablespoons of the sautéed onion and 2 tablespoons parsley. Combine well and pour into a casserole dish. Sprinkle the reserved onion on top and bake for 20 minutes. Sprinkle with the remaining parsley and serve.

Basic Refried Beans

Serves 6

> 6 cups cooked pinto beans
> ½ cup bean water
> ¼ teaspoon garlic powder
> ½ teaspoon onion powder
> ½ teaspoon chili powder
> sea salt or kelp

SUBSTITUTIONS
Pinto: 6 cups cooked small red or black beans
Garlic powder: ½ teaspoon onion powder if garlic is not tolerated
Onion powder: ½ teaspoon garlic powder if onion is not tolerated
Chili powder: ½ teaspoon cayenne powder; 1 minced jalapeño

In a large bowl, mash cooked beans with bean water until desired consistency is reached (or lightly in the blender). Add spices and mix well. Adjust the seasonings. In a saucepan, heat the beans on low heat, stirring often. Serve hot.

CHAPTER 20

Surprising and Different Vegetarian Entrees

VEGETARIAN ENTREES ARE BECOMING more popular, even in restaurants. They are delightful, delicious, and filling. Neither your taste buds nor your tummy will feel cheated. Variety abounds and combinations are almost endless. The various colors will gladden the eye and the rich and interesting flavors will delight your palate. Additional vegetarian entrees of whole-meal salads from various grains, pastas, legumes, nuts, and vegetable combinations can be found beginning on page 247.

Many of the recipes given use butter or oil for sautéing. This step can be omitted or water may be used as a substitute. For the ease of exploring these new experiences, we have broken entrees down into grains, pasta, vegetable combinations, and legumes.

🦋 Hearty Grain Entrees

Moroccan Couscous

Serves 4

1	tablespoon olive or canola oil
⅓	cup chopped yellow onion
½	cup diced red bell pepper
1¼	cups water
⅓	cup raisins (optional)
¼	teaspoon ground cumin
½	teaspoon grated orange peel
⅛	teaspoon cinnamon

  sea salt and black pepper
1 cup quick couscous

SUBSTITUTIONS
Onion: 2 tablespoons minced shallot; ⅓ cup chopped green onion
Bell pepper: ¼ cup diced pimento
Raisins: ⅓ cup currants
Orange peel: ½ teaspoon grated tangerine or tangelo peel
Couscous: 2 cups cooked bulgur wheat or millet

In a saucepan, heat the oil and sauté the onion and bell pepper for 3 to 5 minutes or until onion is transparent. Add water, raisins, cumin, orange peel, cinnamon, and salt and pepper and bring to a boil. Remove from heat and add the couscous. Stir well and cover. Let stand for 5 minutes and serve.

Versatile and Basic Rice

Serves 4

4 cups water
2 cups brown rice
½ teaspoon sea salt
2 tablespoons butter or margarine
1 cup sliced mushrooms
  sea salt and black pepper
2 chopped green onions
2 tablespoons chopped fresh parsley

SUBSTITUTIONS
Butter: 2 tablespoons olive or canola oil
Green onion: ½ cup chopped chives
Parsley: 2 tablespoons chopped fresh cilantro

In a pot with a tight-fitting lid, bring water to a boil. Add rice and salt and reduce heat and simmer with the lid on for 40 minutes. When rice is almost done, melt the butter in a frying pan and sauté the mushrooms with salt and pepper until done. In a serving dish, combine mushrooms with the cooked rice. Sprinkle with green onion and parsley and serve.

VARIATIONS

In a frying pan, heat 1 tablespoon olive or canola oil and sauté 1 diced red bell pepper and ½ cup diced onion for 3 to 5 minutes or until onion is transparent. Add ½ teaspoon oregano and salt and pepper. Add 2 cups of uncooked rice and sauté briefly. Transfer to a pot with a tight-fitting lid, add 4 cups of water, and simmer rice for 40 minutes. Garnish with 2 tablespoons minced red bell pepper and serve.

When rice is almost done, heat 1 tablespoon olive or canola oil in a frying pan and sauté 2 medium diced zucchini (or other summer squash or 1 cup chopped broccoli, green bell pepper, or Brussels sprouts) and 3 cloves minced garlic until tender. Add ½ teaspoon marjoram and salt and pepper. Mix with cooked rice and serve garnished with 2 table-spoons chopped fresh parsley.

When rice is almost done, heat 1 tablespoon olive or canola oil in a frying pan and sauté 2 medium diced Japanese eggplants and ¼ cup diced yellow onion or minced shallots for 3 to 5 minutes or until onion is transparent. Add 1 tablespoon curry powder dissolved in ¼ cup water and salt and pepper. Mix with cooked rice and serve.

Risotto Verte

Serves 4

     2 tablespoons olive or canola oil
     1 cup chopped green onion
     1 cup chopped fresh parsley
  1½ cups finely chopped spinach
     ¼ teaspoon nutmeg
     2 cups rice
     4 cups Vegetable Stock (page 230)
     1 teaspoon sea salt
         black pepper
     ¼ cup grated goat or soy parmesan cheese
     2 tablespoons minced green onion
     2 tablespoons chopped fresh parsley

SUBSTITUTIONS

Green onion: 1 cup chopped yellow onion or leek

Spinach: 1½ cups finely chopped chard or beet greens
Nutmeg: ¼ teaspoon cinnamon
Vegetable stock: 4 cups water

In a large saucepan, heat the oil and sauté the onion, parsley, and spinach until tender and the spinach has wilted. Add the nutmeg and the rice and sauté briefly. Add the stock, salt, and pepper and bring to a boil. Turn down to simmer and cook about 30 minutes or until liquid is absorbed. Place on a serving dish and sprinkle with cheese. Combine the green onion and parsley and sprinkle on top. Serve hot.

Stuffed Greens

Serves 4

    15 large red or green chard leaves
     1 tablespoon olive or canola oil
  1½ cups diced onion
     1 egg
     2 cups cooked rice
    ½ cup chopped parsley
     1 cup goat ricotta cheese
    ½ teaspoon oregano
        sea salt and black pepper

SUBSTITUTIONS
Chard: 15 large spinach, beet, collard, or kale leaves
Egg: 1 teaspoon Egg Replacer or binder (page 140)
Rice: 2 cups cooked millet, kasha, or bulgur wheat
Oregano: ½ teaspoon marjoram or thyme

Preheat oven to 350 degrees F. Wash and dry chard. In a frying pan, heat the oil and sauté the onion for 3 to 5 minutes or until transparent. In a mixing bowl, beat the egg and add the rice, parsley, cheese, oregano, and salt and pepper. Mix well. Place 2 tablespoons of filling inside each leaf. Fold the sides and roll. Place seam side down in an oiled baking dish and add enough water to cover the bottom of the dish. Bake for 25 minutes and serve.

Traditional Kasha

Serves 4

2 cups Vegetable Stock (page 230)
   sea salt and black pepper
1 egg
1 cup kasha
2 tablespoon butter or margarine

In a saucepan, combine the stock and salt and pepper and bring to a simmer. In a small bowl, beat the egg and add the kasha. Mix well. In a frying pan, melt the butter and cook the kasha and egg mixture until the egg is cooked and the kernels are mostly separated. Bring the stock to a boil and add the kasha mixture. Reduce heat to low and cook for 10 to 15 minutes or until the liquid is absorbed. Serve in place of potatoes or rice.

Flavorful Kasha

Serves 4

2 cups water
1 cup kasha
1 tablespoon olive or canola oil
2 cloves minced garlic
1 medium chopped zucchini
1 medium chopped yellow squash
   sea salt and black pepper

SUBSTITUTIONS
Kasha: 1 cup millet or bulgur
Garlic: 1 minced shallot; 1 small minced onion

In a large pot, bring water to a boil and add the kasha. Reduce heat to simmer and cook for 15 minutes. In a frying pan, heat the oil and sauté the garlic, zucchini, and squash until tender. Add salt and pepper and mix with the cooked kasha. Serve hot.

Grain Stuffed Cabbage Rolls

Serves 4

> 1 head green cabbage
> ¾ cup chopped yellow onion
> ¼ cup chopped celery
> 1 tablespoon olive or canola oil
> ¾ cup raw barley
> 2 cups Vegetable Stock (page 230)
> ½ cup chopped almonds
>   sea salt and black pepper
> 1 tablespoon dill
> 1 teaspoon celery seed
> 2½ cups tomato sauce (homemade or prepared)

SUBSTITUTIONS

Cabbage: 1 head Savoy, Chinese, or Napa cabbage
Yellow onion: ¾ cup chopped white or green onion; ½ cup minced shallot
Raw barley: ¾ cup rice, millet, bulgur, quinoa, or kasha
Almonds: ½ cup chopped cashews or pinenuts

Preheat oven to 350 degrees F. Remove core from the cabbage. In a large pot, steam the cabbage for 5 minutes. Separate the leaves and set aside. In another pot, heat the oil and sauté the onion and celery for 3 to 5 minutes or until onion is transparent. Add the grain and sauté briefly. Add the stock, almonds, and salt and pepper and bring to a boil. Simmer until the liquid is absorbed and the grain is done. Add the dill and celery seed and mix well. Place 2 tablespoons of the filling in each leaf, fold the sides and roll. In a lightly oiled baking dish, pour half the sauce and place stuffed leaves seam side down. Pour the rest of the sauce over the leaves and cover with aluminum foil. Bake for 45 minutes and serve.

Grain Pilaf

Serves 4

> 1 cup slivered almonds
> 2 tablespoons butter or margarine
> ½ cup diced carrot

½ cup chopped green onion
¼ cup diced celery
½ cup diced green bell pepper
½ teaspoon oregano
   sea salt and black pepper
4 cups cooked quinoa
¼ cup parsley for garnish

SUBSTITUTIONS

Almonds: 1 cup cashews, pinenuts, or hazelnuts
Green onion: 4 cloves minced garlic; 2 minced shallots
Celery: ¼ cup chopped jicama or chard stems
Oregano: ½ teaspoon marjoram, dill, or cumin; 3 threads saffron
Quinoa: 4 cups cooked rice, millet, amaranth, teff, bulgur wheat, or
   kasha

Preheat oven to 350 degrees F. On a baking sheet, toast the almonds for 10 minutes. In a large pot, melt the butter and sauté the carrot, onion, celery, and bell pepper for 3 to 5 minutes or until onion is transparent. Stir in the oregano and salt and pepper. Add the quinoa, mix well, and sauté until thoroughly heated. Add the almonds to the grain mixture and serve garnished with parsley.

Grain Burger

Serves 4

3 cups water
1 cup teff
1 teaspoon thyme
¼ teaspoon salt
4 chopped green onions
¼ teaspoon black pepper
2 tablespoons olive or canola oil
4 whole grain buns
1 medium sliced onion
2 medium sliced tomatoes
4 large lettuce leaves
   yeast-free pickles or relish

SUBSTITUTIONS
Teff: 1 cup amaranth, quinoa, or millet
Thyme: 1 teaspoon oregano, sage, or marjoram
Green onion: 4 cloves minced garlic; ½ cup chopped onion

In a large pot, bring the water to a boil and add the teff, thyme, and salt.
Reduce heat and simmer for 15 minutes. Cool the grain, mix in the
onion and pepper and form into patties. In a frying pan, heat the oil in
a large frying pan and quickly brown the patties. Place one patty on each
bun and garnish with onion, tomato, lettuce, and pickles.

Classic Crepes

Serves 4

>   1 cup brown rice flour
>   2 large eggs
>   1 cup rice milk
>   ¼ teaspoon sea salt
>   1 tablespoon olive or canola oil

SUBSTITUTIONS
Brown rice flour: 1 cup whole wheat pastry, spelt, buckwheat, barley,
    oat, corn, or millet flour
Eggs: 3 teaspoons Egg Replacer or binder (page 140)
Rice milk: 1 cup soy or goat milk or water

In a blender, combine all the ingredients and blend until smooth. Let
stand for one hour. Batter should be thin and pour easily. If not, add
more milk. Lightly oil a skillet or crepe pan and set it over high heat. Pour
a small amount of batter in the pan and swirl until it barely covers the
bottom of the pan. Cook 2 to 3 minutes until lightly brown. Quickly turn
over and cook the other side for 1 to 2 minutes. Serve immediately or
keep the crepes warm in a 200 degree F oven. Fill with 1 to 2 tablespoons
of filling and roll the crepe. Serve with Basic Cream Sauce II (page 423)
or top with soy or goat cheese. To bake the filled crepes, preheat oven to
350 degrees F. Place crepes in a baking pan and bake for 10 minutes.

FILLING IDEAS
Roll 2 cooked asparagus spears in each crepe and top with grated soy or
goat Parmesan or soy or goat cheese and bake until cheese has melted.

In a frying pan, heat 1 tablespoon olive or canola oil and sauté 1 cup diced zucchini, 2 tablespoons onion, and 1 teaspoon cumin seed for 3 to 5 minutes or until onion is transparent. Salt and pepper to taste. Place 2 tablespoons of mixture in each crepe and roll up. Top with soy or goat cheese and bake until cheese has melted (optional).

Roll cooked broccoli sprinkled with pinenuts in each crepe and top with lemon sauce or soy or goat cheese and bake until cheese has melted.

Steam 3 cups coarsely chopped spinach or other greens. In a frying pan, heat 1 tablespoon butter and sauté ½ cup sliced mushrooms. Add ½ teaspoon nutmeg and salt and pepper. Mix with the well-drained spinach. Place 2 tablespoons of mixture in each crepe and roll up.

In a frying pan, heat 2 tablespoons olive or canola oil and sauté 2 diced Japanese eggplants, 1 large chopped tomato, and 3 tablespoons onion or 2 cloves minced garlic until tender. Place 2 tablespoons of mixture in each crepe and roll up.

Steam 2 cups green beans. Add ½ cup toasted slivered almonds and place 2 tablespoons of mixture in each crepe and roll up. Serve with Almond Cream.

Grain Loaf

Serves 4

> 2 tablespoon olive or canola oil
> ½ cup chopped green onion
> 2 cloves minced garlic
> ¾ cup chopped red bell pepper
> ¼ teaspoon oregano
> sea salt and black pepper
> 2 cups cooked millet
> ¼ cup chopped walnuts

SUBSTITUTIONS

Red bell pepper: ¾ cup chopped green bell pepper; ¾ cup sliced mushrooms; ¾ grated carrot, zucchini, or turnip; ½ cup chopped celery, chard stems, or jicama

Green onion: 2 tablespoons minced shallot; 4 cloves minced garlic; ½ cup chopped onion

Oregano: ¼ teaspoon marjoram or thyme

Millet: 2 cups cooked teff, amaranth, quinoa, kasha, or barley
Walnut: ¼ cup chopped pecans, hazelnuts, or pinenuts

Preheat oven to 400 degrees F. In a frying pan, heat the oil and sauté the onion, garlic, and bell pepper for 3 to 5 minutes or until onion is transparent. Add the oregano and salt and pepper and stir thoroughly. Transfer onion mixture to a mixing bowl and add the millet and walnuts. Mix well. If mixture is too wet, add 1 to 2 tablespoons of millet flour (or same grain flour) to help it bind. Lightly oil and flour a loaf pan. Press the millet mixture into the pan. Bake for 45 minutes to 1 hour. Serve with a nut or tomato sauce.

Basic Polenta

Serves 4

    1   tablespoon olive or canola oil
 1½   cup diced onion
    ¾   cup diced red bell pepper
    ¼   teaspoon thyme
          sea salt and black pepper
    2   cups cooked polenta

SUBSTITUTIONS
Red bell pepper: ½ cup grated zucchini or red, yellow, or green bell pepper
Thyme: ¼ teaspoon oregano or ¼ cup chopped cilantro

In a frying pan, heat the oil and sauté the onion, bell pepper, thyme, and salt and pepper for 3 to 5 minutes or until onion is transparent. Transfer onion mixture to a mixing bowl and add the cooked polenta. Mix well. Pour the polenta into a lightly oiled 9 x 12 baking pan, spreading it evenly. Let cool and become firm. Slice into desired shape. Polenta can be served with a sauce or topped with sautéed or steamed vegetables.

VARIATION
Mexican Polenta
Follow above recipe. Add 1 tablespoon chili powder and 1 minced jalapeño to onion mixture.

❦ Basic Tortillas

Here are some filling ideas for corn and whole wheat tortillas. Combine and create your own delicious concoctions!

Fill tortilla with rice, chopped bell peppers, chopped onion, shredded lettuce, sliced tomato, and sliced avocado. Top with Basic Salsa, mashed avocado, or grated soy or goat cheese.

Fill tortilla with cooked pinto, pink, black, or aduki beans. Add chopped green onion, shredded lettuce or cabbage, sliced tomatoes, chopped bell peppers, sliced avocado, and sliced olives. Top with chopped fresh cilantro, sliced avocado, or grated soy or goat cheese.

Fill tortilla with Lentil Chili. Add chopped onion, sliced tomato, shredded lettuce, and bean or alfalfa sprouts. Top with Basic Salsa or grated soy or goat cheese.

Fill tortilla with Traditional Tabouli. Top with Basic Salsa.

❦ The Pleasures of Pasta

Whole grain pastas are delicious and just as versatile as their refined cousins. Explore them all! The best pasta for any of these dishes (except for the wide flat noodles needed for lasagna) is your favorite pasta.

Basic Pasta

Serves 4

In a large pot, bring 2 to 3 quarts of water to a boil with a little salt. Add 12 ounces of dried or fresh pasta. Cooking times will vary according to the different pastas. Angel hair pasta will require only 2 to 3 minutes, while larger noodles may take 10 to 15 minutes. When possible, cook according to package directions. The best standard for cooking time is individual taste. Drain in large colander and rinse with hot water (so it will stay warm). Serve immediately with your favorite sauce. The following recipes provide different and delicious sauce choices.

Pasta with Fresh Tomatoes

Serves 4

  12 ounces pasta
   2 tablespoons olive or canola oil
   4 cloves minced garlic
   4 medium chopped tomatoes
      sea salt and black pepper
   2 tablespoon chopped fresh basil
   2 tablespoons grated goat or soy Parmesan cheese (optional)

Cook pasta according to directions. In a frying pan, heat the oil and sauté the garlic until browned. Add the tomatoes, salt and pepper. Cook 7 to 10 minutes (tomatoes should still hold their shape but also be cooked). Add the basil. Correct seasonings if needed. Toss or serve with your favorite pasta and sprinkle with cheese.

Lemon Basil Cream Pasta

Serves 4

  12 ounces pasta
   2 tablespoon butter or margarine
   1 tablespoon minced shallots
   2 tablespoons flour
 1–2 cups goat milk
   1 tablespoon lemon juice
   2 teaspoon grated lemon peel
   2 tablespoon dried basil
   2 tablespoons grated goat parmesan cheese (optional)

SUBSTITUTIONS
Shallot: 2 tablespoons minced yellow or white onion
Goat milk: 1–2 cups rice, soy, or nut milk
Goat Parmesan cheese: 2 tablespoons soy Parmesan cheese

Cook pasta according to directions. In a frying pan, melt the butter and sauté the shallots until light brown. Stir in the flour and slowly add the milk, stirring constantly until the sauce is smooth and thick. Add the lemon juice, lemon peel, and the basil. Correct the seasoning with salt and pepper. Toss or serve with your favorite pasta and sprinkle with cheese.

Mushroom Tarragon Pasta

Serves 4

    12 ounces pasta
     2 tablespoon olive or canola oil
     2 cups sliced mushrooms
     1 cup chopped green onions
     1 cup goat milk
     1 tablespoon tarragon
         sea salt and black pepper
     2 tablespoons grated goat or soy parmesan cheese (optional)

SUBSTITUTIONS
Green onion: ¾ cup chopped yellow or white onion plus 1 minced shallot
Goat milk: 1 cup rice, soy, or nut milk
Tarragon: 1 tablespoon oregano or thyme

Cook pasta according to directions. In a frying pan, heat the oil and sauté the mushrooms until soft. Add the green onion, reserving 2 tablespoon for garnish, and sauté for 2 minutes. Slowly add the milk, tarragon, and salt and pepper. Toss or serve with your favorite pasta and sprinkle with cheese. Garnish with reserved green onion.

Vegetable Pasta

Serves 4

    12 ounces pasta
     2 tablespoons olive or canola oil
     4 cloves minced garlic
     2 medium diced zucchini
     2 teaspoons oregano
         sea salt and black pepper
     ¼ cup grated goat Parmesan cheese (optional)

Garlic: 1 minced shallot or small onion
Zucchini: 2 chopped Japanese eggplant; 1 cup chopped green bell pepper; 1 cup chopped broccoli; 2 cups snow peas or chopped summer squash
Oregano: 2 teaspoons basil, marjoram, or dill
Goat Parmesan cheese: ¼ cup grated soy Parmesan cheese

Cook pasta according to directions. In a frying pan, heat the oil and sauté the garlic and zucchini until tender. Add the oregano and salt and pepper. Toss or serve with your favorite pasta and sprinkle with cheese.

Noodles and Cabbage

Serves 4

      8 cups water
      8 ounces buckwheat noodles
     ¼ cup butter or margarine
      1 cup diced yellow onion
      4 cups chopped red cabbage
      1 teaspoon caraway seed
         sea salt and black pepper

SUBSTITUTIONS

Onion: ½ cup minced shallots; 1 cup chopped white onion
Cabbage: 4 cups chopped green, Savoy, Napa, or Chinese cabbage
Buckwheat noodles: 8 ounces whole grain noodles

In a large pot, bring water to a boil with a little salt and add the noodles. Cook for 15 to 20 minutes, until soft but firm, remove from heat and drain. In a frying pan, melt the butter and sauté the onion for 3 to 5 minutes or until onion is transparent. Add the cabbage and sauté for about 6 minutes. Stir in the caraway seed and salt and pepper. Add the noodles, stir well, and serve immediately.

Spinach Lasagna

Serves 6

8	cups water
12	ounces spelt lasagna noodles
2	tablespoon olive or canola oil
1	small diced onion
3	cloves minced garlic
1	large bunch chopped spinach
2	cups Real Tomato Sauce (page 443)
2	medium thinly sliced tomatoes
4	tablespoon chopped fresh parsley
3	tablespoon chopped fresh basil
2	cups goat ricotta cheese

SUBSTITUTIONS

Spelt lasagna noodles: 12 ounces whole wheat, corn, or rice lasagna noodles

Garlic: 1 small diced onion; 3 minced shallots

Onion: 4 cloves minced garlic; 2 minced shallots

Spinach: 1 large bunch chopped chard or beet greens

Basil: 2 teaspoons oregano or marjoram

Preheat oven to 350 degrees F. In a large pot, bring water to a boil with a little salt and add the noodles. Cook for 15 to 20 minutes, until soft but firm, remove from heat and drain. In a frying pan, heat the oil and sauté the onion and garlic for 3 to 5 minutes or until onion is transparent. Add the chopped spinach and cook briefly (do not wilt). In a lightly oiled 9 x 12 baking dish, spoon ⅓ of the sauce on the bottom of the dish. Add a layer of noodles, spinach mixture, sliced tomatoes, and 1 tablespoon each of parsley, basil, and ricotta. Repeat 2 more layers. Finish with a layer of noodles. Garnish with 1 tablespoon of parsley and sliced tomatoes if desired. Bake for 45 minutes.

VARIATION

For a richer lasagna add 1 cup grated goat jack cheese. Add the cheese after the parsley and basil and put a final layer of cheese on top of the last layer of noodles.

Zucchini Tofu Lasagna

Serves 6

  1 pound tofu
  2 tablespoons lemon juice
 ½ teaspoon salt
 ¼ teaspoon nutmeg
  1 teaspoon oregano
  1 tablespoon olive or canola oil
 12 ounces corn lasagna noodles
  2 tablespoons olive or canola oil
  3 diced medium zucchini
  1 diced medium onion
  1 diced red bell pepper
 ½ tablespoon oregano
     sea salt and black pepper
 ¼ cup chopped fresh parsley
  1 cup soy mozzarella cheese
 ¾ cup soy Parmesan cheese

SUBSTITUTIONS

Onion: 2 minced shallots; 1 cup chopped green onion
Corn lasagna noodles: 12 ounces spelt, whole wheat, or rice lasagna
    noodles
Zucchini: 3 cups diced summer squash

In a blender or food processor, combine the tofu, lemon juice, salt, nutmeg, first measure of oregano, and first measure of oil. Blend until
smooth and set aside. Refrigerating for one hour before using will
improve the flavor.

Preheat oven to 350 degrees F. In a large pot, bring water to a boil
with a little salt and add the noodles. Cook for 15 to 20 minutes, until
soft but firm, remove from heat and drain. In a frying pan, heat the oil
and sauté the zucchini, onion, and bell pepper for 3 to 5 minutes or until
onion is transparent. Add the oregano and salt and pepper. Mix well. In
a lightly oiled 9 x 12 baking dish, place a layer of noodles. Spoon ⅓ of
tofu mixture, zucchini mixture, parsley, and cheeses. Repeat 2 more lay-

ers. Finish with a layer of noodles. Garnish with remaining parsley and bake for 45 minutes.

🦋 Vegetable Combinations

Eggplant Pizza

Serves 6

> 1 eggplant
> sea salt and black pepper
> ½ cup Basic Tomato Sauce (page 422)
> ½ teaspoon oregano
> ½ cup grated goat mozzarella cheese

SUBSTITUTIONS
Goat mozzarella cheese: ½ cup grated soy mozzarella or jack cheese
Oregano: ½ teaspoon marjoram or basil

Peel and slice the eggplant. Place on a paper towel or plate and sprinkle with salt. Let it sit for 20 minutes. Preheat broiler. Salt and pepper the eggplant and arrange the slices on a baking sheet or broiler pan. Spoon 1 tablespoon of tomato sauce on each slice, sprinkle with oregano, and place 1 tablespoon grated cheese on top. Cook under broiler 10 to 15 minutes or until the cheese melts and the eggplant is tender.

Grain Pizza Crust

Serves 6

> 2 cups polenta
> 1 cup cold water
> 1 cup boiling water
> ¼ teaspoon sea salt
> 2 eggs
> 1 cup grated soy cheese (optional)

SUBSTITUTIONS
Polenta: 2 cups cooked millet or quinoa
Soy cheese: 1 cup grated goat cheese

Preheat oven to 450 degrees F. In a mixing bowl, combine the polenta with the cold water. Stir in the boiling water with a fork or whisk. Beat the eggs, add with the salt and cheese, and combine thoroughly. Press the mixture evenly into a lightly oiled 10-inch pizza pan and bake for 10 to 15 minutes.

Vegetable Crust

Serves 6

¾ cup grated zucchini
½ cup minced green bell pepper
½ cup grated carrot
¼ teaspoon sea salt
2 eggs
1 cup grated soy cheese
½ teaspoon oregano

SUBSTITUTIONS
Zucchini: ¾ cup grated yellow or patty pan squash
Soy cheese: 1 cup grated goat cheese
Oregano: ½ teaspoon marjoram, thyme, or basil

Preheat oven to 375 degrees F. In a mixing bowl, combine zucchini, bell pepper, carrot, and salt. Mix well. Squeeze the vegetables in order to remove the liquid and allow to drain for 10 minutes in a colander. Beat the eggs and add with cheese and oregano to zucchini mixture. Lightly oil a 10-inch pizza pan and press the mixture into the pan. Bake for 15 minutes.

Liz and Joanna's Pizza

Serves 6

1 recipe Grain Pizza Crust (page 327)
1½ cups Basic Tomato Sauce (page 422)
1 teaspoon oregano
¾ cup grated goat mozzarella cheese
¼ cup grated goat jack cheese
¾ cup sliced mushrooms

¹⁄₃ cup chopped onion
¹⁄₂ cup chopped green bell peppers
¹⁄₄ cup sliced olives (optional)

SUBSTITUTIONS

Grain pizza crust: 1 recipe Vegetable Crust (page 328)
Goat mozzarella: ³⁄₄ cup grated soy mozzarella
Goat jack: ¹⁄₄ cup grated soy jack cheese
Green bell pepper: ¹⁄₂ cup sliced tomato; ³⁄₄ cup grated or sliced zucchini;
    ¹⁄₂ cup grated carrot; ³⁄₄ sliced Japanese eggplant
Onion: 3 cloves minced garlic; ¹⁄₂ cup chopped green onion

Preheat oven to 450 degrees F. Spread the tomato sauce on the pizza crust. Sprinkle the oregano over the sauce. Evenly spread the cheese. Top with mushrooms, onion, bell pepper, and olives. Bake for 15 minutes. Slice and serve.

Basic Quiche

Serves 6

1 baked Basic Pie Crust (page 373)
1 tablespoon butter or margarine
1¹⁄₂ cups chopped spinach
2 minced shallots
3 eggs
¹⁄₄ teaspoon nutmeg
    sea salt and black pepper
1¹⁄₂ cups goat milk
1¹⁄₂ cups grated goat cheese

SUBSTITUTIONS

Butter: 1 tablespoon olive or canola oil
Shallots: ¹⁄₂ cup chopped green onions; 2 cloves minced garlic; ¹⁄₂ chopped
    onion
Goat milk: 1¹⁄₂ cups soy milk
Goat cheese: 1¹⁄₂ cups grated soy cheese

Preheat oven at 375 degrees F. In a frying pan, melt the oil and sauté the spinach and shallots, leaving them slightly undercooked. In a mixing bowl, beat the eggs and add the spinach and shallots, nutmeg, salt and pepper, and milk. Beat well. Fold in the grated cheese, reserving 3 tablespoons. Pour the egg mixture into the baked pie shell and sprinkle with the remaining cheese. Bake for 40 to 45 minutes or until the center is firm.

VARIATIONS

Follow above recipe. Replace the spinach, shallots, and nutmeg with:

1 cup sliced zucchini, ½ cup chopped red onion, and ¼ teaspoon dry mustard.

1 cup sliced green bell peppers, ¾ cup chopped yellow onion or 2 minced shallots, and ¼ teaspoon paprika.

1½ cups sliced mushrooms, 2 cloves minced garlic, and ¼ teaspoon nutmeg.

1 cup sliced tomato, ½ cup chopped leek, and ¼ teaspoon Dijon or dry mustard and ½ teaspoon oregano.

1 cup sliced asparagus, ½ cup chopped leek, and ¼ teaspoon tarragon.

🦋 Legume Entrees

Lentil Chili

Serves 4

2	cups lentils
4	cups water
¼	teaspoon salt
1	bay leaf
2	tablespoons chili powder
1	cup chopped tomatoes
½	cup chopped onion
1	teaspoon cumin seed (optional)
	sea salt and black pepper

SUBSTITUTION

Onion: ¼ cup minced shallots

In a large pot, combine the lentils, water, salt, and bay leaf. Cook on medium heat for about 45 minutes or until lentils are tender. Remove the bay leaf. In a small bowl, mix the chili powder with 1 tablespoon of juice from the tomatoes. In a frying pan, heat 2 tablespoons of water and sauté the tomatoes, lentils, cumin, salt and pepper, and chili mixture. Heat through and serve.

Vegetarian Chili

Serves 4

2½ cups dried pinto beans
2 tablespoons olive or canola oil
1 chopped onion
4 cloves minced garlic
1 teaspoon cumin seed
3 tablespoons sweet chili powder
1 tablespoon flour
4 cups chopped tomatoes
3 bay leaves
1 teaspoon oregano
1 teaspoon sea salt

SUBSTITUTIONS
Pinto beans: 2½ cups small red, black, aduki, pink, or kidney beans
Onion: 2 chopped shallots; 4 cloves minced garlic
Garlic: 4 minced shallots; 1 chopped onion
Oregano: 1 teaspoon marjoram

Rinse and soak the beans for 6 hours or overnight. Drain, transfer to a large pot, and cover with 1-inch of water. Cook for 1½ hours, stirring occasionally, and adding more water if needed. In a frying pan, heat the oil and sauté the onion, garlic, and cumin seed in the oil. In a small bowl, combine the chili powder and flour with a little water and mix well to form a paste. Drain the beans only if they are very moist; be sure to leave some liquid. Add the onion mixture, chili mixture, tomatoes, bay leaves, oregano, and salt. Let simmer for 1 to 2 hours. Adjust the seasonings with extra chili powder, cumin, oregano, or a pinch of cayenne pepper and serve.

Curried Garbanzo Stew

Serves 4

    2   tablespoons olive or canola oil
    1   cup minced onion
    4   cloves minced garlic
    1   medium peeled, diced eggplant
    1   sliced zucchini
    2   cups sliced red cabbage
    1   cup cooked garbanzos
    2   tablespoons curry powder
    ½   teaspoon cinnamon
        sea salt and black pepper
    ⅔   cup raisins (optional)

SUBSTITUTIONS

Onion: 1½ cups chopped green onion; 6 cloves minced garlic
Garlic: ½ cup chopped green onion
Zucchini: 1 sliced summer squash
Red cabbage: 2 cups sliced green cabbage
Raisins: ⅔ cup currants

In a large pot, heat the oil and sauté the onions and garlic for 3 to 5 minutes or until onion is transparent. Add the eggplant, zucchini, cabbage, garbanzos, curry powder, and cinnamon and cook for 15 minutes. Salt and pepper to taste and serve garnished with raisins.

Mexican Casserole

Serves 4

    2½ cups kidney beans
     5 cups water
     1 tablespoons olive or canola oil
     1 medium diced onion
     1 diced green bell pepper
     1 cup cooked corn niblets
     ⅓ cup diced green chilies
     1 teaspoon cumin seed

    1 tablespoon chili powder
       sea salt and black pepper
    ½ cup grated or sliced soy cheese
    1 peeled, pitted, sliced avocado
    ¼ cup chopped fresh cilantro

SUBSTITUTIONS

Kidney beans: 2½ cups aduki, Anasazi, small red, pinto, pink, or black
    beans
Green chilies: 1 seeded, minced jalapeño
Soy cheese: ½ cup grated or sliced goat cheese

Rinse and soak the beans for 6 hours or overnight. Drain. In a large pot,
cover with 1-inch of water and simmer the beans with a little salt until
tender, about 1½ to 2 hours. Preheat oven to 350 degrees F. In a frying
pan, heat the oil and sauté the onion and bell pepper for 3 to 5 minutes
or until onion is transparent. Stir in corn, chilies, cumin, and chili powder and let cook for 5 minutes. Add to beans, salt and pepper to taste,
and mix well. Pour mixture in a 9 x 12 baking dish and top with cheese.
Bake for 45 minutes and serve garnished with sliced avocado and cilantro.

Lentil Loaf

Serves 4

    2 cups lentils
    4 cups water
    6 stalks diced celery
    ¼ teaspoon sea salt or kelp
    2 tablespoons butter or margarine
   2½ cups diced onion
    2 eggs
    ½ cup grated carrot
    1 cup rolled oats
    1 teaspoon thyme
    1 teaspoon oregano
    1 tablespoon lemon juice

SUBSTITUTIONS

Celery: ½ cup grated zucchini, jicama, or carrot

Onion: ¾ cup minced shallots; 1½ cups chopped leek; 6 cloves minced
     garlic

Eggs: 2 teaspoons Egg Replacer or binder (page 140)

Rolled oats: 1 cup wheat, rye, spelt, kamut, or barley flakes

Thyme: 1 teaspoon sage, oregano, or rosemary

In a large pot, combine the lentils, water, celery, and salt and cook on
medium heat for about 40 minutes or until lentils are tender. Drain off
any excess water. Preheat oven to 400 degrees F. In a frying pan, melt
the butter and sauté the onion for 3 to 5 minutes or until transparent.
Transfer lentils and onions to a large mixing bowl. Beat the eggs and
add with the carrot, oats, thyme, oregano, and lemon juice. Add to lentils
and mix well. In a lightly oiled loaf pan, press the mixture and bake for
1 hour. Serve either plain or with a sauce.

Nutloaf

Serves 4

     2 cups almonds
     1 medium diced onion
     3 stalks diced celery
     2 eggs
     1 cup rolled oats
     ½ teaspoon chopped fresh rosemary
     ¼ teaspoon sage
     ½ teaspoon sea salt

SUBSTITUTIONS

Almonds: 2 cups walnuts, cashews, or pecans

Celery: 1½ cups diced jicama or chard stems

Rolled oats: 1 cup wheat, rye, spelt, kamut, or barley flakes; 1 cup cooked
     brown rice

Preheat oven to 350 degrees F. Using a blender, grind the almonds to a
fine powder. In a large mixing bowl, combine the almonds, onion, celery, eggs, oats, rosemary, sage, and salt and mix well. In a lightly oiled

loaf pan, press the mixture and bake for 40 minutes. Serve with a complementary nut sauce.

VARIATION

Both the Lentil Loaf and the Nut Loaf can be used to stuff bell peppers. Take 4 bell peppers, remove the stem and seeds, then fill with mixture. Place the stuffed peppers on a lightly oiled baking sheet and bake in an oven preheated to 350 degree F for 45 minutes.

To stuff summer or winter squash, precook 4 squash on a lightly oiled baking sheet in an oven preheated to 350 degrees F for 40 minutes. Remove and let cool. Remove seeds and fill with mixture. Return to oven and bake for another 40 minutes.

CHAPTER 21

Meat, Poultry, and Fish

RED MEAT (BEEF, LAMB, PORK) should be used in moderation; two to three times a month is sufficient. The healthiest diet is still vegetarian. If you choose to eat meat, trim as much fat as possible from the meat and only purchase meat free of chemicals, steroids, and antibiotics. Some health food stores carry clean, organic meat. Three to four ounces uncooked meat is sufficient for grams of protein and amino acids. The healthiest way to cook meat is to bake, steam, or broil it. Some barbecue methods are also acceptable.

Meat Recipes

Pork Brochettes

Serves 6

1½	pounds pork cut into 2-inch cubes
2	green bell peppers cut into large pieces
½	pound mushrooms
18	boiling onions

Marinade:

2	tablespoons olive or canola oil
¼	cup red wine vinegar
1	teaspoon minced garlic
½	teaspoon cumin
¼	teaspoon red pepper flakes
½	teaspoon tarragon
	sea salt and black pepper

SUBSTITUTIONS

Pork: 1½ pounds beef, cut into 2-inch cubes

Green bell peppers: 2 cubed zucchini

Red wine vinegar: ¼ cup lemon or lime juice

Garlic: 2 teaspoons minced boiling onion

Tarragon: ½ teaspoon oregano, thyme, or rosemary

In a mixing bowl, combine the oil, vinegar, garlic, cumin, pepper flakes, tarragon, and salt and pepper and mix well. Add the pork, making sure all the pieces are covered, and let marinate overnight or at least 1 hour. Preheat the oven broiler to 500 degrees F or prepare a grill or barbecue. Drain the meat and arrange on skewers, alternating the bell peppers, mushrooms, and boiling onions with the meat. Baste with the marinade as it cooks. Cook until done.

VARIATION

Another marinade can be made by combining 1 cup pineapple juice, ¼ cup soy sauce, 4 cloves minced garlic, ½ teaspoon ginger, and black pepper. Follow above recipe.

Summer Minted Lamb

Serves 4

    1 pound cubed lamb
    1 cubed zucchini
    1 red bell pepper, cut in large pieces
   12 boiling onions
Marinade:
    1 minced garlic clove
    ¼ cup lemon juice
    2 tablespoons chopped fresh mint (2 teaspoons dried mint)
       sea salt and black pepper

SUBSTITUTIONS

Zucchini: 1 cubed summer squash or kohlrabi

Red bell pepper: 1 cup cubed turnip

Garlic: 1 chopped boiling onion

Lemon juice: ¼ lime juice or raspberry vinegar

In a mixing bowl, combine the garlic, lemon juice, mint, and salt and pepper and mix well. Add the lamb, making sure all the pieces are covered, and let marinate for 30 minutes to 2 hours. Preheat the oven broiler to 500 degrees F or prepare a grill or barbecue. Drain the meat and arrange on skewers, alternating the zucchini, bell pepper, and boiling onions with the meat. Baste frequently with marinade for 5 minutes on a side, turning a few times. Serve hot.

Greek Style Lamb

Serves 6

  2 teaspoons olive or canola oil
  2 pounds cubed lamb
      sea salt and black pepper
  1 cup chopped onion
  2 cups minced tomato
  1 large slice lemon
  1 teaspoon thyme
  1 cup water
  1 large head chopped cauliflower
  2 teaspoons grated lemon peel
  2 tablespoons chopped fresh parsley
 18 black olives (optional)

SUBSTITUTIONS
Onion: 3 minced shallots; 1 large chopped leek
Cauliflower: 1 bunch chopped broccoli, turnip greens, mustard greens, brocoflower, bok choy, or broccoli-rabe
Thyme: 1 teaspoon rosemary or oregano
Water: 1 cup vegetable broth

In a large pot, heat the oil. Season the lamb with salt and pepper and add to pot. Brown the lamb, turning several times, then remove. Add the onion, tomatoes, lemon, thyme, and water. Let simmer for a few minutes. Return meat to pot and continue cooking until the broth is reduced. Add the cauliflower, lemon peel, parsley, and olives. Steam for 10 minutes and serve.

Stir Fry

Serves 4

   2 tablespoons olive or canola oil
   1 pound beef
   2 cloves minced garlic
   4 cups asparagus
   ½ cup sunflower seeds
   1 recipe Pork Brochette Marinade (page 337) (optional)
   1 tablespoon arrowroot

SUBSTITUTIONS

Beef: 1 pound pork, lamb, chicken, turkey, shrimp, scallops, or tofu

Asparagus: 4 cups snow peas, sliced water chestnuts, chopped broccoli, chopped jicama, chopped bell peppers, chopped onion, chopped cauliflower, chopped Bok choy, string beans, peas, sliced mushrooms, mung or soy bean sprouts, sliced carrots, or sliced celery

Sunflower seeds: ½ cup pumpkin seeds, sesame seeds, cashews, almonds, or pinenuts

Marinade: 1 recipe Summer Minted Lamb Marinade (page 338); ¼ cup soy sauce and ½ teaspoon dry or grated ginger

Arrowroot: 1 tablespoon cornstarch

In a wok or large frying pan, heat the oil over high heat. When hot, add beef, garlic, and salt and pepper. Stir frequently until the beef is almost done. Add the asparagus (if using a combination of vegetables, add the longest cook-time vegetables first). Keep stirring 2 to 3 minutes. Add the sunflower seeds and cook for 1 minute. In a small bowl, combine the arrowroot and marinade. Mix well and pour over the ingredients in the wok. Stir briefly and serve.

🦋 Poultry Recipes

Poultry includes turkey, chicken, duck, goose, game hen, and duck and chicken eggs. We have provided several recipes, both basic and different. Poultry is versatile and adapts itself to interesting combinations and ethnic cooking. Also included in this section are stuffing recipes. Explore other cookbooks for additional ideas. Buy organic poultry, as other poultry can be contaminated with antibiotics, steroids, and other chemicals.

To cook turkey, chicken, or game hen, thoroughly wash the bird and remove the giblets and neck. The bird can be stored in the refrigerator for several hours or overnight, provided that it is completely covered.

Stuff the bird as desired and sew it with string or skewers. Season the outside of the bird by sprinkling generously with salt, pepper, garlic or onion powder, thyme, sage, and paprika. These are traditional herbs used for poultry. If you need to replace them, try rosemary, marjoram, oregano, dill, cayenne, tarragon, celery seed or salt, or a combination of cumin, garlic powder, salt, and pepper. To bake the bird on a rack, cover with a lid or foil, and bake in a preheated oven at 325 degrees F for turkey and 350 degrees F for chicken and game hens. Allow 20 minutes per pound for baking time. Baste the turkey once an hour with the broth and the drippings in the pan. Let the turkey sit for 20 minutes before carving. Prepare gravy from the drippings or use a thickener with the strained broth and correct the seasonings. The chopped giblets may be added to the gravy.

Giblet Broth

Makes 4 cups

> giblets and neck from bird(s)
> 1 stalk chopped celery plus leaves
> ¼ cup fresh chopped parsley
> ½ chopped onion
> ¼ teaspoon thyme
> ¼ teaspoon sage
> sea salt and black pepper
> 1 quart water

In a large pot, combine all the ingredients. Bring to a boil and then reduce heat and simmer for at least 1 hour. Use to season stuffing, baste the bird, and flavor the gravy.

Parts of the Poultry

Serves 4

> 3 pounds poultry parts (chicken wings or legs, and turkey wings)
> ¼ teaspoon sage

¼ teaspoon thyme
¼ teaspoon onion powder
¼ teaspoon paprika
   sea salt and black pepper

SUBSTITUTION
Onion powder: ¼ teaspoon garlic powder

Preheat oven to 350 degrees F (325 degrees F for turkey). Wash the poultry parts. In a small bowl, combine the sage, thyme, onion powder, paprika, and salt and pepper and mix well. Rub the seasoning mixture into the poultry. Bake for about 1 hour for the chicken and about 2½ hours for turkey wings. Any leftover poultry can be used to make a broth for soup or a casserole.

Poultry Casserole

Serves 4

2 tablespoons olive or canola oil
1 chopped onion
2 stalks diced celery
1 cup sliced mushrooms
2 cups rice
4 cups Poultry Stock (page 230)
2 cups leftover poultry
1 teaspoon thyme
½ teaspoon sage
   sea salt and black pepper

SUBSTITUTIONS
Onion: 1 cup chopped green onions or leeks; 2 minced shallots
Celery: 2 chopped carrots; ½ chopped red bell pepper
Mushrooms: 1 cup snow peas, peas, chopped broccoli, or green beans
Rice: 2 cups millet, bulgur, kasha, quinoa, or amaranth
Thyme: 1 teaspoon marjoram
Sage: ½ teaspoon rosemary

In a large frying pan, heat the oil and sauté the onion and celery for 3 to 5 minutes or until onion is transparent. Add the mushrooms and sauté for about 5 minutes. Stir in the rice and sauté briefly. Add the stock, poultry meat, thyme, sage, and salt and pepper. Bring to a boil, then reduce heat, cover, and simmer for the required length of time (40 minutes for long-grain brown rice). Serve hot.

VARIATION

Sauté the vegetables as directed above. Add 1 tablespoon flour or other thickener to 1 cup of stock, mix well, then return to remaining stock. Combine with the vegetables to make a gravy. Add the meat and serve over cooked rice, other grain, or noodles.

Herbed Turkey Legs

Serves 4

    2 turkey drumsticks
    1 large chopped onion
    2 cups apple juice
    2 teaspoons rosemary
    1 teaspoon tarragon
    1 teaspoon sage
       sea salt and black pepper

SUBSTITUTIONS

Turkey drumsticks: 4 other poultry parts
Apple juice: 2 cups pear juice
Rosemary: 2 teaspoons thyme
Tarragon: 1 teaspoon marjoram
Sage: 1 teaspoon oregano
Onion: 10 cloves minced garlic; 4 minced shallots; 1½ cups chopped
    green onion

Wash and skin the drumsticks. In a bowl, combine the onion, apple juice, rosemary, tarragon, sage, and salt and pepper. Mix well and add turkey legs, making sure the pieces are covered. Cover and refrigerate for 2 hours. Preheat oven 350 degrees F. Transfer the turkey and marinade to a baking dish. Bake for 2 hours, turning and basting at least once. Any vegetable or potato may be added for the last half hour.

Ginger Chicken
Serves 4

    4 boneless chicken breasts
    1 tablespoon olive or canola oil
    2 cloves minced garlic
    ¼ cup orange juice
  1½ cups snow peas
    ½ cup cashews
    2 teaspoons grated ginger
    ½ teaspoon cardamom
       sea salt and black pepper

SUBSTITUTIONS
Garlic: 1 minced shallot; ¼ cup chopped green onions or white onion
Orange juice: ¼ cup apricot, apple, or pineapple juice
Snow peas: 1½ cups sugar snap peas or green beans
Cashews: ½ cup almonds, walnuts, or pecans
Cardamom: ½ teaspoon cinnamon; ¼ teaspoon allspice

Wash, skin, and cut chicken breasts in half. In a frying pan, heat the oil and sauté the garlic briefly. Add the chicken and cook 4 to 5 minutes each side for small pieces, or until done. Add the orange juice, ginger, snow peas, cashews, ginger, cardamom, and salt and pepper. Stir until well blended and cook for 10 to 15 minutes. If desired, thicken the sauce with 1 tablespoon arrowroot or cornstarch.

Joanna's Chicken Curry
Serves 2

    2 boneless chicken breasts
    1 tablespoon olive or canola oil
    2 chopped green onions
    1 julienne red bell pepper
    1 teaspoon arrowroot
    1 cup rice milk
    1 tablespoon curry powder
       sea salt and black pepper

SUBSTITUTIONS

Green onion: 1 minced shallots; 2 tablespoons minced yellow onion

Arrowroot: 1 teaspoon cornstarch or flour

Rice milk: 1 cup soy or goat milk

Wash, skin, and cut chicken breasts in half. In a frying pan, heat the oil and sauté the green onion and red pepper in the oil until very tender. Add the chicken breasts, cooking for 20 minutes or until done. In a small bowl, combine the arrowroot, rice milk, and curry powder. Mix well and pour over the chicken, stirring constantly until thickened. Correct the seasoning with salt and pepper. Add more milk or arrowroot as desired.

Melissa's Tangy Chicken

Serves 3

- 3 boneless chicken breasts
- ¼ cup flour
- ½ teaspoon thyme
- ½ teaspoon sea salt
- ¼ teaspoon black pepper
- 2 tablespoons olive or canola oil
- 2 cups chopped tomatoes
- 1 cup sliced mushrooms
- ½ cup sliced green onion
- ⅓ cup apple juice
- 2 tablespoons lemon juice

SUBSTITUTIONS

Thyme: ½ teaspoon oregano, basil, or marjoram

Mushrooms: 1 cup sliced jicama or carrots

Green onion: 1 cup chopped chives; ½ cup chopped yellow onion; ½ cup minced shallots

Apple juice: ⅓ cup pear juice

Lemon juice: 2 tablespoons lime juice

Wash, skin, and cut chicken breasts in half. In a shallow dish, combine the flour, thyme, salt, and pepper and mix well. Dredge the chicken in the flour mixture. In a large frying pan, heat the oil and cook the chicken until lightly browned. Add the tomatoes, mushrooms, green onion, apple juice, and lemon juice and cook covered for 40 minutes. Serve over rice.

Mexican Chicken

Serves 4

- 4 chicken thighs
- 1 tablespoon olive or canola oil
- 1 medium minced onion
- 1 cup chopped zucchini
- 1 cup corn niblets
- 2 tablespoons chopped fresh cilantro
- 2 chopped, seeded green chilies
- 1 teaspoon cumin
- ½ cup water
     sea salt and black pepper

SUBSTITUTIONS

Onion: 1 cup chopped green onions; 4 cloves minced garlic; ½ cup minced shallots
Zucchini: 1 cup chopped jicama or summer squash; 1 cup green beans
Corn niblets: 1 cup chopped green bell pepper or carrot
Cumin: ½ teaspoon cinnamon; 1 teaspoon chili powder

Wash and skin chicken thighs. In a frying pan, heat the oil and sauté the onion for 3 to 5 minutes or until transparent. Add the chicken, zucchini, corn, cilantro, chilies, cumin, water, and salt and pepper. Cover and cook 40 minutes or until done.

Rosemary Game Hens

Serves 3

- 3 game hens
- ½ cup water
- 2 tablespoons olive or canola oil
- 5 cloves minced garlic

        juice of 1 lemon
2 tablespoons rosemary
        sea salt and black pepper

SUBSTITUTION

Garlic: ½ cup minced shallots; 1 cup chopped green onion

In a mixing bowl, combine the water, oil, garlic, lemon juice, rosemary, and salt and pepper and mix well. Add the game hens, making sure all the pieces are covered, and let marinate for 1 hour, turning often. Preheat the oven broiler to 500 degrees F or prepare a grill or barbecue. Drain the hens and place in broiler pan or on grill. Broil for 7 to 8 minutes a side and baste frequently with marinade. Serve hot.

Roast Duck

Serves 4

1 5-pound duck
1 halved lemon
1 sliced yellow onion
1 cup chopped celery leaves
    sea salt and black pepper
1½ cups pineapple juice
1 tablespoon honey

SUBSTITUTIONS

Yellow onion: 1 sliced white onion; 3 halved shallots
Pineapple juice: 1½ cups apple or apricot juice
Honey: 1 tablespoon maple syrup

Preheat oven to 325 degrees F. Wash duck and rub cavity with the lemon. Place the onion and celery leaves in the cavity. Sprinkle the duck outside with salt and pepper. Transfer to a baking pan and bake breast side down for 30 minutes. Drain the fat from the pan and pour into a bowl. Add the pineapple juice to the pan and mix well. Baste the duck with the juice and drippings every 20 minutes and continue cooking for 1½ hours. For a crisp skin, brush the duck with the honey 15 minutes before removing from the oven. Do not baste again.

Traditional Stuffing for One Large Chicken or Four Game Hens

Serves 4

- ¼ cup butter or margarine
- 1 medium chopped onion
- 2 stalks chopped celery plus leaves
- 1 cup sliced mushrooms (optional)
- 2 cups cooked millet
- ¼ cup chopped fresh parsley
- 1 teaspoon thyme
- ½ teaspoon sage
  sea salt and black pepper

SUBSTITUTIONS

Butter: ¼ cup olive or canola oil
Onion: ½ cup minced shallots; 1 cup chopped green onion
Celery: ½ cup chopped red or green bell pepper; ½ cup grated carrot
Millet: 2 cups cooked rice, quinoa, kasha, or bulgur
Parsley: ½ chopped fresh cilantro
Thyme: 1 teaspoon marjoram
Sage: ½ teaspoon rosemary

In a frying pan, melt the butter and sauté the onion and celery for 3 to 5 minutes or until onion is transparent. Add the mushrooms and sauté briefly. Add the millet, parsley, thyme, sage, and salt and pepper. Stir well and use as desired. Yields ¾ cup stuffing mix per pound of bird.

Millet (or other grain) may be cooked in Poultry Stock when used with poultry, or with Vegetable Stock for added flavor.

Sweet and Spicy Stuffing

Serves 4

- 1 tablespoon olive or canola oil
- 1 medium chopped onion
- 2 cups cooked quinoa
- 1 cup currants

juice of ½ lemon
¼ cup chopped fresh parsley
⅓ cup pinenuts
¼ teaspoon cumin
¼ teaspoon cinnamon
1 teaspoon grated lemon peel (optional)
sea salt and black pepper

SUBSTITUTIONS

Olive oil: 1 tablespoon butter or margarine
Onion: ½ cup shallots; 1 cup chopped green onion
Quinoa: 2 cups cooked amaranth, millet, rice, or kasha
Currants: 1 cup raisins
Lemon: 2 tablespoons lime, grapefruit, orange, or kumquat juice
Parsley: ¼ cup chopped fresh cilantro
Pinenuts: ⅓ cup sliced almonds, pecans, or walnuts
Cumin: ¼ teaspoon allspice
Cinnamon: ¼ teaspoon cardamom

In a frying pan, heat the oil and sauté the onion for 3 to 5 minutes or until transparent. Add the quinoa, currants, lemon juice, parsley, pinenuts, cumin, cinnamon, lemon peel, and salt and pepper. Stir well and use as desired. Yields ¾ cup stuffing mix per pound of bird.

Also excellent as a cold grain salad.

🦋 Rabbit

Rabbit Stew

Serves 4

1 rabbit
2 tablespoons olive or canola oil
1 sliced carrot
3 cloves minced garlic
1 cup Poultry Stock (page 230)
1 tablespoon lemon juice
2 bay leaves

1   teaspoon rosemary
    sea salt and black pepper
1   tablespoon flour

SUBSTITUTIONS
Olive oil: 2 tablespoons butter or margarine
Carrot: ½ cup chopped jicama or red bell pepper
Garlic: 2 minced shallots; ½ cup chopped onion; ½ cup chopped green
    onion
Poultry stock: 1 cup vegetable stock or water
Lemon juice: 1 tablespoon lime or kumquat juice
Rosemary: 1 teaspoon thyme or tarragon
Flour: 1 tablespoon arrowroot or cornstarch

Wash and salt and pepper the rabbit. In a frying pan, heat the oil and
briefly sauté the carrot and garlic. Add the rabbit and brown lightly. Add
the stock, lemon juice, bay leaves, rosemary, and salt and pepper. Cover
and simmer for 30 minutes or until the rabbit is tender. In a small bowl,
combine the flour with a little of the liquid. Add to the pot and stir until
slightly thickened. Serve hot.

🦋 Fish

Fish is enjoyed for its delicate flavor and health benefits. Unfortunately,
fish can be contaminated with heavy metals like mercury, pesticides,
antibiotics, and other chemicals. Organic fish is available. There are
many varieties of fish (deep sea and fresh water) and shellfish which can
be found in your local area. Remember, if it smells, it's not fresh. Excellent frozen varieties are available.

Basic Fish
Serves 4

1   pound halibut
¼   cup olive or canola oil
¼   cup water
    juice of 1 lemon
1   chopped green onion
1   teaspoon rosemary

    1 tablespoon chopped fresh parsley
        sea salt and black pepper

SUBSTITUTIONS

Halibut: 1 pound swordfish, salmon, cod, snapper, or orange roughy

Lemon: juice of 2 limes

Green onion: 1 tablespoon minced shallot; 1 clove minced garlic; 1 tablespoon chopped chives

Rosemary: 1 teaspoon tarragon or dill

Preheat oven to 400 degrees F. Rinse halibut. In a bowl, combine the oil, water, lemon juice, green onion, rosemary, parsley, and salt and pepper. Place halibut in a baking dish and pour the sauce over the fish and bake for 20 minutes. To steam the halibut, cover the baking dish with aluminum foil and bake for 15 minutes, depending on the thickness of the fish. To broil or barbecue, place on the grill and baste frequently. Cook for 15 minutes, or until done, turning once. If barbecued, adding soaked wood chips for smoking greatly enhances the flavor.

Summer Squash Fillets

Serves 4

    6 sole fillets
  ½ chopped onion
    2 sliced yellow squash
    1 chopped zucchini
    1 cup sliced mushrooms (optional)
  ½ teaspoon oregano
    1 cup vegetable broth
    1 tablespoon arrowroot
    1 teaspoon red pepper flakes
        sea salt and black pepper

SUBSTITUTIONS

Sole fillets: 6 flounder, perch, haddock, sea trout, or cod fillets

Onion: 3 cloves minced garlic; ½ cup chopped green onion; 1 tablespoon minced shallots

Yellow squash: 2 chopped patty squash; 1 chopped carrot

Zucchini: ½ chopped green bell pepper
Oregano: ½ teaspoon marjoram or basil
Vegetable broth: 1 cup water
Red pepper flakes: ⅛ teaspoon cayenne

Steam or bake the sole for about 10 to 15 minutes. In a wok or large frying pan, heat the oil over high heat. Add onion, yellow squash, zucchini, mushrooms, and oregano and cook until tender, stirring constantly. Reduce heat to medium. In a small bowl, combine the broth and arrowroot and mix well. Add broth mixture to the vegetables. Add the red pepper flakes and salt and pepper. Pour mixture over fish and serve.

Moroccan Flavors

Serves 4

    4 thick tuna steaks
    1 teaspoon paprika
    ½ teaspoon cumin
    ½ teaspoon turmeric
    ¼ teaspoon ground anise
    ½ teaspoon powdered ginger
    ⅛ teaspoon cardamom
    ⅛ teaspoon cayenne
       sea salt and black pepper
    2 tablespoons olive or canola oil
    1 tablespoon lemon juice
       Chopped fresh cilantro for garnish

SUBSTITUTIONS
Tuna: 4 thick salmon, shark, halibut, or swordfish steaks
Cumin: ¼ teaspoon ground anise seed
Turmeric: ½ teaspoon powdered ginger
Ginger: ½ teaspoon turmeric
Anise: ¼ teaspoon cumin
Cardamom: ⅛ teaspoon cinnamon
Cayenne: ⅛ teaspoon red pepper flakes
Lemon juice: 1 tablespoon lime juice
Cilantro: chopped fresh parsley

Rinse tuna steaks. In a small bowl, combine the paprika, cumin, turmeric, anise, powdered ginger, cardamom, cayenne, and salt and pepper and blend well. Rub the spice mixture on the fish. Sprinkle fish evenly with the lemon juice and oil. Transfer to a shallow dish and cover and marinate for at least one hour. If broiling or barbecuing, use a very hot heat about 4 inches from the broiler. Cook about 4 minutes on each side. The fish can also be pan fried in a very hot pan (no additional oil is necessary) for about 3 to 4 minutes per side. Garnish with cilantro and lemon wedges. Serve with a sweet grain dish, rice, or couscous.

Basil Tomato Fish

Serves 6

- 6 cod fillets
- ⅓ cup tomato juice
- 1 tablespoon olive or canola oil
- ⅓ cup lemon juice
- 2 tablespoons chopped fresh basil
  sea salt and black pepper
- 1 thinly sliced onion
- ¾ cup halved cherry tomatoes

SUBSTITUTIONS
Cod: 6 flounder, haddock, perch, sole, or sea trout fillets
Lemon juice: ⅓ cup lime or grapefruit juice

Preheat oven to 375 degrees F. Rinse the fillets. In a mixing bowl, combine the tomato juice, oil, lemon, basil, and salt and pepper and mix well. In a baking dish, place the fillets and pour the tomato juice on top. Top fillets with the onion slices and cherry tomatoes. Bake for 15 to 20 minutes.

Fish Kebobs

Serves 4

- 1 pound sea bass
- ¼ cup water
- 1 tablespoon olive or canola oil

    1 clove minced garlic
¼ cup lemon juice
    1 tablespoon chopped fresh parsley
    1 teaspoon ground cumin
      sea salt and black pepper
    3 small summer squash, cut in ½ inch slices
    1 large red bell pepper, cut in ¾ inch pieces

SUBSTITUTIONS

Sea bass: 1 pound halibut, swordfish, tuna, or mahi-mahi

Lemon juice: ¼ cup lime, grapefruit, or kumquat juice

Parsley: 1 tablespoon chopped fresh cilantro

Garlic: 1 chopped green onion; 1 teaspoon minced shallot; 1 tablespoon
    chopped chives; 2 teaspoons minced boiling onion

Summer squash: 1 cup sliced mushrooms; ½ head chopped cauliflower

Red bell pepper: 1 large green bell pepper, cut in ¾-inch pieces; 1 cup
    halved cherry tomatoes; 12 whole boiling onions

Rinse the sea bass and cut into 1-inch cubes. In a mixing bowl, combine
the water, oil, garlic, lemon juice, parsley, cumin, and salt and pepper.
Transfer sea bass to a shallow dish and pour marinade over the fish.
Cover the dish and let sit for 1 hour. Steam the squash and bell pepper
for 2 to 3 minutes or until tender, yet crunchy. For crisper vegetables,
do not steam them. Drain the sea bass and arrange on skewers, alternating the squash and bell pepper with the fish. Lightly oil a broiler pan
and broil under a high heat for 3 to 5 minutes per side, basting frequently
with the marinade. Or grill on the barbecue over medium-hot coals,
basting with the marinade.

Chinese Sea Scallops

Serves 4

    1 pound sea scallops
    2 tablespoons olive or canola oil
    1 teaspoon minced garlic
    2 cubed red bell peppers
    1 cup chopped zucchini
¼ teaspoon red pepper flakes

        sea salt and black pepper
    1 tablespoon lemon juice
    4 tablespoons chopped fresh basil
    1 teaspoon anise seed (optional)
    ½ teaspoon thyme
   1–2 tablespoons flour (optional)

SUBSTITUTIONS

Sea scallops: 1 pound shelled prawns
Garlic: 1 minced shallot; 1 chopped green onion
Red bell peppers: 2 large cubed carrots
Zucchini: 1 cup sliced mushrooms; 1 cup snow peas; 1 cup chopped
    celery
Basil: 4 tablespoons chopped fresh parsley or cilantro
Red pepper flakes: ⅛ teaspoon cayenne
Thyme: ½ teaspoon oregano

Rinse the scallops. In a wok or large frying pan, heat one tablespoon of
oil over medium heat and sauté the garlic, bell peppers, and zucchini.
Stir constantly and cook about 4 minutes. Add the pepper flakes, and
salt and pepper. Add another tablespoon of oil and turn the heat to high.
Add the scallops, lemon juice, basil, anise, and thyme. Correct the seasonings and stir for about 2 to 3 minutes. Make sure the scallops are
heated through, but do not overcook. Remove from heat and stir in flour
to thicken sauce, if desired.

🦋 Whole Meal Salads

Whole meal salads are easy to prepare, utilize leftovers, and are refreshing on a hot summer day. For vegetarian whole meal salad ideas, see
Colorful and Creative Salads.

Seafood Salad

Serves 4

    ½ pound shrimp
    2 chopped green onions
    2 chopped stalks celery

½ chopped, peeled cucumber
6 cups torn red leaf lettuce
2 chopped tomatoes
2 sliced hard-boiled eggs (optional)
¼ cup sliced olives (optional)
¼ cup Close-to-Thousand Island Dressing (page 411)

SUBSTITUTIONS
Shrimp: ½ pound crab, lobster, or tuna
Green onions: ½ sliced red onion; ½ chopped white onion; 1 minced
    shallot
Celery: ½ cup chopped jicama or zucchini
Cucumber: 1 chopped carrot; ½ cup sliced radishes; ½ cup snow peas
Red leaf lettuce: 6 cups romaine, green leaf, or butter lettuce or spinach
Tomatoes: 1 chopped red or green bell pepper

Rinse shrimp. In a salad bowl, combine all ingredients and mix well.
Toss with the dressing and serve.

Oriental Salad

Serves 4

½ cup sliced cooked chicken
2 chopped green onions
1 cup cooked or fresh green peas
½ cup cooked green beans
½ cup blanched broccoli
1 cup sliced water chestnuts (optional)
3 tablespoons toasted sesame seeds
¼ cup Sesame Seed Dressing (page 414)
3 cups torn romaine lettuce
4 to 8 whole leaves lettuce for serving

SUBSTITUTIONS
Chicken: ½ cup sliced cooked turkey, duck, pork, or tofu
Green peas: 1 cup cooked or fresh snow peas; 1 cup sliced green bell
    pepper
Green beans: ½ cup cooked asparagus; 1 cup sugar snap peas

Broccoli: ½ cup sliced celery or jicama
Sesame seeds: 3 tablespoons sunflower or flax seeds
Dressing: ¼ cup Chinese Pasta Salad dressing (page 268)
Romaine lettuce: 3 cups torn red leaf, green leaf, or butter lettuce

In a salad bowl, combine all the ingredients except the lettuce and mix well. Toss with the dressing. On serving plates, arrange the whole leaves. Add the torn lettuce and then the vegetables tossed with the dressing.

Mexican Salad

Serves 4

- ½ cup sliced cooked pork
- 1 medium thinly sliced onion
- 2 cups chopped tomatoes
- ½ cup corn niblets
- 1–2 seeded, minced chilies
- 2 tablespoons chopped fresh cilantro
- ¼ teaspoon cumin
- ½ cup black olives (optional)
  sea salt and black pepper
- 4 corn tortilla shells
- 2 cups shredded lettuce
- 1 peeled, pitted, sliced avocado

Dressing:
- 2 tablespoons olive or canola oil
- 2 tablespoons lime juice
- ½ teaspoon cumin

SUBSTITUTIONS
Pork: ½ cup sliced cooked beef or chicken
Onion: 1 cup chopped green onion
Tomatoes: 2 cups chopped red bell pepper
Corn niblets: ½ cup chopped jicama
Lettuce: 2 cups shredded cabbage or spinach
Cilantro: 2 tablespoons chopped fresh parsley
Lime juice: 2 tablespoons lemon juice

In a small bowl, combine the oil, lime juice, and cumin, mix well and set aside. In a large bowl, combine the pork, onion, tomatoes, corn, chilies, cilantro, cumin, olives, and salt and pepper. Add dressing and mix well. In each tortilla shell, place ¼ cup shredded lettuce. Evenly divide the pork mixture, place on top of lettuce, garnish with avocado slices and serve.

CHAPTER 22

Desserts

DID YOU EAT ALL of your dinner? Now it's time for dessert! Known sugar addicts have tried the following desserts and not been disappointed. Desserts can be delicious, rich in flavor, and satisfy your sweet tooth without the use of sugar. Many of these recipes use safe sweeteners in a quantity that is not appropriate for those with Candida or severe blood sugar problems. Later on, when these issues are under control, these desserts will be a wonderful addition to your diet. Some recipes use a minimum amount of safe sweetener, others use none. One of the ingredients that help to make desserts taste good and have a rich flavor, is butter or fat. Some recipes will use a standard amount of butter or fat and others will not use any, making them fat free. To convert a recipe to fat free, substitute 1 cup of pureed banana, prune, apple, pear, or peach for 1 cup of fat. We have indicated on which recipes this substitution will work.

Just because a different sweetener is added and whole grains and other wholesome ingredients are used does not mean that the desserts are any lower in calories than their white flour and white sugar cousins. Desserts are meant to be treats. Used in moderation they are a delightful enrichment to life. As with other chapters and recipes, we have incorporated traditional favorites with healthy substitutes. We are also including some new and interesting taste treats. See pages 133–138 for more information on the use of sweeteners.

Some recipes will contain old-fashioned whipping cream. When cream is taken from cow's milk, it will produce two different products. If it is cold and whipped it becomes whipped cream, and if it is warm and churned it becomes butter. Often those with dairy allergies do not react to the butter, making the cream also acceptable. If you can use cream, check the labels because dextrose and chemicals are often added to whipping cream.

🦋 Cookies

Oatmeal Cookies

Makes 3 dozen cookies

⅔ cup oat flour
⅓ cup oat bran
½ teaspoon baking soda
½ teaspoon sea salt
⅔ cup butter or margarine
1½ cups date sugar
1 egg
1 teaspoon vanilla extract
¼ cup water
3 cups oatmeal
1 cup chopped walnuts
1 cup raisins (optional)

SUBSTITUTIONS
Date sugar: 1½ cup grape/rice granular concentrate; ¼ cup vegetable glycerin
Vanilla extract: 2 teaspoons vanilla liquid (page 205)
Walnuts: 1 cup chopped pecans or almonds
Raisins: 1 cup currants or dates

Preheat oven to 350 degrees F and grease the cookie sheets. In a mixing bowl, combine the oat flour, oat bran, baking soda, and salt and sift together 2 to 3 times. In another bowl, cream the butter and date sugar until light and fluffy. Add the egg and vanilla extract, mixing well. Blend in the flour mixture and water. Stir in the oats and nuts and raisins. Drop by teaspoon on the cookie sheet and bake for 12 to 15 minutes.

Nut Butter Cookies

Makes 3 dozen cookies

   1¾ cup whole wheat pastry flour
   ¾ teaspoon baking soda
   ½ teaspoon baking powder
   ⅛ teaspoon sea salt
   ½ cup butter or margarine
   ½ cup honey
   1 tablespoon blackstrap molasses (omit if not using honey)
   ½ cup almond butter
   ½ teaspoon vanilla extract

SUBSTITUTIONS

Whole wheat pastry flour: 1¾ cup spelt or brown rice flour; 1½ cups oat flour and ¼ cup oat bran
Honey: ½ cup rice syrup or grape or apple juice concentrate
Almond butter: ¼ cup hazelnut, pistachio, or peanut butter
Vanilla extract: 1 teaspoon vanilla liquid (page 205)

Preheat the oven to 375 degrees F and grease the cookie sheets. In a mixing bowl, combine the flour, baking soda, baking powder, and salt and sift together 2 to 3 times. In another bowl, cream the butter, honey, and molasses until light and fluffy. Add the almond butter and vanilla extract. Blend in the flour mixture and mix well. Drop by teaspoon on the cookie sheet. Press cookies with a floured fork to make a criss-cross pattern and bake for 10 to 12 minutes.

Carob Chip Honey Cookies

Makes 3 dozen cookies

   1¼ cups whole wheat pastry flour
   ½ teaspoon baking soda
   ¾ teaspoon sea salt
   ⅓ cup butter or margarine
   ½ cup honey
   1 tablespoon blackstrap molasses (omit if not using honey)
   1 egg

1 teaspoon vanilla extract
¾ cup carob chips
1 cup chopped walnuts

SUBSTITUTIONS

Whole wheat pastry flour: 1¼ cups spelt or brown rice flour; 1 cup oat
    and ¼ cup oat bran
Honey: ½ cup barley malt or apple or grape juice concentrate; ¾ cup
    date sugar
Egg: 1 teaspoon Egg Replacer or binder (page 140)
Vanilla extract: 2 teaspoons vanilla liquid (page 205)
Walnuts: 1 cup chopped pecans or hazelnuts

Preheat the oven to 375 degrees F and grease the cookie sheets. In a mixing bowl, combine the flour, baking soda, and salt and sift together 2 to
3 times. In another bowl, cream the butter, honey, and molasses until
light and fluffy. Add the egg and vanilla extract. Blend in the flour mixture and mix well. Stir in the carob chips and nuts. Drop by teaspoon
on the cookie sheet and bake for 12 minutes.

Traditional Chocolate/Carob Chip Cookies

Makes 4 dozen cookies

2¼ cups whole wheat pastry flour
1 teaspoon baking soda
½ teaspoon sea salt
1 cup butter or margarine
1¼ cups date sugar
1 teaspoon vanilla extract
2 eggs
1 cup carob chips
1 cup chopped pecans (optional)

SUBSTITUTIONS

Whole wheat pastry flour: 2¼ cups spelt, or brown rice flour, or 2 cups
    oat and ¼ cup oat bran
Date sugar: 1½ cups grape/rice granular concentrate
Vanilla extract: 2 teaspoons vanilla liquid (page 205)

Eggs: 2 teaspoons Egg Replacer or binder (page 140)
Carob chips: 1 cup chocolate chips (health food store variety or Baker's Semi-Sweet)
Pecan: 1 cup chopped walnuts, hazelnuts, or almonds

Preheat oven to 375 degrees F. In a mixing bowl, combine flour, baking soda, and salt and sift together 2 to 3 times. In another bowl, cream butter, sugar, vanilla extract, and eggs until light and fluffy. Blend in the flour mixture and mix well. Stir in the chips and nuts. Drop by teaspoon on the cookie sheet and bake for about 10 to 12 minutes.

Be sure to read the labels for any chocolate or carob chips. Baker's chips are recommended because they have no chocolate liqueur in the ingredients (but they do include sugar). Check out the health food store variety.

Ginger Snaps

Makes 4 dozen cookies

    2 cups whole wheat pastry flour
    2 teaspoons baking soda
    1 teaspoon powdered ginger
    1 teaspoon cinnamon
    1 teaspoon cloves
    ¼ teaspoon sea salt
    ¾ cup butter or margarine
    1 cup date sugar
    ¼ cup blackstrap molasses
    1 egg

SUBSTITUTIONS

Whole wheat pastry flour: 2 cups spelt or brown rice flour; 1¾ cups oat and ¼ cup oat bran
Cinnamon: 1 teaspoon cardamom
Date sugar: 1 cup grape/rice granular concentrate

In a mixing bowl, combine the flour, baking soda, powdered ginger, cinnamon, cloves, and salt and sift together 2 to 3 times. In another bowl, cream the butter, sugar, and molasses until fluffy. Add the egg and mix well. Blend in the flour mixture and mix well. Refrigerate for 1 hour or until chilled. Preheat the oven to 350 degrees F and grease cookie sheets. Shape into 1-inch balls and roll in date sugar. Place on cookie sheet 2 inches apart and bake for 12 to 15 minutes.

Gingerbread Persons

Makes 16 cookies

2¾ cups whole wheat pastry flour
3 teaspoons baking powder
¼ teaspoon baking soda
1 teaspoon cloves
1 teaspoon powdered ginger
1 tablespoon cinnamon
¼ teaspoon allspice
½ cup butter or margarine
½ cup honey
⅔ cup blackstrap molasses
1 egg

SUBSTITUTIONS
Whole wheat pastry flour: 2¾ cups spelt or brown rice flour
Honey: ½ cup barley malt

Preheat oven to 350 degrees F and grease the cookie sheets. In a mixing bowl, combine the flour, baking powder, baking soda, cloves, powdered ginger, cinnamon, and allspice and sift together 2 to 3 times. In another bowl, cream the butter, honey, and molasses until light and fluffy. Add the egg and mix well. Blend in the flour mixture and mix the dough (using the hands if necessary) until all the flour has been worked in. Divide the dough into small, workable amounts and roll out on a floured board until ¼ to ⅓ inch thick. Use a floured cookie cutter to cut the cookies. Transfer the cookies to greased sheets. Use pieces of raisins, fruit, or nuts to make the face. Bake the gingerbread for about 12 minutes or until lightly browned.

Apricot Bars

Makes 2 dozen bars

   1 cup oat flour
   ½ teaspoon cinnamon
   ½ cup oat bran
 1½ cups oatmeal flakes
   ¾ cup butter or margarine
   ½ cup chopped pecans

Filling:
 1¼ cups apricots
 1¾ cups water
   ½ teaspoon cinnamon
   1 teaspoon lemon juice
      grated peel of 1 lemon
   ¾ cups chopped pecans
   ¼ teaspoon sea salt

SUBSTITUTIONS

Oat flour: 1½ cups barley, whole wheat pastry, or spelt flour
Cinnamon: ½ teaspoon cardamom
Oatmeal: 1½ cups barley, spelt, or wheat flakes
Pecans: ½ cup chopped walnuts or hazelnuts
Apricots: 1¼ cups figs or dates
Cinnamon: ½ teaspoon cardamom
Pecans: ¾ cups chopped walnuts or hazelnuts

Preheat the oven to 375 degrees F and grease a 9 x 9 baking pan. In a saucepan, combine apricots and water and bring to a boil. Reduce heat to medium and cook until tender. Mash the apricots and stir until the mixture thickens. Add the cinnamon, lemon juice, lemon peel, pecans, and salt and mix well. Set aside. In a mixing bowl, combine the flour and cinnamon and sift together 2 to 3 times. Add the oat bran and oatmeal and the mix well. Work the butter and pecans into the flour mixture until crumbly. Press one-half the flour mixture into the bottom of the pan. Spread the apricot mixture on top and then place the remaining flour mixture on top of the apricots. Press down and bake for about 25 minutes or until lightly brown. Cut into pieces.

Fat Free Carob Brownies

Makes 16 brownies

    1½ cups whole wheat pastry
     1 cup roasted carob powder
     ¼ teaspoon sea salt
     ¾ cups date sugar
     2 cups sugarless applesauce
     1 teaspoon vanilla extract
    1½ cups chopped walnuts

SUBSTITUTIONS

Whole wheat pastry: 1½ cups spelt or brown rice flour; 1¼ cups oat
    flour and ¼ cup oat bran
Date sugar: ½ cup honey and 1 tablespoon blackstrap molasses; ¾ cup
    apple juice concentrate; ¾ cup barley malt
Vanilla extract: 2 teaspoons vanilla liquid (page 205)
Walnuts: 1½ cups chopped almonds, pecans, or hazelnuts

Preheat the oven to 350 degrees and grease a 9 x 9 baking dish. In a mixing bowl, combine the flour, carob, salt and sift together 2 to 3 times. In
another bowl, combine the date sugar, applesauce, and vanilla extract,
mix well, then add to flour mixture. Add the nuts and blend well. Place
the mixture in the pan and bake for 45 minutes.

Fat Free Apple Crisp

Makes 1 crisp

     4 peeled, sliced sweet apples
     1 cup oatmeal
     1 tablespoon oat flour (or matching flour)
     1 teaspoon cinnamon
     ¼ teaspoon nutmeg (optional)
     ¼ to ½ cup apple juice or puree
     1 tablespoon honey and 1 drop of blackstrap molasses (optional)
     ½ cup chopped walnuts

Apples: 4 peeled, pitted, sliced peaches, nectarines, pears; 10 to 15 peeled,
    pitted, sliced apricots
Oatmeal: 1 cup barley, spelt, kamut, or wheat flakes
Cinnamon: 1 teaspoon cardamom
Apple juice: ¼ to ½ cup peach, nectarine, pear, or apricot juice or puree
    (match to fruit)
Honey: 1 tablespoon barley malt or rice syrup; 2 tablespoons date sugar
Walnuts: ½ cup chopped almonds, pecans, or hazelnuts

Preheat the oven to 350 degrees. Grease a 9 x 9 square or 9-inch round
pan and arrange the apple slices. Sprinkle with a little cinnamon and a
dash of nutmeg. In a mixing bowl, combine the oatmeal, flour, cinnamon, nutmeg, apple juice, honey, and walnuts and spoon on top of the
apples. Bake for 40 minutes, 20 minutes for softer fruits. Cover it after
it has browned and continue baking.

🦋 Candy Treats

Carob Nut Bars

Makes 2 dozen bars

    ⅔ cup peanut butter
    ⅔ cup honey
    ⅔ cup sifted roasted carob powder
    ⅓ cup peanuts
    ¾ cup carob chips

SUBSTITUTIONS
Peanut butter: ⅔ cup almond, hazelnut, or pistachio butter
Honey: ⅔ cup rice syrup or maple syrup

Grease a 8 x 8 pan. In a saucepan, heat the peanut butter and honey
together. Add the carob powder, peanuts, and carob chips and mix well.
Press into pan and refrigerate for 2 hours or until chilled. Slice and serve.

Natural Candy

Makes 5 dozen balls

- 1 cup peanut butter
- ¼ cup sifted roasted carob powder
- ¼ cup mashed banana
- 2 teaspoons vanilla extract
- 1 teaspoon cinnamon

SUBSTITUTION
Peanut butter: 1 cup almond, cashew, hazelnut, or pistachio butter
Vanilla extract: 4 teaspoons vanilla liquid (page 205)

In a mixing bowl, combine the peanut butter, carob powder, banana, and vanilla extract and mix well. Shape into balls, and roll in cinnamon. If desired, press nuts (matching the nut butter) on top. Refrigerate for 2 hours or until chilled.

🦋 Puddings and Mousse

Blueberry Pudding

Serves 4

- 2½ cups blueberries
- 4 cups water
- ½ cup oat flour
- 1 cup grape juice concentrate
- 1 teaspoon lemon juice

SUBSTITUTIONS
Blueberries: 2½ cups huckleberries
Oat flour: ½ cup brown rice, whole wheat pastry, spelt, or millet flour
Grape juice concentrate: 1 cup apple juice concentrate, grape/rice granular concentrate, or rice syrup; ¼ vegetable glycerin

In a saucepan, combine the blueberries and the water. Bring to a boil, then reduce heat to simmer for 15 minutes. Drain the juice and set aside. In a mixing bowl, add the berries and mash them. Add the flour and mix well. In another bowl, combine the berry water, grape juice concentrate, and lemon juice. Blend berry water mixture into the flour mixture and mix well. If lumps become a problem, add a bit more water and continue to stir. Place mixture in sauce and bring to a simmer, stirring constantly until thick. Add more grape juice concentrate to taste. Let cool and serve garnished with whole berries.

Apple and Sweet Potato Pudding

Serves 4

- 1 baked sweet potato
- 1 cup sliced apple
- 1 tablespoon raisins (optional)
- ½ cup orange juice
- 2 teaspoons grape juice concentrate
- ½ cup crushed crackers

SUBSTITUTIONS
Sweet potato: 1 baked yam, squash, or small pumpkin
Apple: 1 sliced pear; 1 cup crushed pineapple
Raisin: 1 tablespoon currants
Orange juice: ½ cup tangerine, pineapple, apple, or pear juice
Grape juice concentrate: 2 teaspoons maple syrup, rice syrup, or honey
Crushed crackers: ½ cup crushed cookies or rice cakes

Preheat the oven at 350 degrees F and grease 9-inch baking dish. Arrange the cooked potato and sliced apples. Sprinkle with the raisins, orange juice, apple juice concentrate, and crushed crackers. Bake for 30 minutes.

Rice Pudding

Serves 4

- 2 cups cooked brown rice
- 1½ cups rice milk
- 1 cup raisins
- 4 teaspoons rice syrup
- 1 teaspoon cinnamon
- 1 teaspoon vanilla extract (optional)

Raisins: 1 cup apple, apricots, or currants
Rice syrup: 4 teaspoons barley malt; 2 teaspoons honey
Cinnamon: 1 teaspoon cardamom; ½ teaspoon nutmeg
Vanilla: 2 teaspoons vanilla liquid (page 205)

In a saucepan, combine all the ingredients and mix well. Cook on medium heat until the ingredients are warm and blended well. Serve with chopped nuts sprinkled on top.

Corn Pudding

Serves 4

- ⅔ cup cornmeal
- 5 cups goat milk
- ½ cup grape juice concentrate
- ¼ cup blackstrap molasses
- ½ teaspoon powdered ginger
- 1 teaspoon cinnamon
- 2 eggs
- ½ cup chopped nuts (optional)

SUBSTITUTIONS
Goat milk: 5 cups nut, soy, or rice milk
Grape juice concentrate: ½ cup rice syrup; ¼ cup honey; ⅓ cup maple syrup
Molasses: ¼ cup sorghum or barley malt
Cinnamon: 1 teaspoon cardamom
Eggs: 2 teaspoons Egg Replacer or binder (page 140)
Nuts: ½ cup raisins or currants

Preheat the oven to 350 degrees F. In a mixing bowl, combine the cornmeal with one cup of the milk and stir until smooth. Add the grape juice concentrate, molasses, powdered ginger, and cinnamon and mix well. Beat the eggs and add to the cornmeal mixture. Add the nuts and mix well. Pour cornmeal mixture into a 9 x 12 baking pan. Pour the remaining milk over the cornmeal and bake for 45 minutes.

Old-Fashioned Pudding

Serves 4

    2 cups nut milk
    ½ cup rice syrup
    3 tablespoons arrowroot
    1 teaspoon vanilla extract

SUBSTITUTIONS

Nut milk: 2 cups goat or soy milk
Rice syrup: ½ cup apple or grape juice concentrate, maple syrup; ½ cup
    grape/rice granular concentrate; 2 tablespoons vegetable glycerin
Arrowroot: 3 tablespoons agar flakes or cornstarch
Vanilla extract: 2 teaspoons vanilla liquid (page 205)

In a saucepan, combine the milk, rice syrup, and arrowroot and cook
on medium heat, stirring constantly until thickened. Remove from the
heat, stir in the vanilla extract and refrigerate for 2 hours or until chilled.

VARIATIONS

Lemon Pudding
Follow above recipe. Omit the vanilla extract and add 2 tablespoons
lemon juice and 1 teaspoon grated lemon rind when you add the rice
syrup.
Carob Pudding
    Follow above recipe. Add ¼ cup sifted, roasted carob powder to the
nut milk, mixing well, along with either ½ cup date sugar, ¼ cup honey
and 2 teaspoon blackstrap molasses, or ½ cup barley malt.
Chocolate Pudding
    Follow above recipe. Melt one square of pure baking chocolate in ½
cup of the milk, then proceed as directed.

Ginger Pumpkin Mousse

Serves 4

    1 package unflavored gelatin
    ¼ cup water
    ¾ cup pureed pumpkin

⅓ cup honey
 1 tablespoon blackstrap molasses (omit if not using honey)
¼ teaspoon powdered ginger
¼ teaspoon cinnamon
¼ teaspoon nutmeg
¼ teaspoon sea salt
½ cup almond milk
 1 egg yolk
 3 egg whites
¼ teaspoon cream of tartar
⅓ cup chopped toasted almonds

SUBSTITUTIONS
Unflavored gelatin: 3 tablespoons agar flakes or arrowroot
Pumpkin: ¾ cup pureed squash, sweet potato, or yam
Honey: ½ cup date sugar, barley malt; ⅓ cup maple syrup
Cinnamon: ¼ teaspoon cardamom
Nutmeg: ¼ teaspoon allspice
Egg: ¼ cup Egg Replacer or binder (page 140)
Almonds: ⅓ cup chopped, toasted hazelnuts

In a saucepan, sprinkle gelatin over the water to soften. Cook over medium heat, stirring constantly until the gelatin dissolves. (If using the another thickener, stir into the water and blend well.) Stir in the pumpkin, honey, molasses, powdered ginger, cinnamon, nutmeg, salt, spices, nut milk and the egg yolk. Increase heat just to boiling, stirring constantly. Refrigerate until the mixture mounds slightly when dropped from a spoon. In a mixing bowl, beat the egg whites and cream of tartar in a bowl until stiff. Fold the egg whites gently into the pumpkin mixture. Divide into dessert dishes, top with the nuts and refrigerate for about 3 hours or until chilled.

🦋 Pie Crusts and Pies

Basic Pie Crust

Makes 2 crusts

- 2 cups whole wheat pastry flour
- ⅔ cup butter or margarine
- 7 tablespoons cold water
- ¼ teaspoon sea salt
- ¼ teaspoon cinnamon (optional)

SUBSTITUTION

Whole wheat pastry flour: 2 cups spelt, barley, oat, rice, or millet flour

Preheat oven to 450 degrees F. In a mixing bowl, combine the flour and salt and sift together 2 to 3 times. Cut in butter with the hands until the mixture is like oatmeal, not sticky. Add the cold water with a fork. Add more water if necessary. The mixture should clear the sides of the bowl and stick together. Do not knead or over mix. Wrap in waxed paper and refrigerate for at least ½ hour. Lightly flour both the rolling pin and the rolling surfaces, and roll out dough. Line pie plates with dough and crimp edges. To prebake crust, prick the shell with a fork and bake for 10 to 12 minutes or until lightly browned.

Nut Pie Crust

Makes 1 crust

- ¼ cup butter or margarine
- 1 cup chopped walnuts
- ½ teaspoon cinnamon (optional)

SUBSTITUTION

Walnuts: 1 cup chopped almonds, pecans, or hazelnuts

Preheat oven to 350 degrees F. In a saucepan, melt the butter and remove from heat. Transfer butter to a mixing bowl and add walnuts and cinnamon. Mix well and spoon into an 8-inch pie dish, pressing the mixture into the bottom and sides of the dish. To prebake crust, bake for 10 minutes. Crust can also be filled, then baked.

VARIATION
Follow recipe above. Add 2 tablespoons coconut to nuts. Proceed as directed.

Cookie Pie Crust

Makes 1 crust

   2½ tablespoons butter or margarine
   1½ cups crushed lemon cookies

SUBSTITUTION
Lemon cookies: 1½ cups crushed ginger cookies

Preheat oven to 350 degrees F. In a saucepan, melt the butter and remove from heat. Transfer butter to a mixing bowl and add crushed cookies. Mix well and spoon into an 8-inch pie dish, pressing the mixture into the bottom and sides of the dish. To prebake crust, bake for 10 minutes. Crust can also be filled, then baked.

Pumpkin Pie

Makes 1 pie

   2 cups cooked, pureed pumpkin
   1⅔ cups goat milk
   ¼ cup honey
   1 tablespoon blackstrap molasses (omit if not using honey)
   2 eggs
   1 teaspoon cinnamon
   ½ teaspoon powdered ginger
   ¼ teaspoon cloves
   ¼ teaspoon sea salt
   1 9-inch unbaked Basic Pie Crust (page 373)

SUBSTITUTIONS
Pumpkin: 2 cups cooked, pureed squash, sweet potato, or yam
Goat milk: 1⅔ cups nut, rice, or soy milk
Honey: ½ cup date sugar or rice syrup; 1 tablespoon vegetable glycerin; or ⅓ cup maple syrup
Eggs: 2 teaspoons Egg Replacer or binder (page 140)
Cinnamon: 1 teaspoon cardamom

Preheat the oven to 450 degrees F. In a mixing bowl, combine the pumpkin, goat milk, honey, and molasses. Lightly beat the eggs and add with the cinnamon, powdered ginger, cloves, and salt. Mix well and pour into pie shell. Bake for 40 minutes.

Apricot Pie

Makes 1 pie

- 1 recipe Basic Pie Crust (page 373)
- 4 cups peeled, pitted, sliced apricots
- 1 teaspoon nutmeg
- ¼ cup honey
- 2 tablespoons flour (same as used for crust)
- 2 tablespoons butter or margarine

SUBSTITUTIONS

Apricots: 4 cups peeled, pitted, sliced peaches or nectarines
Nutmeg: 1 teaspoon powdered ginger or cinnamon
Honey: ⅓ cup rice syrup or grape or apple juice concentrate; 1 tablespoon vegetable glycerin

Preheat oven to 425 degrees F. Roll out ½ of the dough to fit the pie dish. Fill with the apricots. Sprinkle lightly with the nutmeg. Evenly spread the honey. Sprinkle a light layer of flour over the top. Dot with the butter. Roll out the rest of the pastry and cover with either a full or a lattice work top for the pie. Crimp the edges. Bake for 15 minutes, then reduce heat to 375 degrees for 30 minutes or until lightly browned. With apricot use nutmeg; with peaches or nectarines, use cinnamon or ginger.

Apple Pie

Makes 1 pie

- 1 recipe Basic Pie Crust (page 373)
- 6 peeled, cored, sliced green apples
- 1 teaspoon cinnamon
- ½ teaspoon nutmeg
- ½ cup raisins (optional)
- 4 tablespoons flour (same as used for crust)
- ⅓ cup honey

2 tablespoons blackstrap molasses (omit if not using honey)
3 tablespoons butter or margarine

SUBSTITUTIONS
Raisins: ½ cup currants or dates
Honey: ¾ cup apple juice concentrate or date sugar

Preheat oven to 350 degrees F. Roll out ½ of the pie dough. Put a layer of sliced apples in the bottom of the dish. Sprinkle generously with the cinnamon and lightly with the nutmeg. Add ½ of the raisins. Dust lightly with the flour. Evenly spread the honey and molasses over it and dot with about ½ of the butter. Prepare another layer the same way. It should mound nicely. Roll out the rest of the pastry and cover with either a full or a lattice work top for the pie. Sprinkle lightly with cinnamon and nutmeg. Bake for 15 minutes and then reduce heat to 375 degrees for 30 minutes or until lightly browned.

Berry Pie

Makes 1 pie

1 recipe Basic Pie Crust (page 373)
4 cups blueberries
¾ cup grape juice concentrate
1 teaspoon lemon juice
3 tablespoons cornstarch
3 tablespoons butter or margarine (optional)

SUBSTITUTIONS
Blueberries: 4 cups blackberries, boysenberries, raspberries, or huckleberries
Grape juice concentrate: ¾ cup apple juice concentrate, rice syrup, or
  grape/rice granular concentrate
Cornstarch: 3 tablespoons arrowroot; 4 tablespoons flour (same as used
  for crust)

Preheat oven to 425 degrees F. Roll out ½ of the dough to fit the pie dish. In a mixing bowl, combine the blueberries, grape juice concentrate, lemon juice, and cornstarch and mix well. Fill the crust with the berry mixture. Dot with the butter. Roll out the rest of the pastry and cover with either a full or a lattice work top for the pie. Crimp the edges. Bake for 10 minutes, then reduce heat to 350 degrees for 25 to 30 minutes or until lightly browned.

VARIATION

Cherry Pie

Follow above recipe. Replace the berries with 4 cups pitted cherries. Omit the lemon juice and add ½ teaspoon almond extract or 1 teaspoon almond liquid (page 206). Bake as directed.

Lemon Meringue Pie

Makes 1 pie

- 1 unbaked Basic Pie Crust (page 373)
- 3 large eggs
- 1¼ cups sifted grape/rice granular concentrate
- 4 tablespoons arrowroot
- 1½ cups water
- ¼ cup lemon juice
   grated peel of 2 lemons
- 1 tablespoon butter or margarine (optional)

SUBSTITUTIONS

Grape/rice granular concentrate: 3 tablespoons vegetable glycerin for filling and 1 tablespoon for meringue
Arrowroot: 4 tablespoons cornstarch
Lemon juice: ¼ cup lime juice
Grated lemon peel: grated peel of 4 limes

Preheat oven to 450 degrees F. Weigh down pie shell with beans and bake for 15 minutes. Remove pie crust and lower heat to 350 degrees F. Separate the eggs. In a saucepan, heat the water. Gradually stir in 1 cup of the grape/rice granular concentrate (if using the glycerin, add it after you have removed saucepan from the heat) and the arrowroot in the water and blend until smooth. If the granular does not fully dissolve, raise the heat and continue stirring. Add the egg yolks and blend well. Stirring constantly, bring to a boil for 1 minute. Remove from heat and stir in the lemon juice, lemon rind, and butter. Set aside and let cool.

Turn into the pie shell. In another bowl, whip the egg whites until foamy. Gradually beat in the remaining ¼ cup of the sifted sweetener (use only the fine granular). Continue beating until stiff peaks are formed. Spread the meringue, starting from the outside edge, filling in the center. Bake for 15 minutes, until lightly browned.

Tart Shell

Makes 1 large tart shell or 3 small tart shells

- 1⅓ cups whole wheat pastry flour
- ¼ teaspoon cinnamon (optional)
- ¼ teaspoon sea salt
- ⅓ cup canola or safflower oil
- 2 tablespoons ice water
- 2 teaspoons grape juice concentrate (minus equal water)

SUBSTITUTIONS
Whole wheat pastry flour: 1⅓ cups spelt, rice, or oat flour
Grape juice concentrate: 2 teaspoons rice syrup

Preheat oven to 375 degrees F. In a mixing bowl, combine the flour, cinnamon, and salt and sift together 2 to 3 times. Add oil, water, and grape juice concentrate (for a sweet crust). Mix until barely blended and forms a ball. It should not be sticky and do not overmix. Let rest for 30 minutes. Flour the working surface and roll dough with a rolling pin. Roll out the dough to fit the pie dish and crimp edges. To cook the shell, bake for 15 minutes. Fill baked tart shell with pudding filling (lemon custard from the Lemon Meringue Pie recipe) and layer with fresh kiwi, raspberries, strawberries, or nuts.

Apple Tart

Makes 1 pie

- 1 baked Tart Shell or 3 small Tart Shells (page 378)
- ¼ cup apple sauce (enough to cover bottom of tart shell)
- 3 large sweet apples
- ½ teaspoon cinnamon
- ¼ teaspoon nutmeg
- 2 tablespoons sugarless apricot jam

Preheat oven to 375 degrees F. Cover the bottom of the tart shell with apple sauce. Sprinkle lightly with cinnamon and nutmeg. Arrange the sliced apple in a pattern. Sprinkle again with cinnamon and nutmeg. Bake for 20 minutes for small tarts and 40 minutes for pie. Remove from oven. In a saucepan or microwave oven, melt the apricot jam and pour over the tart to glaze.

Boysenberry Tart

Makes 1 pie

- 1 unbaked Tart Shell or 3 small Tart Shells (page 378)
- ⅓ cup sugarless boysenberry jam
- ¾ cup boysenberries
- 2 tablespoons grape juice concentrate
- 1 teaspoon flour (same as used for crust)

SUBSTITUTIONS
Boysenberries: ¾ cup blackberries
Grape juice concentrate: 2 tablespoons apple juice concentrate or grape/rice granular concentrate; 1 teaspoon vegetable glycerin

Preheat oven to 375 degrees F. In a saucepan, melt jam and combine with boysenberries, grape juice concentrate, and flour and mix well. Pour into tart shell and bake for 15 minutes for small tarts and 30 minutes for pie.

Pear Tart

Makes 1 pie

- 1 unbaked Tart Shell or 3 small Tart Shells (page 378)
- 3 sliced pears
- 2 tablespoons chopped walnuts
- ⅓ cup sugarless red raspberry jam

Preheat oven to 375 degrees F. In the tart shell, arrange sliced pears and sprinkle with walnuts. In a saucepan or microwave oven, melt jam and pour over the pears and walnuts. Bake for 15 to 20 minutes for small tarts and 30 minutes for pie.

Pumpkin Tart

Makes 1 pie

　　1　unbaked Tart Shell or 3 small Tart Shells (page 378)
　　1　cup cooked, pureed pumpkin
　　¾　cup rice milk
　　⅓　cup rice syrup
　　1　egg
　　½　teaspoon cinnamon
　　¼　teaspoon powdered ginger
　　⅛　teaspoon cloves
　　¼　teaspoon sea salt

SUBSTITUTIONS

Pumpkin: 1 cup cooked, pureed squash, sweet potato, or yam
Rice milk: ¾ cup goat, soy, or nut milk
Rice syrup: ¼ cup honey and 1 teaspoon blackstrap molasses; ⅓ cup
　　barley malt or maple syrup
Cinnamon: ½ teaspoon cardamom

Preheat oven to 400 degrees F. In a mixing bowl, combine the pumpkin, rice milk, rice syrup, egg, cinnamon, powdered ginger, cloves, and
salt and mix well. Pour into tart shells and bake for 15 minutes for small
tarts and 30 minutes for pie.

🦋 Cakes

French Delight Cake

Makes 1 cake

　　1　cup less 2 tablespoons whole wheat pastry flour
　　4　eggs
　　¼　cup unsalted butter or margarine
　　½　cup grape juice concentrate
　　1　teaspoon lemon juice
　　1　teaspoon grated lemon peel
Filling:
　　1　cup raw milk whipping cream
　　⅓　cup grape juice concentrate

½–2 teaspoons of lemon juice
 ½ teaspoon grated lemon peel
 1 cup sugarless raspberry jam

SUBSTITUTIONS

Whole wheat pastry flour: 1 cup less 2 tablespoons spelt or brown rice
  flour
Grape juice concentrate: ¼ cup honey; ½ cup apple juice concentrate;
  ⅓ rice syrup
Grape juice concentrate: 2 tablespoons honey; ⅓ cup apple juice concentrate or rice syrup
Sugarless raspberry jam: 1 cup sugarless boysenberry or blackberry jam

Preheat oven to 350 degrees F and butter and flour a 9-inch cake pan.
In a mixing bowl, sift the flour 2 to 3 times. In another bowl, separate
eggs and beat the whites until stiff. In a saucepan, melt the butter and
remove from heat. Warm a large mixing bowl (either in the microwave
or by running hot water in it) and beat the egg yolks and grape juice
concentrate until the mixture is very light, fluffy, and almost white. Add
the lemon juice and lemon peel and beat in. Divide the flour into 3 por-
tions and fold into the egg yolk mixture with a spatula. Cut and fold in
the beaten egg whites. Add the butter and gently fold in. Pour the batter into the pan and bake for 25 to 40 minutes or until firm when touched
with fingertip. Turn it out onto a wire rack covered with wax paper to
cool. When cool, split the cake into three layers.

   In a chilled bowl, whip the chilled whipping cream until it begins to
thicken. Slowly add in a steady stream, from 2 tablespoons to ⅓ cup
grape juice concentrate (taste for desired sweetness) and the lemon juice.
Add the lemon peel and continue whipping the cream until thick.

   Assemble the cake by spreading alternate layers with the raspberry
jam and the cream. The top layer and sides should be the cream. Garnish with fresh raspberries and/or almond slices.

Fruit Upside Down Cake

Makes 1 cake

   3 tablespoons butter or margarine
  ¼ cup honey

  2 teaspoon blackstrap molasses
  1 cup unsweetened pineapple slices
 ¼ cup chopped walnuts
1¼ cups whole wheat pastry flour
1½ teaspoons baking powder
 ⅓ cup butter or margarine
 ¼ cup honey
  2 teaspoon blackstrap molasses
  1 egg
  1 teaspoon vanilla extract
 ½ cup reserved pineapple juice

SUBSTITUTIONS

Pineapple: 1 cup sliced pears, peaches, nectarines, or apricots
Walnuts: ¼ cup chopped pecans; ½ whole cherries
Whole wheat pastry flour: 1¼ cup spelt, rice, barley, or oat flour
Egg: 1 teaspoon Egg Replacer or binder (page 140)
Pineapple juice: ½ cup pear, peach, nectarine, or apricot juice

Preheat oven to 350 degrees F. In a saucepan, melt the first measure of butter and transfer to a 9-inch cake pan. Add the first measure of honey and molasses and spread evenly. Drain the pineapple and reserve the juice. Arrange the pineapple slices and walnuts in the bottom of the pan.

In a mixing bowl, combine the flour and baking powder and sift together 2 to 3 times. In another bowl, cream the butter with the honey and molasses. Add egg and vanilla extract and beat well. Alternately add the flour mixture and juice and beat smooth. Pour into the pan and bake for 40 to 45 minutes. Let stand for 5 minutes, then turn out and serve.

Pumpkin Cake

Makes 1 cake

2¼ cups whole wheat pastry flour
  2 teaspoons baking powder
  1 teaspoon baking soda
 ½ teaspoon cinnamon
 ½ teaspoon allspice
 ¼ teaspoon cloves

½ cup butter or margarine
½ cup honey
¼ cup blackstrap molasses
2 eggs
½ teaspoon vanilla extract
½ cup cooked, pureed pumpkin
½ cup soy milk

SUBSTITUTIONS

Whole wheat pastry flour: 2½ cups spelt, rice, soy, or millet flour
Cinnamon: ½ teaspoon cardamom
Allspice: ½ teaspoon powdered ginger
Honey: 1 cup date sugar or apple/rice granular concentrate; ¾ cup rice
    syrup or maple syrup
Vanilla extract: 1 teaspoon vanilla liquid (page 205)
Pumpkin: ½ cup cooked, pureed squash, sweet potato, or yam
Soy milk: ½ cup goat or rice milk or water

Preheat oven to 350 degrees F and butter and flour two 9-inch cake pans.
In a mixing bowl, combine the flour, baking powder, baking soda, cinnamon, allspice, and cloves and sift together 2 to 3 times. In another
bowl, cream the butter with the honey and molasses. Add eggs and beat
until light and fluffy. Add the vanilla extract and pumpkin and mix well.
Alternately add the flour mixture and the soy milk and beat smooth.
Pour the batter into the cake pans and bake for 40 minutes or until firm
when touched with fingertip.

Liz's Soft Gingerbread

Makes 1 cake

3 cups whole wheat pastry flour
3 teaspoon baking powder
1 teaspoon powdered ginger
1 tablespoon cinnamon
1 teaspoon cloves
1 cup olive or canola oil
3 eggs
⅔ cup honey
⅔ cup blackstrap molasses

1 cup water

SUBSTITUTIONS
Whole wheat pastry flour: 3 cups spelt or rice flour; 2½ cups oat flour
    and ½ cup oat bran
Honey: ⅔ cup barley malt; 1 cup date sugar

Preheat oven to 375 degrees F and butter and flour an 8 x 12 cake pan.
In a mixing bowl, combine the flour, baking powder, powdered ginger,
cinnamon, and cloves and sift together 2 to 3 times. In another bowl,
combine the oil, eggs, honey, and molasses and beat well. Alternately
add the flour mixture and water to the egg mixture and beat until smooth.
Pour into the cake pan and bake for 35 to 45 minutes, or until firm when
touched with fingertip.

Yule Log

Makes 1 cake

1 cup hazelnuts
2 tablespoons whole wheat pastry flour
¾ cup grape/rice granular concentrate
¼ teaspoon almond extract
4 eggs

SUBSTITUTIONS
Hazelnuts: 1 cup almonds
Whole wheat pastry flour: 2 tablespoons rice or spelt flour
Grape/rice granular concentrate: 2 tablespoons vegetable glycerin
Almond extract: ½ teaspoon almond liquid (page 206)

Preheat oven to 350 degrees F and butter a 15 x 10-inch baking sheet.
Line the sheet with wax paper and butter the paper. In a blender, grind
the hazelnuts to a fine powder. In a mixing bowl, sift the flour 2 to 3
times and add to the hazelnuts. Add the grape/rice granular concentrate, almond extract, and eggs and blend well. Pour the batter into the
baking sheet and bake for 15 minutes (be careful not to overbake). Cover
the cake with a damp towel for 30 minutes or until cool. Gently loosen
the cake from the baking sheet and turn it over onto a sheet of wax paper,
removing the paper from the bottom. Spread the filling the entire length
of the cake, not quite touching the edges. Carefully roll the cake over on

itself. On the last roll place the cake on an appropriate size serving dish.

DECORATION IDEAS
The following are suggestions for decorating this traditional holiday cake. The idea is to make it look like a log.

Spread with whipped cream to look like snow. Garnish with nuts.

Spread with Carob Cream Frosting (page 385) or Chocolate Butter Cream Frosting (page 386). Create mushrooms out of a little whipped cream. Garnish with chopped or whole nuts.

Add cranberries or Christmas berries to the filling and outside for a colorful touch.

🦋 Frostings

Cream Frosting

Makes 1½ cups

    1 cup raw milk whipping cream
    1 teaspoon vanilla extract
    ¼ cup honey

SUBSTITUTIONS
Vanilla extract: 2 teaspoons vanilla liquid (page 205); 1 teaspoon almond extract; 2 teaspoons almond liquid (page 206)
Honey: 2 tablespoons rice syrup, apple or grape juice concentrate, or grape/rice granular concentrate

In a chilled bowl, whip the chilled whipping cream until it barely starts to thicken. Add the vanilla extract and the honey. Continue beating until thick and solid. It will cover an average size cake.

Carob Cream Frosting

Makes 1½ cups

    1 cup raw milk whipping cream
    1 teaspoon vanilla extract
    ¼ cup honey
    ⅓ cup carob powder

Vanilla extract: 2 teaspoons vanilla liquid (page 205)
Honey: 2 tablespoons rice syrup, apple or grape juice concentrate, or
    grape/rice concentrate

In a chilled bowl, whip the chilled whipping cream until it barely starts
to thicken. Add the vanilla extract and the honey and blend well. Slowly
add the carob powder until desired color and flavor are achieved. Continue beating until thick and solid. It will cover an average size cake.

Traditional Butter Cream Frosting

Makes 2 cups

    1 cup unsalted sweet butter or margarine
    ¼ cup water
    9 tablespoons sifted grape/rice granular concentrate
    5 beaten egg yolks
    ⅛ teaspoon cream of tartar

SUBSTITUTION

Grape/rice granular concentrate: 9 tablespoons rice syrup (omit the
    water)

In a mixing bowl, cream the butter until it is light in color and very fluffy.
In a saucepan, heat the water and slowly stir in the grape/rice granular
concentrate. Bring to a boil and cook for 2 to 5 minutes constantly stirring. If any lumps do not dissolve, continue heating, as they will dissolve at a higher temperature. In another bowl, combine the egg yolks
with the cream of tartar and mix well. Add the syrup in a steady stream
and beat well. Beat with an electric mixer until cool and thickened. Add
the egg yolk mixture to the butter and beat well. Add the flavoring and
mix well. Refrigerate to harden to spreading consistency.

VARIATIONS

Prepare above recipe. Add 1 teaspoon vanilla or almond extract or lemon
juice and 2 teaspoons grated lemon peel.

Prepare above recipe. Add 3 squares or 3 ounces of melted Baker's
pure chocolate mixed in 1 tablespoon water.

Prepare above recipe. Add ⅓ cup sifted carob powder.

Prepare above recipe. Add ⅓ cup ground nuts.

🦋 Bavarian Creams

Berry Cream

Serves 6

2 cups fresh raspberries
   whole berries for topping
2 teaspoons lemon juice
1 envelope unflavored gelatin
⅛ cup cold water
1 cup raw milk whipping cream
⅓ cup grape juice concentrate

SUBSTITUTIONS

Raspberries: 2 cups blackberries, boysenberries, huckleberries, or blueberries
Unflavored gelatin: 2 tablespoons agar flakes or kuzu
Grape juice concentrate: ⅓ cup rice syrup or apple juice concentrate

In a mixing bowl, crush the fruit and strain through a fine sieve. Add the lemon juice and grape juice concentrate and stir until concentrate is completely dissolved. In a saucepan, sprinkle gelatin over the water to soften. Cook over medium heat, stirring constantly until the gelatin dissolves. Add gelatin to the raspberries. Place the mixing bowl in a larger bowl filled with cracked ice and stir until raspberry mixture cools and begins to thicken. In a chilled bowl, whip the chilled whipping cream until it stands in peaks. Fold the whipped cream into the raspberries. Rinse a 1-quart mold in cold water, pour in the raspberry cream and refrigerate for 2 to 3 hours or until chilled. To serve, unmold on a chilled serving dish and garnish with whole raspberries and more whipped cream.

Peach Cream

Serves 6

2 cups peeled, pitted peaches
1 envelope Knox gelatin
2 teaspoons lemon juice
¼ cup honey
1 teaspoon almond extract
1 cup whipping cream

SUBSTITUTIONS
Peaches: 2 cups peeled, pitted apricot or nectarine
Honey: ⅓ cup grape juice concentrate or rice syrup
Almond extract: 2 teaspoons almond liquid (page 206)

In a blender, add the peaches and blend until smooth. In a saucepan, sprinkle gelatin over ¼ cup cold peach pulp to soften. Cook over medium heat, stirring constantly until the gelatin dissolves. Add gelatin mixture to remaining peach pulp. In a mixing bowl, add the peach mixture, lemon juice, honey, and almond extract and mix well. Place the mixing bowl in a larger bowl filled with cracked ice and stir until peach mixture cools and begins to thicken. In a chilled bowl, whip the chilled whipping cream until it stands in peaks. Fold the whipped cream into the peach mixture. Rinse a 1-quart mold in cold water, pour in the peach cream and chill for 2 to 3 hours or until chilled. Garnish with sliced fruit and more cream, and/or add sliced almonds sautéed in butter.

Strawberry Almond Cream

Serves 6

  ½ cup almonds
1½ cups water
  2 cups sliced strawberries
  2 envelopes Knox gelatin
  ⅓ cup grape juice concentrate
  1 teaspoon lemon juice
  ½ teaspoon almond extract
  2 tablespoons grape juice concentrate
  ½ cup sliced strawberries
  ¼ cup slivered almonds
  1 teaspoon butter or margarine (optional)

SUBSTITUTIONS
Grape juice concentrate: ⅓ cup apple juice concentrate or rice syrup
Almond extract: 1 teaspoon almond liquid (page 206)
Almonds: ½ cup cashews or hazelnuts

Grind the almonds to a fine powder in the blender. Add enough water to make 1½ cups of almond milk. Puree the strawberries and pour ½ cup of it into a saucepan. Sprinkle the gelatin on it to soften. Mix the sweetener, lemon, and almond extract and blend. Add to the almond milk. Dissolve the gelatin over heat and add to the mixture. Pour into a ring or other mold. Refrigerate for several hours. Sweeten the strawberries and let them sit. Before unmolding, toast the almonds in butter or in the oven for a few minutes. To serve, unmold onto a serving dish, pour the strawberries into the center of the ring, and garnish with the almonds.

❦ Fruit Fancies and Ices

Pears with Raspberries

Serves 4

> 1 cup raspberry juice
> 4 peeled, sliced or halved pears
> ½ cup raspberries
> 4 sprigs fresh mint

In a saucepan, heat the juice and poach the pears for 5 minutes. Serve with a little juice poured over the fruit and garnish with fresh, whole, or pureed berries and a sprig of mint.

Baked Apple

Serves 4

> 4 cored apples
> 1 cup apple juice
> ½ teaspoon cinnamon
> ½ teaspoon nutmeg
> ¼ cup chopped walnuts

SUBSTITUTION
Walnuts: ¼ cup pecans, almonds, or hazelnuts

Preheat oven to 350 degrees F. In a baking dish, place apples and pour apple juice over them. Sprinkle generously with cinnamon and lightly with nutmeg. Fill centers with nuts. Bake covered for 45 minutes to 1 hour.

Spiced Peaches

Serves 4

  1 cup peach puree
  1 cup water
  4 teaspoons honey
  4 cinnamon sticks
 16 cloves (4 per peach)
  4 pitted, peeled, sliced or halved peaches

SUBSTITUTION

Honey: 4 teaspoons rice syrup, grape or apple juice concentrate, or maple
   syrup
Peach: 4 pitted, peeled, sliced or halved nectarine

In a saucepan, combine the peach puree, water, honey, cinnamon, and
cloves and heat gently over low heat. Add the peaches and simmer for
5 to 10 minutes. Serve each in a bowl with ¼ of the juice and a cinnamon stick.

Fruit Ice

  2 cups watermelon, peach, raspberry, apricot, strawberry, pine-
     apple, nectarine, blackberry, boysenberry, huckleberry, blue-
     berry, cherry, kiwi, mango, or honeydew melon
  2 cups matching juice (for the melons, juice is not required—add
     a little water if needed)

Peel, seed, and coarsely chop the fruit. In a blender, blend the fruit until
smooth, adding a little juice if necessary. Add the remaining juice and
blend.
   Alternative method: add sweetener and lemon juice (see below).
Freeze the ice in a churn freezer or pour into a shallow container, cover,
and freeze. When serving, if the ice needs to be more slushy, cut into
chunks and return to blender and process briefly.

VARIATION

For a sweeter ice, add ¼ to 1 cup rice syrup, honey, maple syrup, or grape
juice concentrate, and 1 teaspoon lemon juice.

Quick Sorbet

Serves 2

> 2 cups of frozen sliced peaches, bananas, nectarines, pears, apricots, or any berry

Take fruit from freezer and defrost briefly. It should still be firm and have ice crystals. In a blender, place the fruit and blend until desired consistency is reached.

Chris's Carob Cream

Serves 4

> 1 cup cashews
> 2–3 cups water
> 1 tablespoon maple syrup
> 1–2 tablespoons carob powder
> Ice cubes

Soak cashews for 6 hours in 2 cups of water. Drain and place the nuts in chilled blender and process to a fine paste. Slowly add the water, maple syrup, and the carob powder. Freeze the cream in a churn freezer or omit the ice cubes and pour into a shallow container, cover, and freeze.

CHAPTER 23

Fruits and Juices

FRUITS ARE DELICIOUS, DELIGHTFUL, and nutritious. Choices are abundant, especially during the summer. Fruits can be fresh, frozen, canned, or dried. Fruits are versatile and great for salads, desserts, fruit drinks, snacks, breakfast, lunch, or dinner.

❧ Alternatives to Fresh

Different varieties of fresh fruit are not always available throughout the year. Some fruits, like berries, can develop molds very quickly. Fruits commercially canned in their own juice (like pineapple), or home-canned in their own juice or with an appropriate sweetener, are an alternative. Fruit frozen without sugar is available in supermarkets or health food stores. Frozen berries are an excellent way to avoid the mold problem; you use only what you need and there is less waste.

If you have tested sensitive to food grade vegetable petroleum, beeswax, or lactase resin base wax and resin, be extra careful about choosing fruit. Organic is always best. Below is list of commercially grown fruits that may contain one or more of these additives.

Fruits That May Contain Additives

Apple	Papaya
Lemon	Passion fruit
Lime	Peach
Grapefruit	Pineapple
Melon	Plum
Nectarine	Pomegranate

❧ Dried Fruit

Dried fruit presents special problems. The dehydration of fruit concentrates the natural fruit sugars. Fruits can become moldy and the sul-
furization, or treatment with sulfur dioxide, will not necessarily destroy
the mold and the fruit will be contaminated with a chemical. Commercially dried fruit may also have other chemicals added. There are
organically dried fruits available, or you could dry your own. Use only
fresh fruit that is without signs of spoilage.

❧ Special Issues

Candida and blood sugar problems, whether hypoglycemia or diabetes,
pose special considerations when it comes to the use of fruit. For those
with severe Candida or blood sugar problems, fruit should be totally
restricted. If the Candida is not too bad, then fruit in moderation (1 to
2 pieces a day, and/or 2 to 4 ounces of juice a day) is suggested. The same
would apply for those with blood sugar problems. Whole fruit contains
fiber and pectin, which aid in the digestion and slows down the absorption of fruit sugar. Fruit juice greatly reduces the amount of fiber and
pectin and contains more sugar and calories. Soft-shelled melons, soft
fruits (like peaches), and berries can develop mold quickly. When you
cut the melons, the mold from the rind can be spread inside the melon.
To avoid the potential problem, select the harder-shelled melons, like
honeydew or watermelon.

❧ Fun Fruits

Following is a list of different taste treats for you to explore and enjoy.
Depending upon your area, they will be available at various times during the year.

Asian pear
These pears are a cross between an apple and a pear.

Casaba melon
This melon has a hard shell with a very pale-green, sweet, juicy flesh.

Cherimoya
It has a thin pale-green skin with a white flesh and the flavor resembles a mix of banana, pineapple, and papaya.

Crane melon
This melon has a soft shell with an orange flesh similar to cantaloupe.

Elderberry
These small, slightly sour, deep blue berries grow in clusters like grapes. They are a very healing food, good in soup and jams.

Guava
It is a small, sweet-smelling, oval fruit with a light pink flesh.

Kiwi
Fuzzy on the outside and green on the inside, a kiwi is an aesthetic delight. The black markings on the green on the inside are beautiful. The flavor is a mixture of tart and sweet.

Kumquat
It is from the citrus family. It is very small, orange fruit and has a sour taste similar to bitter lemon.

Loquat
This small, yellow fruit comes from an Asian evergreen tree.

Mango
This tropical fruit has a beautiful, orange-red skin when ripe and an orange, perfumed, juicy flesh.

Papaya
This tropical fruit has a rich, yellow-orange skin when ripe with a unique flavor. It is known for its ability to aid digestion.

Passion fruit
This tropical fruit has a delicious, sweet, aromatic flavor.

Persian melon
This melon has a thicker skin than the cantaloupe and although the flavor is similar, it really is more delicate and full.

Persimmon
This winter fruit hangs like orange lanterns on the persimmon tree. The taste is bitter, like a lemon. It is delicious in made into persimmon bread.

Pomegranate
The hard fruit has a rose-red skin and juicy seeds. It has a bitter sweet flavor.

Star fruit
When sliced crosswise, the slices of this fruit resembles stars. The color is greenish-gold and the flavor varies from sweet to tangy.

The colors and delicate flavors of fruit add to the beauty of a meal. Following are a few suggested combinations for fruit salads. Expand upon these creations; use your imagination and create your own. Use about 1 cup of fruit per person. Add nuts or seeds, if desired, and extra fruit juice for a dressing. The various mints (from spearmint to lemon mint) are a delightful addition to any salad. Cut-up fruits served with a dip are also a welcome refresher on a hot summer's day.

Fruit Combinations

Any melon, banana, pineapple

Apple, grapes, oranges (or Mandarin orange or tangerine)

Apricots, blackberry

Blueberry or huckleberry, pineapple, cherimoya

Cantaloupe (or crane or Persian), honeydew, and watermelon. Serve cut up or use a melon baller.

Kiwi, Asian pear, tangerine (or tangelo)

Mango, papaya, passion fruit

Nectarine, cherries, plum

Peach, strawberry, banana

Pears, raspberry

Pineapple, banana, apple

Pineapple, grapefruit, red grapes

Star fruit, orange, pomegranate

Serving Ideas

Carve out one half of a watermelon (or both halves of a pineapple) and fill
with any combination of fruits.

Make kebabs of fruit on toothpicks or skewers.

Arrange the fruit by color and texture on a serving dish, plain or with a dip.

Serve on a bed of greens.

Serve fruits sprinkled with coconut.

❧ Fruit and Vegetable Beverages and Juices

There are many delicious juices available made from all types of fruit.
As with other foods, read the labels. Frequently, apple or grape juice
concentrate is added to improve the flavor and sweetness. Vegetable
juices are loaded with nutrition, especially absorbable minerals, and are
very healing for the body.

Lemonade

Serves 2

> ½ cup lemon juice
> 2 cups cold water
> 3 tablespoons honey

SUBSTITUTIONS

Lemon juice: ½ lime juice

Honey: 6 tablespoons grape or apple juice concentrate or rice syrup

Combine all the ingredients and mix well. Adjust honey to your taste
and serve over ice.

Orange-Berry Wake-Up

Serves 2

> 2 cups orange juice
> ½ cup fresh or frozen strawberries
> ½ banana (or increase the berries to ¾ cup)

1 teaspoon grape juice concentrate (optional)
2 sprigs fresh mint

SUBSTITUTIONS

Orange juice: 2 cups tangerine juice

Strawberry: ½ cup fresh or frozen raspberry, blackberry, boysenberry, or loganberry

Grape concentrate: 1 tablespoon apple juice concentrate or rice syrup; 2 teaspoons honey

In a blender, combine all the ingredients and blend until smooth. Serve with sprig of mint.

Sparkling Apple Juice

Serves 6

2 cups apple juice
¼ cup honey (optional)
2 teaspoons blackstrap molasses (omit if using other sweetener)
½ teaspoon nutmeg
½ teaspoon powdered ginger
5 cups seltzer water
1 peeled, seeded, sliced apple

SUBSTITUTIONS

Honey: ¼ cup grape or apple juice concentrate or rice syrup

Nutmeg: ½ teaspoon cinnamon

Powdered ginger: ¼ teaspoon cloves

In a saucepan, combine the apple juice, honey, molasses, nutmeg, and ginger. Cook gently over low heat for 5 to 8 minutes, then set aside and let cool. In a large punch bowl, combine the seltzer with the apple juice mixture and stir well. Garnish individual servings with apple slices and a dash of nutmeg.

Cherry Spice Juice

Serves 8

  2 quarts cherry juice
  1 sliced lemon
  ⅓ cup apple juice concentrate
  6 whole cloves
  1 cinnamon stick
 12 whole allspice
     1-inch piece fresh ginger (½ teaspoon powdered ginger)

SUBSTITUTIONS
Cherry juice: 2 quarts cranberry juice
Lemon: 2 limes; 1 sliced orange
Cinnamon: 4 cardamom pods
Allspice: ½ teaspoon nutmeg
Apple concentrate: ⅓ cup grape juice concentrate or rice syrup; ¼ cup
    honey

In a saucepan, combine the cherry juice, apple juice concentrate, and half the lemon slices. Place the cloves, cinnamon stick, allspice, and ginger in a cheese cloth bag. Place the spice bag in the cherry juice mixture and simmer on low heat for 10 minutes. Discard spice bag. Serve hot or cold. Garnish individual servings with remaining lemon slices.

Very Berry Juice

Serves 1

  1 cup strawberry juice
  ⅓ cup fresh or frozen strawberries
  ⅓ cup fresh or frozen blackberries

SUBSTITUTIONS
Strawberry: 1 cup raspberry or boysenberry juice
Strawberry: ⅓ cup fresh or frozen raspberries or boysenberries
Blackberry: ⅓ cup fresh or frozen raspberries or boysenberries

In a blender, combine all the ingredients and blend until smooth.

Kiwi "UP"

Serves 1

> 1 peeled, chopped kiwi
> 1 cup pineapple
> ¼ cup chopped fresh or canned pineapple

SUBSTITUTIONS
Pineapple: 1 cup papaya or guava juice
Pineapple: ¼ cup papaya or guava

In a blender, combine all the ingredients and blend until smooth.

Passionate Peach Juice

Serves 1

> 1 peeled, chopped peach
> 1 cup peach juice
> 1 tablespoon lime juice
> 1 lime slice for garnish

SUBSTITUTIONS
Peach: 1 peeled, chopped nectarine
Lime juice: 1 tablespoon lemon juice
Lime: 1 lemon slice

In a blender, combine the peach, peach juice, and lime juice and blend until smooth. Serve garnished with a lime slice.

✤ Smoothies

"Milk" Smoothie

Serves 1

> 1 cup vanilla soy milk
> 2 large pitted, chopped dates
> ⅛ teaspoon cinnamon

SUBSTITUTIONS
Vanilla soy milk: 1 cup rice, coconut, or goat milk with a little vanilla
Dates: ¼ cup any chopped fruit

In a blender, combine all the ingredients and blend until smooth.

Fruit Smoothie

Serves 1

1 cup apple juice
1 ripe banana
1 sprig mint

SUBSTITUTIONS
Apple juice: 1 cup any fruit juice
Banana: ½ cup any chopped fruit

In a blender, combine the apple juice and banana and blend until smooth.
Serve garnished sprig of mint.

Nut Smoothie

Serves 2

¼ cup almond
1½ cups apricot juice
¼ cup peeled, pitted, sliced apricots

SUBSTITUTIONS
Almond: ¼ cup cashews or hazelnuts
Apricot juice: 1½ cups peach, pineapple, pear, or nectarine
Apricots: ¼ peeled, pitted, sliced peach, pineapple, pear, or nectarine
(same as the juice)

In a blender, grind the nuts to a fine powder. Add the apricot juice and
apricots and blend until smooth.

✄ Juicer Fun

The following are various vegetable juice combinations. A vegetable juicer is necessary. See page 464 for sources and brands. Also see book list on page 472 for books on this important subject.

Carrot Apple Juice

Serves 1

> 3 carrots
> 1 large apple

In a juicer, process carrots and apple and serve.

Healthy Surprise Juice

Serves 1

> 1 apple
> ¼ green bell pepper
> 2 leaves red cabbage
> 3 chard leaves
> 4 romaine leaves

SUBSTITUTIONS

Apple: 1 pear
Red cabbage: 2 leaves green cabbage, collards, or kale
Chard: 3 leaves spinach or beet greens
Romaine: 4 leaves escarole; 4 watercress stems

In a juicer, process all the ingredients and serve.

Vegetable Juice Combinations

Carrot, beet, celery
Carrot, beet, cucumber
Carrot, cabbage, celery
Carrot, celery, any lettuce
Carrot, celery, parsley, spinach
Carrot, dandelion, turnip
Carrot, radish
Carrot, turnip, watercress
Celery root, parsley, any lettuce
Celery, any cabbage
Celery, any cabbage, beet
Celery, cucumber, spinach
Celery, cucumber, turnip
Celery, dandelion, spinach

Celery, endive, parsley
Celery, green beans
Celery, green or red bell pepper, kohlrabi
Tomato, any onion, any lettuce
Tomato, beet, celery
Tomato, carrot, turnip
Tomato, celery, green bell pepper
Tomato, garlic, celery
Tomato, green beans, turnip
Tomato, jicama, parsley
Tomato, parsley, spinach
Tomato, watercress, cucumber

Other juice ideas: kale, beet greens, collards, chard, potato, parsnip, turnip greens, mustard greens, asparagus, zucchini. Fresh juice may also be extracted from any fruit.

🦋 Hot Drinks

Hot Spiced Apple Juice

Serves 1

    1 cup unfiltered apple juice
    1 cinnamon stick
    6 whole cloves

SUBSTITUTIONS
Cinnamon: 1 cardamom pod
Cloves: 6 whole allspice

In a saucepan, combine all the ingredients and heat slowly. Serve with cinnamon stick.

Mulled Cranberry Juice

Serves 4

> 1   quart cranberry juice
> 1   cup orange juice
> 15 whole cloves
> 1   sliced orange

SUBSTITUTIONS
Orange juice: 1 cup apple or raspberry juice
Cloves: 15 whole allspice; 4 cinnamon sticks

In a saucepan, combine the cranberry juice, orange juice, and cloves and heat slowly. Serve garnished with orange slices.

Hot Carob

Serves 2

> $1\frac{1}{2}$ cups rice milk
> $\frac{1}{4}$ cup carob powder
> 3   tablespoons honey
> $\frac{1}{2}$ teaspoon vanilla extract

SUBSTITUTIONS
Rice milk: $1\frac{1}{2}$ cups soy, goat, or nut milk
Honey: 6 tablespoons apple or grape juice concentrate, rice syrup, maple syrup
Vanilla extract: 1 teaspoon vanilla liquid (page 205); $\frac{1}{4}$ teaspoon almond extract; $\frac{1}{2}$ teaspoon almond liquid (page 206)

In a saucepan, combine the rice milk and the carob powder. Add the honey and the vanilla and heat slowly to desired temperature.

🦋 Alternatives to Coffee and Soda Pop

Coffee and soda pop are not good for you. Coffee is being linked to various medical problems like PMS, fibercystic breast disease, and heart disease. Soda pop is high in sodium and phosphorous (which upsets our mineral balance) and the diet varieties contain questionable artificial sweeteners. What do you do now?

There are good quality, water-processed brands of decaffeinated coffee available through your local health food store. Provided that you are not allergic to coffee itself, used in moderation it should be acceptable. Another alternative is to explore the various grain beverages. Some can be brewed like coffee; often more than one grain is used, so be sure to read the label. Wonderful varieties of herb teas can be found in both the supermarket and the health food store. Their flavors are delicious and delightful with many choices. Some people like a tablespoon of blackstrap molasses heated in a cup of water.

Soda pop can be replaced with seltzer water and juice, or a twist of lemon or lime. There are flavored mineral waters on the market. But be sure to read the label because they frequently contain sugars in different forms. Read all the fine print. Health food store varieties of "cola," "root beer," and "ginger ale" can also be found. But be sure to check the labels.

CHAPTER 24

Dressings, Sauces, and Dips

OUR COMMITMENT is to provide you with interesting foods while maintaining our integrity regarding allergies, addictions, and healthy food choices. Dressings, sauces, and dips pose a special problem because they so frequently contain sugar, yeast, dairy, and other common allergens.

These recipes are what you have been waiting for! Any food can be enhanced with a dressing or sauce. Following are recipes for dressings and sauces made without dairy, sugar, or yeast. Most are easy to make and taste delicious. Enjoy them as they are or add your own special touch. The recipes listed below are free of vinegar, a major source of yeast problems. If vinegar is tolerated, it may be used in the recipes in place of the lemon or lime juice. Choose from the following lists of available vinegars and oils according (for more information on oils, see page 142).

In the Lemonette, Lemon Thyme, Sesame Seed, Poppy Seed and Zesty Mint dressings, the oil can be reduced to half the amount indicated in the recipe. Water can be substituted for the difference. If desired the oil can be eliminated from the Sesame Seed Dressing. In the Zesty Mint Dressing, replace half the oil with water and/or lemonade.

Vinegars

Apple cider vinegar	Red wine vinegar
Balsamic rice vinegar	Rice vinegar
Plum (Umeboshi) vinegar	White wine vinegar
Red raspberry vinegar	

Oils

Monosaturated	Saturated	Polyunsaturated
Canola oil	Butter	Corn oil
Olive oil		Peanut oil
Rapeseed oil		Safflower oil
		Sesame oil
		Soybean oil
		Sunflower seed oil
		Walnut oil

Mayonnaise

The basis for many dressings and sauces is a good mayonnaise. There are good commercial products on the market made from healthy oils and do not contain sugar. For those with allergy restrictions and Candida, the egg and vinegar in mayonnaise remain a problem. The following recipes are egg-free, sugar-free, and yeast-free.

If yeast is not a problem, you can also use vinegar or prepared mustard in the following recipes. If mustard is an allergen, omit from the recipe and experiment with other spices like paprika, dill, or tarragon.

A reminder: All mayonnaise requires refrigeration. These mayonnaise recipes contain no preservatives and we recommend that you use them within five days.

Eggless "REAL" Mayonnaise

Makes 3 cups

> 1 cup cold water
> 3 tablespoons lemon juice
> 1 tablespoon arrowroot
> 1 teaspoon sea salt or kelp
> 1 teaspoon dry mustard
> 2 cups canola oil

SUBSTITUTIONS

Lemon juice: 3 tablespoons lime or kumquat juice
Arrowroot: 1 tablespoon potato starch or corn starch
Canola oil: 2 cups olive or safflower oil

In double boiler, combine the water, lemon juice, arrowroot, and salt. Cook over medium heat, stirring often until the mixture thickens. Set aside and let cool. Transfer mixture to a blender. Add mustard and mix well. With the blender running, add the oil in a steady slow stream and blend until all oil is emulsified. (If you are not using a blender, place mixture in a bowl and whip with a whisk while adding the oil). Blend in 1 tablespoon of hot water to stabilize and either refrigerate in a covered container or serve immediately. The flavor is excellent and comes very close to real mayonnaise!

Soy Eggless Mayonnaise

Makes 1 cup

> ¾ cup tofu
> ½ cup water
> 3 tablespoons canola oil
> 4 tablespoons minced onion
> 2 tablespoons lemon juice
> 1½ teaspoons dry mustard
> ¼ teaspoon white pepper
> ¼ teaspoon tarragon
>   sea salt or kelp

SUBSTITUTIONS

Canola oil: 3 tablespoons olive or safflower oil
Onion: 2 cloves minced garlic; 1 minced shallot
Lemon juice: 2 tablespoons lime or kumquat juice
White pepper: pinch cayenne; ⅛ teaspoon red pepper flakes
Tarragon: ¼ teaspoon marjoram or thyme

In a blender, combine all the ingredients and blend until smooth. This mayonnaise will keep refrigerated in a covered container for 8 to 12 weeks. The flavor will be stronger and not as light.

Cashew Mayonnaise

Makes 2 cups

> ½ cup cashews
> 1 cup water

    1 clove minced garlic
   ⅓ cup lemon juice
   ¼ teaspoon dill
    1 teaspoon sea salt or kelp
    1 cup canola oil

SUBSTITUTIONS
Cashews: ½ cup almonds
Garlic: 1 teaspoon onion powder or chopped chives
Lemon juice: ⅓ lime or kumquat juice
Dill: ¼ teaspoon tarragon, rosemary, or paprika
Canola oil: ⅓ cup olive or safflower oil

In a blender, combine the cashews and water and blend until creamy. Add garlic, lemon, dill, and salt and blend. With the blender running, add the oil in a steady slow stream and blend until all oil is emulsified. Thin with water to desired consistency. Refrigerate in a covered container or serve immediately.

    The flavor is different from regular mayonnaise. It is rich and enhances various recipes.

Egg Mayonnaise

Makes 1½ cups

    1 egg
    1 teaspoon dry mustard
   ½ teaspoon sea salt or kelp
    3 tablespoons lemon juice
    1 cup canola oil

SUBSTITUTIONS
Dry mustard: 1 teaspoon Dijon mustard
Lemon juice: 3 tablespoons lime or kumquat juice
Canola oil: 1 cup olive or safflower oil

In a blender, combine the egg, mustard, salt, and lemon juice and blend well. With the blender running, add the oil in a steady slow stream and blend until all oil is emulsified. (If you are not using a blender, place mixture in a bowl and whip with a whisk while adding the oil). Blend in 1 tablespoon of hot water to stabilize and either refrigerate in a covered container or serve immediately.

🦋 Favorites

Basic Catsup

Makes 1½ cups

> 1 cup tomato puree (fresh or canned)
> ¼ cup canola oil
> 1 tablespoons honey
> 1 tablespoon lemon juice
> ¼ teaspoon onion powder
> ¼ teaspoon oregano
> ⅛ teaspoon celery seed (optional)
>   sea salt or kelp and black pepper

SUBSTITUTIONS
Canola oil: ¼ cup olive or safflower oil
Honey: 2 tablespoons rice syrup or grape juice concentrate
Lemon juice: 1 tablespoon lime juice
Onion powder: ¼ teaspoon garlic powder
Oregano: ¼ teaspoon marjoram or thyme

In a blender, combine all the ingredients and blend until smooth. Refrigerate in a covered container or serve immediately.

Close-to-Thousand Island Dressing

Makes 1½ cups

> 1 cup Eggless "REAL" Mayonnaise (page 408)
> 3 teaspoons tomato paste
> 1 teaspoon lemon juice
> 1 teaspoon onion powder
> ¼ teaspoon dill
> ¼ teaspoon sea salt or kelp

SUBSTITUTIONS
Eggless mayonnaise: 1 cup soy or commercially prepared mayonnaise
Lemon juice: 1 teaspoon lime juice or vinegar

Onion powder: ¼ teaspoon garlic powder
Dill: ¼ teaspoon paprika, oregano, or parsley

In a blender, combine all the ingredients and blend until smooth. Adjust seasonings and refrigerate in a covered container or serve immediately.

Catsup may be used to replace the tomato paste. Make sure it is a sugar-free variety from the health food store. In addition, catsup will usually contain vinegar, which is a yeast.

Almost Ranch Dressing

Makes 1½ cups

> 1 cup Eggless "REAL" Mayonnaise (page 408)
> ½ cup goat milk ricotta cheese
> 2 teaspoons lemon juice
> 1 tablespoon onion powder
> ½ teaspoon dill
> ¼ teaspoon sea salt or kelp
> ¼ black pepper (optional)

SUBSTITUTIONS
Eggless mayonnaise: 1 cup soy or commercially prepared mayonnaise
Lemon juice: 2 teaspoons lime juice
Onion powder: 1 teaspoon garlic powder; 1½ tablespoons chopped chives; 1 tablespoon minced shallot; 1½ tablespoons chopped green onion
Dill: ¼ teaspoon marjoram or tarragon

In a blender, combine all the ingredients and blend until smooth. Adjust seasonings and refrigerate in a covered container or serve immediately.

Practically It "Blue Cheese" Dressing

Makes 2½ cups

> 1 cup Eggless "REAL" Mayonnaise (page 408)
> 2 teaspoons lemon juice
> 1 teaspoon onion powder
> ¼ teaspoon sea salt or kelp

¼ teaspoon black pepper (optional)
1½ cups goat feta cheese

SUBSTITUTIONS

Eggless mayonnaise: 1 cup soy or commercially prepared mayonnaise
Lemon juice: 2 teaspoons lime juice
Onion powder: 1 teaspoon garlic powder, chopped chives; ½ teaspoon
  minced shallot; 2 teaspoons chopped green onion

In a blender, combine all the ingredients, except for ¾ cup feta cheese, and blend well. Add the rest of the crumbled feta cheese, stir well with a spatula, and refrigerate in a covered container or serve immediately.

Lemonette Dressing

Makes ¾ cups

½ cup canola oil
1 clove minced garlic
¼ cup lemon juice
½ teaspoon dry mustard (optional)
¼ teaspoon oregano
  sea salt and black pepper

SUBSTITUTIONS

Canola oil: ½ cup olive or safflower oil
Garlic: ½ teaspoon minced shallot or onion powder; 1 teaspoon chopped
  chive or chopped green onion
Lemon juice: ¼ cup vinegar
Oregano: ¼ teaspoon thyme, tarragon, marjoram, basil, or dill

In a blender, combine all the ingredients and blend until smooth. Adjust seasonings and refrigerate in a covered container. Shake well before pouring on salad.

Lemon Thyme Dressing

Makes 2 cups

1 cup canola oil
1 clove minced garlic

   ½ cup lemon juice
   2 teaspoons grated lemon peel
   ¾ teaspoon thyme
   ⅓ cup chopped fresh parsley
      sea salt and black pepper

SUBSTITUTIONS
Canola oil: 1 cup olive or safflower oil
Garlic: ½ teaspoon chopped chives

In a blender, combine all the ingredients and blend until smooth. Adjust seasonings and refrigerate in a covered container. Shake well before pouring on salad.

Sesame Seed Dressing

Makes 1½ cups

   2 tablespoons sesame seeds
   1 cup Sesame Milk (page 199)
   ¼ cup canola oil
   1 tablespoon lemon juice
   1 tablespoon honey
   1 teaspoon cumin

SUBSTITUTIONS
Canola oil: ¼ cup olive or safflower oil
Lemon juice: 1 tablespoon lime or kumquat juice
Honey: 1 tablespoon apple juice concentrate or brown rice syrup

In a frying pan, place the seeds and toast on medium heat for 2 to 3 minutes. In a blender, combine the toasted seeds and the rest of the ingredients, and blend until smooth. Adjust seasonings and refrigerate in a covered container. Shake well before pouring on salad.

Poppy Seed Dressing

Makes 2 cups

- 1 egg
- ½ cup lemon juice
- 3 tablespoons minced yellow onion
- 1 tablespoon honey
- 3 tablespoons poppy seeds
  sea salt or kelp
- 1 cup canola oil

SUBSTITUTIONS

Lemon juice: ½ cup lime, pineapple, or kumquat juice
Onion: 4 tablespoons green onion; 3 tablespoons minced shallot
Honey: 1 tablespoon apple juice concentrate or rice syrup
Canola oil: 1 cup olive, safflower, or corn oil

In a blender, combine the egg, lemon juice, onion, honey, poppy seeds, and salt and blend well. With the blender running, add the oil in a steady slow stream and blend until all oil is emulsified. (If you are not using a blender, place mixture in a bowl and whip with a whisk while adding the oil). Blend in 1 tablespoon of hot water to stabilize and either refrigerate in a covered container or serve immediately.

Zesty Mint Dressing

Makes 1 cup

- ½ cup canola oil
- ⅓ cup lemonade (sugarless health store variety)
- 4 to 5 fresh mint leaves

SUBSTITUTIONS

Canola oil: ½ cup olive or safflower oil

In a blender, combine all the ingredients and blend until smooth. Refrigerate in a covered container. Shake well before pouring on salad.

This delicious surprise works well with cold grain or pasta salads.

🦋 Oil-Free Dressings

Tangy Citrus Dressing

Makes 1½ cups

    2 tablespoons cornstarch
    4 tablespoons warm water
    1 cup grapefruit juice
    2 cloves minced garlic
    ¼ cup lemon juice
    ¼ teaspoon thyme
    ¼ teaspoon oregano
    1 teaspoon chopped fresh parsley

SUBSTITUTIONS
Cornstarch: 2 tablespoons kuzu or arrowroot
Oregano: ¼ teaspoon tarragon

In a small bowl, combine the cornstarch and water and mix well. Set aside. In a blender, combine the remaining ingredients and blend. Add the cornstarch mixture and blend until smooth. Refrigerate in a covered container. Shake well before pouring on salad.

Salad in a Bottle

Makes 2 cups

    1 cup tomato juice
    ½ cup chopped yellow onion
    ½ peeled, pitted avocado
    ¼ cup chopped celery
    2 tablespoons chopped fresh parsley
    ¼ teaspoon tarragon
       sea salt and black pepper

SUBSTITUTIONS
Onion: ½ cup chopped white onion; ⅓ cup chopped green onion or
    chives; 1 minced shallot
Celery: ¼ cup chopped green bell pepper
Tarragon: ¼ teaspoon basil, thyme, oregano, dill, or marjoram

In a blender, combine all the ingredients and blend until smooth. Refrigerate in a covered container. Shake well before pouring on salad.

Cool as a Cucumber Dressing

Makes 2 cups

- ½ seeded, peeled, cubed cucumber
- 1 cup water
- ½ cup lemon juice
- 1 small onion
- 2 cloves minced garlic
- ½ teaspoon dill
- 1 tablespoon parsley
- ½ teaspoon celery seed
  sea salt and black pepper

SUBSTITUTIONS
Lemon juice: ½ cup lime or kumquat juice
Onion: 2 minced shallots; 3 chopped green onions

In a blender, combine all the ingredients and blend until smooth. Refrigerate in a covered container. Shake well before pouring on salad.

Versatile Garbanzo Dressing

Makes 1 cup

- 1 cup cooked, pureed garbanzo
- 3 tablespoons lemon juice
- 1 chopped green onion
- 1 tablespoon chopped fresh parsley
- ½ teaspoon cumin

SUBSTITUTIONS
Lemon juice: 3 tablespoons lime juice
Green onion: ½ teaspoon onion powder; 1 tablespoon chopped onion;
    2 tablespoons chopped chives; 1 clove minced garlic; ¼ teaspoon
    garlic powder
Parsley: 1 tablespoon chopped fresh cilantro
Cumin: ½ teaspoon coriander

In a blender, combine all the ingredients and blend until smooth. Refrigerate in a covered container. Shake well before pouring on salad.

VARIATION
Add ¼ cup peeled, seeded, chopped cucumber and ½ teaspoon dill to ingredients.

Chive Tofu Dressing
Makes ½ cup

> ½ cup tofu
> 3 tablespoons lemon juice
> ¼ cup chives
> 2 tablespoons chopped fresh parsley
> ½ teaspoon paprika
>   sea salt and black pepper

SUBSTITUTION
Chives: 1 chopped green onion; 2 tablespoons chopped onion

In a blender, combine all the ingredients and blend until smooth. Refrigerate in a covered container. Shake well before pouring on salad.

Creamy Basil Dressing
Makes 1 cup

> ½ cup almonds
> ⅓ cup water
>   juice of ½ large lemon
> ¼ teaspoon minced shallot
> 7 fresh basil leaves
> 1½ teaspoons Parsley Patch
>   sea salt and black pepper
> 2½ tablespoons canola oil

SUBSTITUTIONS
Almonds: ½ cup cashews
Lemon juice: juice of 1 lime or 5 kumquats

Shallot: ¼ teaspoon onion powder; ½ teaspoon minced onion; 1 teaspoon chopped chives
Canola oil: 2½ tablespoons olive or safflower oil

Blanch almonds in boiling water for 2 to 3 minutes. Drain the almonds and remove the skins. In a blender, grind the almonds to a powder. Add the water, lemon juice, shallot, basil, Parsley Patch, and salt and pepper and blend well. With the blender running, add the oil in a steady slow stream and blend until all oil is emulsified. Refrigerate in a covered container or serve immediately.

VARIATION

Follow above recipe. Replace nuts and water with ½ cup soy, goat, or rice milk. The flavor will be excellent but the consistency will be thinner.

Cucumber Dressing

Makes 1 cup

- ½ peeled, chopped cucumber
- ¼ cup canola oil
- 2 tablespoons tahini (optional)
  juice of 1 lemon
- 1 tablespoon chopped green onion
- ¼ teaspoon paprika
  sea salt or kelp

SUBSTITUTIONS

Green onion: ½ tablespoon minced shallot; 1 tablespoon minced onion
Lemon juice: juice of 2 limes; juice of 6 kumquats
Canola oil: ¼ cup olive or safflower oil

In a blender, combine all the ingredients and blend until smooth. Refrigerate in a covered container. Shake well before pouring on salad.

Zesty Tomato Dressing

Makes 1 cup

- 2 chopped tomatoes
- ¼ cup lemon juice

   1 clove minced garlic
   2 tablespoons minced green bell pepper
   1/8 teaspoon cayenne powder
   1/4 teaspoon basil
   1/4 teaspoon oregano
   1/4 teaspoon thyme
   1/4 teaspoon marjoram
   1/4 cup olive oil

SUBSTITUTIONS

Garlic: 1 tablespoon chopped green onion or minced white onion; 1/2
   tablespoon minced shallot
Olive oil: 1/4 cup canola or safflower oil

In a blender, combine the tomatoes, lemon juice, garlic, bell pepper,
cayenne powder, basil, oregano, thyme, and marjoram and blend well.
With the blender running, add the oil in a steady slow stream and blend
until all oil is emulsified. Refrigerate in a covered container or serve
immediately.

   Note: If allergic to any of the herbs or rotating, the dressing will taste
very good with the use of only one herb. Use 1 teaspoon of the individual herb. Adjust amounts if more than one is used.

🦋 Sauces

Orange Delight Sauce

Makes 2 cups

   1 small sweet potato
   1/2 cup Poultry Stock (page 230)
   1/2 cup orange juice
   2 chopped carrots
   2 chopped leeks (white part only)
   1/4 teaspoon thyme

SUBSTITUTIONS

Sweet potato: 1 small yam
Poultry stock: 1/2 cup Vegetable Stock (page 230), Quick Herb Stock
   (page 229), or water

Orange juice: ½ cup tangerine juice
Leeks: 2 tablespoons minced shallot; 1 chopped small onion
Thyme: ¼ teaspoon rosemary; ¼ teaspoon rosemary and ¼ teaspoon
    thyme

Preheat oven to 350 degrees F and bake the sweet potato for 30 minutes
or until tender. Peel the sweet potato and set aside. In a blender, combine the sweet potato with the remaining ingredients and blend until
smooth. Serve with Winter Squash or Grain Pilaf.

Barbecue Sauce

Makes 2½ cups

     ¼ cup olive oil
     1 medium chopped onion
     4 cloves minced garlic
     ⅓ cup diced celery
     1 cup Basic Tomato Sauce (page 422)
    2½ tablespoons honey
     ½ tablespoon blackstrap molasses (omit if using other sweetener)
        juice of 1 large lemon
     1 tablespoon dry mustard
        sea salt and cayenne pepper

SUBSTITUTIONS
Olive oil: ¼ cup canola or safflower oil
Onion: 3 minced shallots
Tomato sauce: 1 cup Basic Catsup (page 411)
Honey: 6 tablespoon rice syrup or grape juice concentrate

In a soup pot, heat the oil and sauté the onion and garlic for 2 to 3 minutes or until onion is transparent. Add the celery, tomato sauce, honey,
molasses, lemon juice, and mustard. Simmer for 35 to 45 minutes. Correct the seasonings with the salt and cayenne pepper. Let cool, transfer
to a covered container, and refrigerate until ready to use. Serve with Pork
Brochettes.

Basic Tomato Sauce

Makes 4 cups

- 2 tablespoons olive oil
- 6 cloves minced garlic
- 3 stalks minced celery plus leaves
- 1 cup sliced mushrooms (optional)
- 3 cups tomato sauce
- ½ teaspoon basil
  black pepper

SUBSTITUTIONS

Olive oil: 2 tablespoons canola or safflower oil
Garlic: 1 small chopped onion
Celery: ½ chopped green bell pepper; 2 chopped zucchini
Tomato sauce: 2 6-ounce cans tomato paste and 2 cans water
Basil: ½ teaspoon oregano, thyme, or marjoram

In a frying pan, heat the oil and sauté the garlic and celery for 2 to 3 minutes. Add the mushrooms and sauté until tender. Add the tomato sauce, basil, and pepper. Correct the seasonings with more basil or garlic powder. Simmer gently for 10 to 15 minutes. Serve with Basic Polenta or Eggplant Pizza.

Basic Cream Sauce I

Makes 1 cup

- 2 tablespoons butter or margarine
- 2 tablespoons whole wheat pastry flour
- 1 cup goat milk
  sea salt and black pepper

SUBSTITUTIONS

Whole wheat pastry flour: 2 tablespoons oat, soy, spelt, brown rice, or
    quinoa flour
Goat milk: 1 cup rice or soy milk

In a frying pan, melt the butter and stir in the flour, letting the mixture cook over low heat for 3 to 4 minutes. Pour in the milk slowly, stirring continually to prevent lumps. Let cook until desired thickness is achieved. Add salt and pepper and serve immediately with Stuffed Greens or Basic Asparagus.

Basic Cream Sauce II

Makes 1 cup

> 2   tablespoons butter or margarine
> 1½ tablespoons cornstarch
> 1   cup goat milk
>   sea salt and black pepper

SUBSTITUTIONS
Cornstarch: 1½ tablespoons arrowroot or kuzu
Goat milk: 1 cup rice or soy milk

In a frying pan, melt the butter. In a small bowl, combine the cornstarch with 3 tablespoons and mix well. Add remaining milk to the butter and slowly heat. When hot (not boiling), add the cornstarch mixture and stir until desired thickness is achieved. Add salt and pepper and serve immediately with Classic Crepes or any steamed vegetable.

VARIATIONS
Double either Basic recipe and sauté ½ cup chopped green bell pepper (or red or yellow or a combination of bell peppers) in the butter. Add ½ cup grated Monterey Jack goat cheese and serve immediately. This sauce is good with pasta or cauliflower and other vegetables.

Use either Basic recipe and add any of the following for an herb cream sauce: 1 teaspoon dill, tarragon, oregano, parsley, marjoram, thyme, or curry, 2 teaspoons paprika, or ¼ to ½ teaspoon nutmeg. Wonderful with vegetables!

Double either Basic recipe and add 1 tablespoon shallot and 2 table-spoons dried basil or 7 leaves of fresh basil. Sauté the minced shallot in the butter and continue with recipe. Add basil with the salt and pepper. Great with pasta, fish, or grain dishes.

Use either Basic recipe and add one of the following: 2 cloves minced garlic, 1 large chopped green onion, 2 tablespoons chopped yellow onion,

2 tablespoons chopped leek, or 2 teaspoons shallot. Sauté in the butter and proceed with the basic recipe.

Pesto

Makes 2 cups

> 2 cups fresh basil leaves
> 4 cloves garlic
> ½ cup pinenuts
>   sea salt and black pepper
> ½ cup olive oil

SUBSTITUTIONS
Pinenuts: ½ cup almonds or walnuts
Olive oil: ½ cup canola or safflower oil

In a blender, combine the basil, garlic, pinenuts, and salt and pepper and blend until smooth. With the blender running, add the oil in a steady slow stream and blend until all oil is emulsified. Refrigerate in a covered container or serve immediately with Basic Pasta or spread on Basic Polenta.

Nut White Sauce

Makes 2½ cups

> ½ cup cashews
> 2 cups water
> 2 tablespoons butter
> 2 tablespoons minced onion
> 3 tablespoons arrowroot
>   sea salt and black pepper

SUBSTITUTIONS
Cashews: ½ cup almonds or walnuts
Arrowroot: 3 tablespoons cornstarch or kuzu
Onion: 2 teaspoons onion powder
Butter: 2 tablespoons olive or canola oil

In a blender, grind the cashews to a fine powder. Add the water in a steady stream, blend until smooth, and set aside. In a frying pan, melt the butter and sauté the onion for 2 to 3 minutes or until onion is transparent. Add the arrowroot to the butter and stir well. Slowly add the cashew mixture, stirring constantly over a medium flame until desired thickness is achieved. Add salt and pepper and serve immediately with Nutloaf or any steamed vegetable.

VARIATIONS

Add one or more of the following: 1 teaspoon curry, tarragon, dill, marjoram, oregano, paprika, thyme, or parsley, or ⅛ to ¼ teaspoon cayenne.

Add one or more of the following: ½ teaspoon paprika, ¼ teaspoon thyme, and ½ cup chopped pimento. This sauce can be chilled and used as a dip for crackers, chips, or vegetables.

Add ½ diced red pepper or ½ cup sliced mushrooms or both. Add ½ teaspoon of your favorite herb.

Walnut Sauce

Makes ½ cup

½ cup walnuts
2 cloves minced garlic
1½ tablespoons butter
1½ tablespoons flour
½ cup water

SUBSTITUTIONS

Walnuts: ½ cup pecans
Garlic: ¼ chopped onion; ½ minced shallot
Butter: 1½ tablespoons olive or canola oil

In a blender, grind the walnuts to a fine powder and set aside. In a frying pan, melt the butter sauté the garlic for 2 to 3 minutes. Stir in the flour, letting the mixture cook over low heat for 3 to 4 minutes. Slowly add the walnuts and water. Let cook until desired thickness is achieved. Garnish with chopped walnuts or parsley. Serve with Noodles and Cabbage.

Quick Walnut Sauce
To cut down the percentage of fat, blend the walnuts and the garlic in the blender until smooth. Add water or vegetable broth to desired consistency. Heat in saucepan and serve garnished with chopped walnuts or parsley.

Dill Soy Cucumber Sauce

Makes 1½ cups

    1 peeled, seeded cucumber
    1 cup soy sour cream
    ¼ cup minced onion
    3 tablespoons lemon juice
    ½ teaspoon dill weed
       sea salt and black pepper

SUBSTITUTIONS
Soy sour cream: 1 cup goat sour cream
Onion: 2 tablespoons minced shallot; ¼ cup chopped green onion
Lemon juice: 3 tablespoons lime juice

In a mixing bowl, grate cucumber. In another bowl, combine the sour cream, onion, lemon juice, dill, and salt and pepper. Add cucumber and mix well. Serve with Fish Kebobs, as a dip for vegetables, or even as a salad dressing.

Split Pea Sauce

Makes 1 cup

    ½   cup yellow split peas
    1½ cups vegetable stock
    1   teaspoon onion powder
    ¼   teaspoon nutmeg
        sea salt and black pepper
    1   tablespoon fresh chopped cilantro

SUBSTITUTIONS
Onion powder: ½ teaspoon garlic powder
Cilantro: 1 tablespoon chopped fresh parsley

In a saucepan, combine the split peas, vegetable stock, onion powder, nutmeg, and salt and pepper. Bring to a boil, then reduce heat and simmer gently for 45 minutes to one hour. Transfer to a blender, add the cilantro, and blend until smooth. Great on potatoes, carrots, or cauliflower.

Lentil Sauce

Makes 1 cup

- ½ cup lentils
- 1 cup Vegetable Stock (page 230)
- ½ chopped onion
- 1 stalk chopped celery plus leaves
- ¼ teaspoon thyme
- 2 tablespoons chopped fresh parsley
  sea salt and black pepper

SUBSTITUTION
Onion: 1 minced shallot; 1 chopped leek

In a saucepan, combine all the ingredients and bring to a boil. Reduce heat and simmer gently for 45 minutes to one hour. Transfer to a blender and blend until smooth. Serve with Lentil Loaf or Basic Rice.

Basic Bean Sauce

Makes 1 cup

- 2 tablespoons canola oil
- 2 cloves minced garlic
- ½ chopped green bell pepper
- 1½ cups cooked pinto beans
- ⅓ cup water
- 1 teaspoon cumin

SUBSTITUTIONS
Canola oil: 2 tablespoons olive or safflower oil
Garlic: ½ minced onion; 2 minced shallots
Green bell pepper: ½ cup seeded, chopped green chilies
Pinto beans: 1½ cups cooked black, red, or aduki beans
Water: ⅓ cup vegetable stock
Cumin: 1 teaspoon marjoram or oregano; 2 tablespoons chopped fresh
    cilantro

In a frying pan, heat the oil and sauté the garlic and bell pepper for 2 to
3 minutes until tender. Set aside. In a blender, combine the beans, water,
cumin, and bell pepper mixture and blend well. Serve with Grain Loaf.
Also good with quinoa, millet, buckwheat, corn, and rice.

VARIATION
For extra spice add ¼ teaspoon cayenne, 1 teaspoon chili powder, ½ teaspoon red pepper flakes, or ½ chopped and seeded jalapeño.

Spicy Pepper Sauce
Makes ½ cup

    1 red bell pepper
    ¼ cup water
    1 chopped green onion
    ½ seeded, minced jalapeño
        sea salt and black pepper

SUBSTITUTIONS
Red bell pepper: 1 yellow bell pepper
Water: ¼ cup vegetable stock
Green onion: 1 tablespoon chopped chives
Jalapeño: ¼ teaspoon cayenne or red pepper flakes

Roast red pepper directly over gas flame or under the broiler until charred.
Place pepper to steam in a paper bag for 10 minutes. Remove pepper
from bag, scrape off the skin, and seed and chop. In a blender, combine
pepper with water, green onion, jalapeño, and salt and pepper and blend
well. Serve with Steamed Potatoes or Basic Polenta.

Garlic Sauce

Makes ½ cup

    8 cloves minced garlic
    3 tablespoons butter or margarine
    1 tablespoon spelt flour
    ¾ cup water
    1 tablespoon chopped fresh parsley

SUBSTITUTIONS
Spelt flour: 1 tablespoon rice, oat, quinoa, whole wheat pastry or soy
    flour
Water: ¾ cup vegetable stock

In a frying pan, melt the butter and sauté the garlic until tender. Stir in
the flour, letting the mixture cook over low heat for 3 to 4 minutes. Pour
in the water slowly, stirring continually to prevent lumps. Let cook until
desired thickness is achieved. Add the parsley and serve immediately.
The sauce may also be pureed in a blender for a smooth sauce. Serve
with Nutloaf or any steamed vegetables.

Dips

Basic Salsa

Makes 2 cups

    4 diced tomatoes
    1 small chopped red onion
    1 seeded, minced jalapeño
    1 clove minced garlic (optional)
    4 tablespoons chopped fresh cilantro
    1 tablespoon lemon juice
       sea salt and black pepper

SUBSTITUTIONS
Red onion: ½ medium chopped white onion; 2 minced shallots; 4
    chopped green onions
Jalapeño: 1 seeded, minced serrano chili
Lemon juice: 1 tablespoon lime juice or cold water

In a mixing bowl, combine all the ingredients and mix well. Refrigerate in a covered container or serve immediately. Great with chips, tortillas, rice, black beans, and eggs.

Green Salsa

Makes 3 cups

- 2 cups chopped tomatillos
- 1 chopped white onion
- 2 cloves minced garlic
- 1½ serrano chilies
- ½ peeled, pitted, chopped avocado
     sea salt and black pepper
- 1 cup water
- 4 tablespoons chopped fresh cilantro

SUBSTITUTIONS
White onion: 3 minced shallots
Serrano chilies: 1 seeded, minced jalapeño

In a blender, combine the tomatillos, onion, garlic, chilies, avocado, and salt and pepper and blend. Add the water and blend until smooth. Pour into a serving dish and garnish with the cilantro.

Guacamole

Makes 1 cup

- 2 pitted, peeled, chopped avocados
- ½ small chopped red onion
- 1 seeded, chopped jalapeño
- 3 tablespoons chopped fresh cilantro
- 2 tablespoons lemon juice
- ½ small chopped tomato (optional)
     sea salt and black pepper

SUBSTITUTIONS
Red onion: 3 chopped green onions; 1 minced shallot
Jalapeño: 1½ seeded, chopped serrano chilies

Cilantro: 3 tablespoons chopped fresh parsley
Lemon juice: 2 tablespoons lime juice

In a mixing bowl, combine all the ingredients and mix well. Refrigerate in a covered container or serve immediately.

Bean Dip

Makes 1½ cups

- 1 cup cooked black beans
- 2 tablespoons water
- 2 cloves minced garlic
- ¼ cup chopped yellow onion
- ½ chopped red bell pepper
- 1 teaspoon lemon juice
- 1 teaspoon oregano
   sea salt and black pepper

SUBSTITUTIONS
Black beans: 1 cup pinto or red beans
Lemon juice: 1 teaspoon lime juice
Oregano: 1 teaspoon thyme or marjoram

In a blender, combine all the ingredients and blend until smooth. Garnish with chopped onion, tomato, or parsley. Refrigerate in a covered container or serve immediately.

Spicy Bean Dip

Makes 1 cup

- 1 cup cooked red beans
- 2 tablespoons water
- 2 cloves minced garlic
- ¼ teaspoon cumin seed
- ½ teaspoon chili powder
- ¼ teaspoon red pepper flakes
- 1 teaspoon lemon juice
   sea salt and black pepper

SUBSTITUTIONS

Red beans: 1 cup cooked black, aduki, or pinto beans

Red pepper flakes: ½ seeded, minced jalapeño or serrano chile; ⅛ teaspoon cayenne pepper

Lemon juice: 1 teaspoon lime juice

In a blender, combine all the ingredients and blend until smooth. Garnish with chopped parsley or chilies. Refrigerate in a covered container or serve immediately.

Sesame Eggplant Dip

Makes 1½ cups

- 1 eggplant
- 1 whole clove garlic
- 1 tablespoon canola oil
- 1 clove minced garlic
- 1 chopped green bell pepper
- 1 chopped tomato
- 1 tablespoon lemon juice
  sea salt or kelp and black pepper
- 1 tablespoon chopped fresh parsley
- 1 tablespoon sesame seeds

SUBSTITUTIONS

Canola oil: 1 tablespoon olive or safflower oil

Garlic: ½ chopped onion; 1 minced shallot

Green bell pepper: 1 chopped red or yellow bell pepper

Lemon juice: 1 tablespoon lime juice

Parsley: 1 tablespoon oregano or marjoram

Sesame seeds: 1 tablespoon sunflower or flax seed

Preheat the oven to 375 degrees F. Chop the whole garlic clove and insert in the eggplant. Bake the eggplant for 1 hour or until soft. In a frying pan, heat the oil and sauté the minced garlic and the bell pepper for 2 to 3 minutes or until tender. Set aside. Cool and peel the eggplant. In a mixing bowl, mash eggplant and add bell pepper mixture, tomato, lemon juice, and salt and pepper. Mix well. In a frying pan, lightly toast the sesame seeds. Garnish dip with parsley and sesame seeds.

VARIATION
For a completely smooth dip, combine all the ingredients in the blender and blend until smooth. Garnish as above.

🦋 Creamy Dips

Basic Cream Dip
Makes 1½ cups

> 1 cup soy sour cream
> 2 tablespoons lemon juice
> ¼ cup chopped onion
> 1 clove minced garlic (optional)
>   sea salt and black pepper

SUBSTITUTIONS
Soy sour cream: 1 cup goat ricotta cheese
Lemon juice: 2 tablespoons orange juice
Onion: 1 large chopped green onion; 1 tablespoon chopped chives
If allergic to garlic and onion, substitute: 1 tablespoon red or green bell
    pepper and 1 tablespoon celery.

In a blender, combine all the ingredients and blend until smooth. Add more lemon juice if needed for desired consistency. Refrigerate in a covered container or serve immediately.

VARIATIONS
Omit the garlic and add another ¼ cup chopped onion and 1 teaspoon chopped fresh parsley. Blend well.

Omit the onion and add 2 cloves of garlic and 1 teaspoon oregano or marjoram. Blend well.

Add 2 teaspoons dill. Blend well.

Add 1½ teaspoons curry powder. Blend well. Homemade chutney, is delightful addition.

After blending the basic recipe, add ¼ cup crumbled goat feta or herbed soy cheese

Omit the garlic and add ½ cup cooked pureed spinach, watercress, or carrot and ¼ teaspoon nutmeg. Blend well. Add a little more onion at the very end for a little texture. Sprinkle with nutmeg as garnish.

🦋 Fruit Dips

Basic Fruit Dip I

Makes 1 cup

- 1 cup plain goat yogurt
- 2 teaspoons lemon juice
- ¼ teaspoon cinnamon

SUBSTITUTIONS

Goat yogurt: 1 cup soy yogurt

Lemon juice: 2 teaspoons orange, pineapple, raspberry, boysenberry, peach, blueberry, or papaya juice

Cinnamon: ¼ teaspoon nutmeg

In a blender, combine all the ingredients and blend well. Add more lemon juice for a thinner consistency. Refrigerate in a covered container or serve immediately.

Basic Fruit Dip II

Makes 1½ cup

- 1 cup plain goat or soy yogurt
- 1 teaspoon lemon juice
- ½ banana
- ⅛ teaspoon ground or fresh ginger

SUBSTITUTIONS

Goat yogurt: 1 cup plain soy yogurt

Lemon juice: 1 teaspoon orange juice

In a blender, combine all the ingredients and blend well. Add more lemon juice for a thinner consistency. Refrigerate in a covered container or serve immediately.

Use either Basic recipe and add ¼ cup pureed mango, papaya, raspberry, or kiwi. Blend well.

Use either Basic recipe and add ¼ cup chopped dates, currants, coconut, minced nuts, minced fruit, figs, or sunflower or other seeds. Blend well.

Almond Cream Surprise

    1 cup almonds
    ¼ cup water
    1 tablespoon lemon juice
    1 tablespoon honey
    ¼ teaspoon almond extract (optional)
    ¼ teaspoon cinnamon

SUBSTITUTIONS
Almonds: 1 cup cashews or hazelnuts
Lemon juice: 1 tablespoon orange juice
Almond extract: ½ teaspoon almond liquid (page 205)
Cinnamon: ¼ teaspoon nutmeg
Honey: 2 tablespoons rice syrup or barley malt

Blanch the almonds in boiling water for 2 to 3 minutes. Drain the almonds and remove the skins. In a blender, coarsely grind the almonds. Remove about 2 tablespoons of nuts, then continue grinding to a fine powder. Add the water, lemon juice, honey, almond extract, and cinnamon and blend until smooth. Stir in the nuts and refrigerate in a covered container or serve immediately.

VARIATIONS
Add ¼ cup pureed peach or raspberry. Garnish with the fresh fruit.

    Omit the honey and stir in 2 tablespoons any melted and cooled sugarless jam.

    Omit the nutmeg or cinnamon and add ¼ teaspoon ground or fresh ginger.

    Add ¼ cup minced dates, currants, sunflower seeds, figs, or coconut.

CHAPTER 25

Canning Hints, Helps, and Recipes

BESIDES "CANNING" FRUITS, VEGETABLES, and other products in jars, canning also includes freezing and dehydrating. To adequately cover the subject of canning would require a whole book. The following information is provided to clarify a few misconceptions. A major misconception regarding canning is the presumed need for sugar. Only in very large amounts can sugar act as a preservative; other alternative sweeteners can be used for canning, jams, and jellies. Foods can also be canned in water or in their own juice. The results will be just as good, if not better. For more information regarding canning, see page 472 for some excellent books on the subject.

There are several advantages to canning or preserving your own food, especially if it is from your chemical-free garden. You will know what is in the food; it makes use of what you have available; you control the amount of sweetener, if any; and the nutrients are captured right out of the garden. Another wonderful advantage of preserving your own food is that it tastes closer to fresh. Fruits canned in honey are beautiful to look at and do not lose their color as quickly as fruits preserved in sugar. Honey enhances and sustains the flavor of most fruit—peaches will taste like real peaches. When you are making sugar-free jams and jellies, the fruit has to be either frozen or processed in canning jars that can be sealed.

🦋 Sweeteners for Canning Syrups

Fruit Concentrates
Concentrated fruit juice is an excellent sweetener. Some can be purchased at the store or you can make your own. Frozen "pure" apple,

orange, pineapple, and grape juice is available in the freezer section of
your local supermarket. Be sure to check the label! Liquid white grape
juice concentrate can be found at the health food store. Other fruit concentrates, like apple, should become available as the demand increases—
watch your local stores and keep asking. Concentrates can be made from
juice by gently simmering (slow cooking prevents flavor changes and
prevents scorching) and reducing the volume by one half. You can also
create your own juice concentrates by using the discarded portion of
apples (peel and core as you would in preparing for apple jelly only keep
simmering it down), or simmering dried fruits, like raisins, pineapple,
dates, and apricots.

Honey

Light, local honey will provide the best flavor. Honey used in moderation will complement your favorite fruit. It enhances the flavor, adds to
the beauty, and creates a richness to the product. It works well in the
canning of fruit, jams, and jellies, and even in preserves like relishes,
pickles, and chutney.

Other Sweeteners

Alternative "safe" sweeteners that are appropriate for canning are: rice
syrup, maple syrup used as a light syrup, grape or apple juice concentrate, grape/rice granular concentrate, and date sugar in preserves. Experiment with vegetable glycerin as a sweetener before using it.

❧ Canning

There is nothing like the feeling of satisfaction after a day of canning,
seeing the shelves lined with your hard work. Fruits present the biggest
problem because they are normally canned in a heavy sugar syrup. Unless
you are using one to two times as much sugar as fruit, it will not preserve it. The canning process itself, seals, protects and preserves the fruit.
The most sugar can do is improve the flavor, which it doesn't.

Sugar Alternatives in Canning

Can the fruit in water. This is the most healthful, but not necessarily the
most palatable.

Can the fruit in juice processed from the same fruit. Select riper, slightly bruised fruit. Make sure all "bad spots" are removed and process in your juicer or blender (bottled juice will also work). Replace juice amount in the same proportions as the syrup. A little lemon juice will enhance the flavor.

Use juice combinations (like apple juice with pears) for canning.

Use a syrup made from fruit juice.

Make a honey syrup and proceed as usual.

Make a syrup from an alternative sweeteners and proceed as usual.

Syrups for Canning

When choosing one of these sweeteners and syrups, the actual sweetness of the fruit should be considered. These syrups can be used for canning or freezing.

Syrups for Canning
(4 Cups of Fruit)

	Honey	Other Sweetener *(grape or apple juice concentrate,* *rice syrup, maple syrup)*	Water
Light	½ cup	1 cup	3 cups
Medium	½ cup	1 cup	2 cups
Heavy	½ cup	1 cup	1 cup

Grape or Apple Fruit Juice Syrup (not concentrate)

	Fruit Juice	Lemon Juice	Water
Light	⅓ cup	1 teaspoon	1 cup
Medium	⅔ cup	1½ teaspoons	1 cup
Heavy	1 cup	2 teaspoons	0 cup

Sweetener/Fruit Combinations

Fruits	Honey	Other Sweeteners
Soft/sweet fruits	Yes	Yes
Sour or hard fruits	Yes	Yes
Berries	No	Yes (grape or apple juice concentrate, rice syrup)

🦋 Jams and Jellies

Making your own fresh jams or jellies can be rewarding and fun. Because there is no sugar, the fruit needs to be processed in an open kettle method or steamer, for 10 minutes after it has returned to a boil or steam. Use the half pint or pint size canning jars with the sealable lids. See the chart for jelling agents. The amount of sweetener used will depend upon the sweetness of the fruit used and your own personal taste.

Jelling Agents for Jams and Jellies
(4 Cups of Fruit)

Sweetener	Agar	Gelatin	Pectin
¾ cup honey	2-3 tablespoons	2 tablespoons	3 ounces liquid
1½ cup syrup/ concentrate	3 tablespoons	3 tablespoons	4 ounces liquid
1½ cup grape/rice concentrate	2-3 tablespoons	2 tablespoons	3 ounces liquid

Low-Methoxyl Pectin

Low-methoxyl pectin will gel unsugared jams and jellies. This type of pectin is necessary when you are not using sugar. It can be used with any type of sweetener or even pure juice. It is activated by the calcium naturally present in most fruits. Extra calcium is sometimes required. Below is a conversion chart.

Calcium (di-calcium phosphate) works with low methoxyl pectin.

Use ⅛ teaspoon to ¼ cup water and shake before using. This mixture will store well.

For sweeteners, see the chart on page 138 to convert to other sweeteners.

Low-Methoxyl Pectin Conversion Chart

Fruit Type (4 cups)	Lemon Juice	Sweetener	Low-Methoxyl Pectin	Calcium
Berries	4 tablespoons	1 cup grape juice concentrate	2 teaspoons	2 teaspoons
Soft/sweet	¼ cup	¾ cup honey plus ½ cup water	1 tablespoon	4 teaspoons
Sour/hard	¼ cup	¾ cup plus 2 tablespoons honey plus ½ cup water	1 tablespoon	4 teaspoons

General Directions

After preparing the fruit for jam or jelly, follow these general directions.

Low-Methoxyl Pectin
Stir the pectin into the sweetener. Add the mixture to the fruit heated to a rolling boil. Bring to a rolling boil again and boil for the appropriate time for that specific fruit. Add the calcium solution and stir well. Remove from heat, skim if necessary, pour into sterilized jars, and process in canner or freeze.

Agar
Combine the sweetener with the fruit, reserving ½ cup. Bring the sweetener and fruit to a boil for 2 minutes and then reduce heat to simmer. Stir the agar into the reserved ½ cup, mix well, and add to the simmering jam. Remove from heat, skim if necessary, pour into sterilized jars, and process in canner or freeze.

Gelatin
Follow the directions for agar.

Pectin
Use a high pectin and high acid fruit. High pectin and high acid fruits include apples, plums, grapes, blackberries, cherries, raspberries, cranberries, loganberries, guava, and quince. Stir the pectin into the fruit. Bring to a boil. Add the sweetener and bring to rolling boil. Boil 4 minutes for jam and 1 minute for jelly. Remove from heat, skin if necessary, pour into sterilized jars, and process in canner or freeze.

🦋 Dehydrating

Dehydrating the produce from your garden or marketplace is an excellent way to preserve foods. Some foods, like apricots, will have an increase in their nutritional value. For others, some of the nutrients may be lost. In general it is fun, simple, and nutritious. Most foods can be cut and placed on the racks without any other process involved. Sulfur and other chemicals are not necessary. Store in a hard, safe plastic or safe metal or glass container. Do not store in plastic bags for any length of time. There are several good commercial dehydrators on the market. For information about dehydrators or further instructions on how to dehydrate, see pages 464–472.

🦋 Canning Recipes

Catsup

Makes 3 quarts

> 5 quarts chopped tomatoes
> 5 medium sliced onions
> 1 chopped red bell pepper (optional)
> ¼ scant cup honey
> 1 tablespoon blackstrap molasses (omit if using other sweetener)
> 1 spice bag containing:
>   1 cinnamon stick
>   1 teaspoon whole cloves

2 teaspoons allspice
1 teaspoon mace
¼ teaspoon nutmeg
1 teaspoon dill seed
2 teaspoons celery seed
¼ teaspoon dry mustard
½ clove garlic
1 bay leaf
2 cups apple cider vinegar
sea salt and cayenne pepper

SUBSTITUTIONS
Red bell pepper: 1 chopped green bell pepper
Honey: ½ cup rice syrup, apple or grape juice concentrate
Apple cider vinegar: 2 cups lemon juice

In a large soup pot, combine the tomatoes, onions, and red pepper and simmer until soft. Transfer tomato mixture to a blender and blend until smooth. Return mixture to soup pot and bring to a boil. Add the spice bag and boil until liquid is reduced by half. Remove the spice bag and add the vinegar. Reduce heat and simmer for 8 to 12 minutes. Add salt and cayenne pepper to taste. Pour into sterile pint or half-pint canning jars and seal.

Real Tomato Sauce

Makes 3½ quarts

1¼ cups olive or canola oil
3 cups chopped onion
5 quarts chopped tomatoes
1 cup salt-free tomato paste
4 tablespoons basil
6 teaspoons oregano
15 cloves minced garlic
8 cups water
sea salt and black pepper

SUBSTITUTIONS
Onion: 3 cups chopped green onion; ½ cup minced shallots; 30 cloves
    minced garlic
Oregano: 6 tablespoons marjoram

In a soup pot, heat the oil and sauté the onions for 2 to 3 minutes or
until transparent and have a little color. Add the tomatoes, tomato paste,
basil, oregano, and some salt and pepper. Simmer for 5 minutes, stirring occasionally. Add the minced garlic cloves. Stir briefly and add the
water. Simmer sauce over low heat for 1 to 2 hours. If too thick, add
more water. If too thin, add more tomato paste. Pour into sterile pint
or half-pint canning jars and seal.

Chili Sauce

Makes 2 quarts

        4   quarts peeled, quartered tomatoes
        3   diced green chili peppers
        2   large chopped onions
        2   tablespoons honey
        1   teaspoon blackstrap molasses (omit if using other sweetener)
    1½   cups apple cider vinegar
        1   tablespoon sea salt
        1   teaspoon dry mustard
        2   teaspoons black pepper
    1½   teaspoon allspice
        1   teaspoon celery seed
        ½   teaspoon cinnamon
        ¼   teaspoon ginger
        ¼   teaspoon nutmeg
        ¼   teaspoon cloves

SUBSTITUTIONS
Onion: 6 minced shallots; 2 bunches chopped green onion
Honey: 4 tablespoons rice syrup or apple juice concentrate
Apple cider vinegar: 1½ cups lemon juice

In a soup pot, combine all the ingredients and simmer slowly for 2 hours, stirring occasionally, or until mixture is very thick. Transfer mixture to a blender and blend until smooth. Pour into sterile pint or half-pint canning jars and seal.

Zucchini Bread and Butter Pickles

Makes 5 quarts

 4 quarts thinly sliced zucchini
 4 thinly sliced yellow onions
 ½ cup sea salt
 4 cups apple cider vinegar
 3 cups grape or apple juice concentrate (cooked down from 6 cups)
 1 cup water
 2 tablespoons mustard seed
 1½ teaspoon turmeric
 1 teaspoon whole cloves
 1 teaspoon celery seed

SUBSTITUTIONS

Yellow onions: 4 thinly sliced white onions; 12 minced shallots
Grape juice concentrate: 3 cups apple juice concentrate (cooked down from 6 cups)
Apple cider vinegar: 4 cups lemon juice

In a mixing bowl, combine the zucchini, onions, and salt and cover with ice for 3 hours. Drain and rinse. Transfer zucchini mixture to a soup pot and add vinegar, grape juice concentrate, water, mustard seed, turmeric, cloves, and celery seed and bring to a boil for 4 minutes. Pack in hot, sterilized jars and process in boiling water bath or steamer for 15 minutes.

Green Tomato Chutney

Makes 1 quart

 2¼ cups chopped green tomatoes
 2¼ cups peeled, cored, chopped tart apples
 1 cup minced onion

1 thinly sliced lemon
½ cup honey
½ cup apple cider vinegar
½ cup water
1 tablespoon mustard seed
1 teaspoon ginger
¾ teaspoon sea salt
¼ teaspoon allspice
⅛ teaspoon cayenne powder
1½ cups currants or raisins (optional)

SUBSTITUTIONS
Onion: 3 minced shallots; 3 cloves minced garlic
Honey: ¾ cup rice syrup; 1 cup apple juice concentrate
Apple cider vinegar: ½ cup lemon juice

In a soup pot, combine all the ingredients and simmer for 20 minutes or until the fruit is soft and the flavors are well blended. Pack in hot, sterilized jars and process for 5 minutes in the boiling water bath or a steamer.

Appendix I

Food Family Lists

The following foods are broken down into botanical families. Frequently, people are allergic or addicted to one or more members of the same family. This list will assist you in understanding the connection between allergens and the addiction process, and their location in a food family. For example, chocolate, cola, and cocaine are all in the same family. This list also gives you further information regarding other possible food choices and can help to clarify your questions and choices.

If you are allergic to most of the grains in the grass family, by searching the list you will find that the grain buckwheat is in the buckwheat family and not related to wheat, making this grain safe to eat.

Banana

Arrowroot
Banana
Plantain

Bellflower Thistle

All lettuce
Artichoke
Dandelion
Endive
Escarole
Jerusalem artichoke
Romaine lettuce

Safflower
Sunflower
Tarragon

Birch

Hazelnut (filbert)

Brassica

Broccoli
Brussels sprout
Cauliflower
Chinese cabbage
Collards
Green cabbage

Horseradish
Kale
Kohlrabi
Mustard greens
Mustard seed
Radish
Red cabbage
Rutabaga
Turnip
Watercress

Buckthorn

Cream of tartar
Grape

Buckwheat

Buckwheat
Garden sorrel
Rhubarb

Carica

Papaya

Carrot

Anise
Caraway
Carrot
Celery
Celery root
Chervil
Coriander
Cumin
Dill
Fennel
Parsley
Parsnip

Cashew

Cashew
Mango
Pistachio
Poison oak
Poison ivy
Poison sumac

Crustacean

Crab
Crayfish
Lobster
Prawn
Shrimp

Cyperacese

Water chestnut

Dillenia

Kiwi
Passion flower
Passion fruit

Ebony

Persimmon

Farinosa

Pineapple

Fish

Bass
Butterfish
Catfish
Cod
Flounder
Halibut
Herring
Perch
Salmon
Sardine
Shark
Sole
Swordfish
Trout
Tuna
Whitefish

Flax

Flaxseed

Fungus

Baker's yeast
Brewer's yeast
Mushroom
Truffle

Ginger

Cardamom
Ginger
Turmeric

Gourd

All summer squash
All winter squash
Cantaloupe
Casaba
Chayote
Crane
Crenshaw
Cucumber
Gherkin
Honeydew
Muskmelon
Persian melon
Pumpkin
Watermelon

Grasses

Bamboo shoots
Barley
Cane sugar
Corn
Corn sugar
Lemon grass
Millet
Oats

Rice
Rye
Sorghum
Triticale
Wheat
Wild rice

Heath

Bearberry
Bilberry
Blueberry
Cranberry
Huckleberry

Honeysuckle

Elderberry

Laurel

Avocado
Bay leaf
Cinnamon

Legume

Alfalfa
All beans
All peas
Carob
Fenugreek
Guar gum
Gum acacia
Jicama
Kudzu
Lentils
Lupine
Peanut
Soy

Split pea
String bean

Lily

Aloe vera
Asparagus
Chive
Garlic
Leek
Onion
Sarsaparilla
Shallot

Madder

Coffee

Mallow

Cottonseed oil
Okra

Mammal

Beef
Bison
Butter
Cow's milk
Goat
Goat dairy
Goat yogurt
Hard cow cheese
Lamb
Ox
Pork
Rabbit
Soft cow cheese
Yogurt

Maple

Maple sugar
Maple syrup

Mollusk

Abalone
Clam
Cockle
Mussel
Octopus
Oyster
Scallop
Snails
Squid

Mulberry

Breadfruit
Fig
Mulberry

Myristicase

Allspice
Clove
Guava
Jamaica pepper
Mace
Nutmeg

Myrtle

Allspice
Clove
Eucalyptus
Guava

Nightshade

Cayenne
Chili pepper
Eggplant
Garden peppers
Paprika
Pimento
Potato
Sesame
Sweet potato
Tobacco
Tomatillo
Tomato
Yam

Nightshade Mint

All mints
Basil
Marjoram
Oregano
Rosemary
Sage
Thyme

Orchid

Vanilla

Palm

Coconut
Date

Pepper

Black pepper
White pepper

Pink

Beet
Beet sugar
Lamb's quarters
Spinach
Swiss chard

Poppy

Poppy seed

Poultry

Chicken
Chicken egg
Cornish hen
Duck
Duck egg
Game hem
Goose
Pheasant
Quail
Turkey
Turkey egg

Protea

Macadamia

Purgel

Curry
Tapioca

Rose

Almond
Apple
Apricot
Blackberry

Boysenberry
Crabapple
Cherry
Dewberry
Loganberry
Loquat
Nectarine
Peach
Pear
Plum
Prune
Quince
Raspberry
Rose hips
Strawberry
Wild cherry

Rue

Grapefruit
Kumquat
Lemon
Lime
Orange
Tangelo
Tangerine

Sapucala

Brazil nut

Saxifrage

Currant
Gooseberry

Soapberry

Lychee nut

Stercullia

Chocolate

Cocaine

Cola nut

Gum karay

Theobromine

Walnut

Black walnut

Butternut

Chestnut

Hickory nut

Pecan

Walnut

🦋 Toxin List

The list below provides names of some of the more common toxins to be found in our environment–air, water, food, and at home or office. The information will assist you in your label reading and awareness of products that may contain one or more of the toxins listed below. As many of the toxins as possible should be eliminated from your diet and environment as they contribute to the weakening of the immune system and the disease process.

There are two lists, one is of common toxins found in the air, water, food, and home and office. The second list is of food grade toxins commonly used on fresh produce. This additional information can assist those with severe allergies. If you are severely allergic to dairy products, lactase based wax may contribute to your difficulty. If you are severely allergic to molds, then dairy or meat products containing antibiotics should be avoided. READ! READ! READ!

Common Toxins

Aflatoxins	Benzene	Endrin
Alcohol	Chlordane	Epoxides
Aldrex	Chlorine	Ethyl paraben
Amidox 50	Cyclamic acid	Food additives
Amine 50	Dacamine 4-d	Food coloring
Antibiotics	DDT	Food preservatives
Aspartame (nutrasweet)	Dieldrin	Formaldehyde
Ban-oxalis	Diethyl pyrocarbamate	Grammexane
Banex	Dioctyl sodium endopest	

Common Toxins, *continued*

Heavy metals
  Aluminum
  Cadmium
  Lead
  Mercury
Heptachlor
Hydrocarbons
Latex
Lindane
Metabisulfites
Methoxone
Molds
  Aspergillus
  Fusarium
  Penicillium
  Phoma
MSG
Organophosphate
Ozone
Parasites
PCP
Petrochemicals
Pharmaceutical drugs
Phenol
Polyurethane
Propyl paraben
Radon
Recreational drugs
Saccharin

Smog
Steroids
Sulfosusccinate
Sulfur dioxide
TCA
Thiodan
Tobacco
Tordon
Trichloroethylene
Trihalomethanes
Weedone

Aluminum Sources

Air-borne contamination
  Air conditioner
  Corrosion
  Clay dust
Any cans
Baking powder
Cookware
  Pans
  Pots
Dialysis
Foil
Food additives
Hot water supplies
  Cathodic corrosion
  prevention

Infant formulas
  Emfamil Neonatal
  Emfamil Premature
  Emfamil with Iron
  Formula
  Osterfeed
  Similac (20k and 24k
  calorie ounce)
  Similac PM 60/40
  Similac Special Care
  SMA
  Wysoy
Intravenous fluids for
  infants and adults
Pharmaceutical
  preparations
  Aluminum hydroxide
  gels
  Antacid
  Antiperspirants
  Aspirin
  Deodorants
Spices
Water supplies
  Aluminum
  flocculating agents

The above information was compiled from *Food Chemical Sensitivity* by Robert A. Buist, Ph.D. (Garden City Park, NY: Avery Publishing Group, 1988).

Food Grade Toxins

Commercially grown foods that may contain vegetable petroleum, beeswax, lactase resin base wax, or resin.

Apple	Eggplant	Peas	Sugar cane
Avocado	Melon	Pineapple	Sweet potato
Bell pepper	Nectarine	Plums	Tomato
Chili pepper	Papaya	Pomegranate	Turnip
Citrus fruit	Passion fruit	Rutabaga	Yucca
Cucumber	Peach	Squash	

🦋 Guide to Questionable Additives in Common Foods

The following list is a general guide through the maze of common food additives. Read and beware–if you can't pronounce it, don't buy it. The list is not all inclusive; thorough label reading is your best assurance of good health. Products may differ and not all items of the same variety will contain identical additives.

Baby Food

Carrageenan
Modified starch
Salt
Sweetener

Cakes, Cookies, and Pastries

Artificial color
Artificial flavor
BHA
BHT
Salt
Sulfites
Sweetener

Canned Fruits and Vegetables

Artificial color
Calcium salt
EDTA
Salt
Sulfites
Sweetener

Cereal

Artificial color
Artificial flavor
BHA
BHT
Propyl gallate
Salt
Sweetener

Condiments

Artificial color
Benzoate
EDTA
GMP
IMP
Modified starch
MSG
Polysorbate
Salt
Sulfites
Sweetener

Dairy Products

Artificial color
Artificial flavor
Carboxymethylcellulose
Carrageenan
GMP
Hydrolyzed vegetable protein
IMP
MSG
Phosphate
Salt
Sweetener
Vegetable gum

Flour Products–Baked Goods

Artificial flavor
Calcium peroxide
Chlorine
Corn syrup
Dextrin
Hydroxylated lecithin
Modified starch
Mono and diglycerides

Propionate
Salt
Sulfites
Sweetener

Frozen Desserts

Artificial color
Artificial flavor
Carrageenan
Mono and diglycerides
Salt
Sweetener
Vegetable gum

Jams and Jellies

Agar
Artificial color
Artificial flavor
Benzoate
Carboxymethylcellulose
Carrageenan
Propionates
Solvent
Sweetener
Vegetable gum

Oils, Spreads, and Shortenings

Artificial color
Artificial flavor
BHA
BHT
Dimethylpolysiloxane
ETDA
Oxystearin
Polysorbate
Propyl gallate
Salt

Pasta

Disodium phosphate
Salt
Sulfites

Pies

Artificial color
Artificial flavor
BHA
BHT
Modified starch
Salt
Sweetener

Powdered Mixes

Artificial color
Artificial flavor
DSS (dioctyl sodium
sulfo succinate)
Hydrolyzed vegetable protein
Salt
Sweetener
Vegetable gum

Prepared/Convenience Foods

Artificial color
Artificial flavor
Carrageenan
GMP
Hydrolyzed vegetable protein
IMP
Modified starch
Mono and diglyceride
MSG
Phosphate
Salt
Sweetener
Vegetable gum

Processed Meats

Artificial color
Artificial flavor
BHA
BHT
MSG
Nitrate
Nitrite
Phosphate
Propyl gallate
Salt
Sweetener

Puddings and Gelatins

Artificial color
Artificial flavor
BHA
Carrageenan
Mono and diglycerides
Polysorbate
Salt
Sweetener

Salad Dressing (Mayonnaise)

Artificial color
Artificial flavors
BHA
BHT
Carboxymethylcelluose
EDTA
GMP
IMP
Modified starch
Mono and diglycerides
Salt
Sweetener
Vegetable gum

Sauces and Gravies

Benzoate
Hydrolyzed vegetable protein
Salt
Sweeteners
Texturized vegetable protein

Snack/Junk Food

Artificial color
Artificial flavor
BHA
BHT
Brominated vegetable oil
Caffeine
GMP
Hydrolyzed vegetable protein
IMP
Modified starch
Mono and diglycerides
Propyl gallate
Salt
Sulfites
Sweetener

Soups and Mixes

Artificial color
Artificial flavor
BHA
BHT
GMP
Hydrolyzed vegetable protein
IMP
Modified starch
MSG
Propyl gallate
Salt

Sulfites
Texturized vegetable protein

Soft Drinks

Artificial color
Artificial flavor
Caffeine
Phosphoric acid
Sweeteners

Toppings and Icings

Artificial color
Artificial flavor
Carrageenan
Modified starch
Mono and diglycerides
Polysorbate
Sweetener
Vegetable gum

Yogurt

Agar
Artificial color
Artificial flavor
Carrageenan
Gelatin
Modified starch
Pectin
Sweetener
Vegetable gum

Appendix II

🦋 Sources

The purpose of this chapter is to supply you with the names and addresses of suppliers of quality products. These products have been searched out and tested. None of these companies have solicited to have themselves included. Except for some whole grain bread with yeast that might be included, these products are yeast free (no yeast, vinegar, or sugar). It is broken down into categories for easy reference. Also included in this appendix are resources for product aids for health, general information, and allergy testing laboratories.

Bean Products

ANASAZI BEANS: Adobe Milling Co., PO Box 596, Dove Creek, CO 81324

BEAN DIPS: Fantastic Foods, 1250 North McDowell Street, Petaluma, CA 94954

BEAN FLOUR: Arrowhead Mills, PO Box 2059, Hereford, TX 79045
Ener-G Foods Inc., PO Box 84487, Seattle, WA 98124

BEAN PASTA: Orgran Natural Food Products, 53-55 Lavinia Street, Athol Park, South Australia 5012

Community Mill and Bean, 267 Route 89 South, Savannah, NY 13146

Eagle Organic and Natural Food, 4007 Church Avenue, Huntsville, AR 72740

Condiments

AGAR, KUZU, KELP/DULSE: Eden Foods, 701 Clinton-Tecumseh Highway, Clinton, MI 49236

EGG REPLACER: Ener-G Foods Inc., PO Box 84487, Seattle, WA 98124

Filigree Farms, Route 2, Box 162, Okanogan, WA 98840

HERBS: Cottage Garden Herbs/ Wind River Farm, PO Box 312, Merlin, OR 97532

NO VINEGAR PICKLES AND SAUERKRAUT: Cascadian Farms, 719 Metcalf, Rockport, WA 98283

SPICES: Spice of Life, PO Box 1287, Fallbrook, CA 92028
Whitney Spice Co., PO Box 147, Duncan Mills, CA 95430

SPICES AND HERBS: Nature's Herb Co., 1010 46th Street, Emeryville, CA 94608

YEAST FREE DRESSING: The Grape Leaf, 4031 Balboa Street, San Francisco, CA 94121

"Dairy" Products

ALMONDRELLA (almond cheese): Sharon's Finest, PO Box 5020, Santa Rosa, CA 95402-5020

FRUIT SORBET: Cascadian Farms, 719 Metcalf Street, Sedro Wooley, WA 98284

GOAT CHEESE: Laura Chenel, 1550 Ridley Avenue, Santa Rosa, CA 95401
Sonnet Farms, Spectrum Marketing, 133 Copeland Street, Petaluma, CA 94952

GOAT FETA CHEESE: Domestic Cheese Co., 450 Toland Avenue, San Francisco, CA 94125

GOAT MILK AND YOGURT: Redwood Hill Farm, 10855 Occidental Road, Sebastopol, CA 95472

GOAT MILK RECIPES: California Goat Dairyman's Association, PO Box 934, Turlock, CA 95380

ORGANIC GOAT AND COW: Morningland Dairy, Route 1, Box 188B, Mountain View, MO 65548

RICE MILK AND ICE CREAM: Imagine Foods, Inc., 299 California Avenue, Palo Alto, CA 94306

SILKEN TOFU: Morinaga Milk Co., Shiba #5-33-1 Minato-Ku, Tokyo, 108 Japan

SOY CHEESE: Tofu Rella, Sharon's Finest, PO Box 5020, Santa Rosa, CA 95402

Soya Kaas Inc., 6029 La Grange Street, Atlanta, GA 30336

SOY MILK: Edensoy, Eden Food Co., 701 Clinton-Tecumseh Highway, Clinton, MI 49236

Westbrae Natural Foods, PO Box 48006, Gardenia, CA 90248

SOY PARMESAN: Soyco Foods, PO Box 5181, Newcastle, PA 16105

SOY YOGURT: Soya Latee', Soyeh Natural Inc., 29528 Union City Boulevard, Union City, CA 94587

Grain Products: Breads

ESSENE BREAD (yeast free): Lifestream, 9100 Van Horne Way, Richmond, BC, V6X 1W3 Canada

KAMUT BAGELS (yeast free): Pacific Bakery, 514 South Hill Street, Oceanside, CA 92049

RYE BREAD (yeast free): Rudolph's Specialty Bakery, 200 Rittenhouse Circle, Bristol, PA 19007

SPELT BREAD: Rudi's, 3640 Walnut Street, Boulder, CO, 80301

SPELT AND WHOLE WHEAT BREADS (yeasted): Great Harvest, 170-4 Farmers Lane, Santa Rosa, CA 95405

WHEAT FREE BREAD: Food for Life Baking Co., 299 East Doherty Street, Corona, CA 91719

WHOLE WHEAT BREAD: Alvarado Street Bakery, 500 Martin Avenue, Rohnert Park, CA 94928

Grain Products: Cereals

Eagle Organic and Natural Food, 4007 Church Avenue, Huntsville, AR 72740

CREAM OF BUCKWHEAT: Pocono, Birkette Mills, Penn Yan, NY 14527

CREAM OF RICE: Erewhon US Mills Inc., 4301 N. 30th Street, Omaha, NE 68111

CREAM OF RYE: Roman Meal, PO Box 1126, Tacoma, WA 98411

KAMUT: Kamut Association of North America, 2161 Meyers Avenue, Escondido, CA 92029

KASHA (buckwheat groats): Kashi Co., PO Box 8557, La Jolla, CA 92038-8557

PUFFED KAMUT, MILLET, RICE, AND WHEAT: Arrowhead Mills, PO Box 2059, Hereford, TX 79045

RYE AND RICE: American Prarie Mercantile Food Co., PO Box 55,
Philmont, NY 12565

VITA-SPELT (whole grain flakes): Purity Foods Inc., 2871 West Jolly
Road, Okemos, MI 48864

QUINOA, AMARANTH, WHEAT, RYE, MILLET, TEFF, WHEAT,
CRACKED WHEAT, BARLEY, OAT, RYE, AND TRITICALE
FLAKES: Arrowhead Mills, PO Box 2059, Hereford, TX 79045

Grain Products: Flour

Baker's Catalogue, PO Box 876, Norwich, VT 05055

Community Mill and Bean, 267 Route 89 South, Savannah, NY 13146

Eagle Organic and Natural Food, 4007 Church Avenue, Huntsville,
AR 72740

KAMUT FLOUR: Kamut Association of North America, 2161 Meyers
Avenue, Escondido, CA 92029

Montana Flour and Grains, PO Box 808, Okemos, MI 48864

QUINOA FLOUR: Quinoa Corporation, PO Box 1039, Torrance, CA
90506

SOY, WHEAT, RYE, TEFF, BARLEY, OAT, MILLET, AMARANTH,
BUCKWHEAT, CORN, RICE, AND KAMUT FLOUR: Arrowhead
Mills, PO Box 2059, Hereford, TX 79045

SPELT FLOUR: Vita-Spelt, Purity Foods, 2871 West Jolly Road, Big
Sandy, MT 59520

Grain Products: Pasta

BARLEY AND BARLEY AND SPINACH PASTA: Orgran Natural
Food Products, 53-55 Lavinia Street, Athol Park, South Australia
5012

BUCKWHEAT PASTA (soba) : Westbrae Natural Foods, PO Box
48006, Gardenia, CA 90248

CORN PASTA: De Boles, Nutritional Foods, Inc., Garden City Park,
NY 11040

KAMUT PASTA: Eden Food Co., 701 Clinton-Tecumseh Highway,
Clinton, MI 49236

QUINOA AND CORN PASTA: Quinoa Corporation, PO Box 1039,
Torrance, CA 90506

RICE PASTA: Pastariso Products Inc., 55 Ironside Crescent, Unit 6 & 7, Scarborough, Ontario, M1X 1N3, Canada

RICE, MILLET, AMARANTH, AND WHEAT PASTA: Health Valley Foods, 16100 Foothill Boulevard, Los Angeles, CA 90061

SPELT PASTA: Vita-Spelt, Purity Foods Inc., 2871 West Jolly Road, Okemos, MI 48864

Grain Products: Snacks

AMAZAKI PUDDING AND LIQUID: Grainaissance, 1580 62nd Street, Emeryville, CA 94608

BROWN RICE WAFERS (unsweetened): Westbrae Natural Foods, PO Box 48006, Gardenia, CA 90248

COOKIES: Health Valley Foods, 16100 Foothill Boulevard, Los Angeles, CA 90061

CORN CHIPS AND TORTILLAS: La Tortilla Factory, 3654 Standish Avenue, Santa Rosa, CA 95407

GRAIN DRINK: Barley Brew, Sundance Roasting Co., PO Box 1886, Sandpoint, ID 83865

RICE CAKES: Airin, Empress Foods, Inc., 3064 Main Street, Rancho Dominguez, CA 90221

Lundberg Family Farms, PO Box 369, Richvale, CA 95974

RYE CRACKERS: Wasa Light Rye, Sandoz Nutrition Corporation, 5100 Gamble Drive, Saint Paul, MN 55416

WHEAT CRACKERS: Hol*Grain, Parco Foods, Inc., 2200 West 138th Street, Blue Island, IL 60406

WHEAT TORTILLAS: Alvarado Street Bakery, 500 Martin Avenue, Rohnert Park, CA 94928

Jams and Jellies

APPLE CONCENTRATE: Kozlowski Farms, 5566 Gravenstein Highway, Forestville, CA 95436

GRAPE CONCENTRATE: Sorrell Ridge Farm, 100 Market Street, Port Reading, NJ 07064

LOW-METHOXYL PECTIN: Pomona's Universal Pectin, PO Box 1083, Greenfield, MA 01302

Juices

Country Fresh, PO Box 1324, Sonoma, CA 95476
R.W. Knudsen Sons, PO Box 369, Chico, CA 95927
Santa Cruz Natural Juices, PO Box 1510, Freedom, CA 95019
Westbrae Natural Foods, PO Box 48006, Gardenia, CA 90248

Nuts And Nut Butters

Kettle Foods, PO Box 664, Salem, Oregon 97308-0664
Nature's Best, 105 South Puente Street, Brae, CA 92621
Omega Nutrition USA, 6505 Aldrich Road, Ferndale, WA 98248
Sharon's Finest, PO Box 5020, Santa Rosa, CA 95402-5020
Westbrae Natural Foods, PO Box 48006, Gardenia, CA 90248

Oils

Hain Pure Food Co., 16100 Foothill Boulevard, Los Angeles, CA
    90061
Spectrum Naturals, 133 Copeland Street, Petaluma, CA 94952
Omega Nutrition USA, 6505 Aldrich Road, Ferndale, WA 98248

Organic Meat And Poultry

D'Artagnan, 399-419 Saint Paul Avenue, Jersey City, NJ 07306

Organic One-Stop Shopping

Allergy Resources, Inc., 195 Huntington Beach Drive, Colorado
    Springs, CO 80921
Green Earth, 2545 Prairie Avenue, Evanston, IL 60201
Organic Foods Express, 11003 Emack Road, Beltsville, MD 20705
Rising Sun Organic Food, PO Box 627, PA 150 & 1-80, Milesburg, PA
    16853
Specialty Organic Source, PO Box 1628, Champaign, IL 61824-1628
Trading Company, 120 South East Avenue, Fayetteville, AR 72701
Walnut Acres Organic Farms, Walnut Acres Road, Penns Creek, PA
    17862

Processed Foods

CANNED FRUITS: Nutradiet, S & W Fine Foods Inc., 3160 Crow Canyon Road, San Ramon, CA 94583

CANNED SOUPS: Hain Pure Food Co., 16100 Foothill Boulevard, Los Angeles, CA 90061
Health Valley Foods, 16100 Foothill Boulevard, Los Angeles, CA 90061

CANNED VEGETABLES: Cascadian Farms, 719 Metcalf Street, Rockport, WA 98283

FALAFEL AND PILAF: Fantastic Foods, 1250 North McDowell Boulevard, Petaluma, CA 94954

FROZEN VEGETABLES AND FRUITS: Cascadian Farms, 719 Metcalf Street, Rockport, WA 98283

Produce

Covalda Date Company, PO Box 908, Coachella, CA 92236-0908

Diamond Organics, PO Box 2159, Freedom, CA 95019

Forever Green Farms, PO Box 2976, Petaluma, CA 94953

Ronniger's Seed Potatoes, Star Route, Moyie Springs, ID 83845

Seaside Banana Garden, 6823 Santa Barbara Avenue, Ventura, CA 93001

Starr Organic Produce, PO Box 561502, Miami, FL 33256-1502

Sweeteners

BARLEY MALT: Eden Foods Inc., 701 Clinton-Tecumseh Highway, Clinton, MI 49236

BLACKSTRAP MOLASSES: Plantation, Allied Old English Inc., 100 Market Street, Port Reading, NJ 07064

DATE SUGAR: Nature's Cuisine, Nature's Best, 105 South Puente Street, Brae, CA 92621

GRAPE AND APPLE JUICE CONCENTRATE: Benard Jensen, PO Box 8, Solano Beach, CA 92075

GRAPE JUICE CONCENTRATE: Cascadian Farm, 719 Metcalf Street, Rockport, WA 98283

GRAPE AND RICE CONCENTRATE: FruitSource Associates, 445 Vick Drive, Santa Cruz, CA 95060

MAPLE SYRUP: Shady Maple Farms, 786 8th Street East, La Guadeloupe, Quebec, G0M 1G0, Canada

RICE SYRUP: Lundberg Family Farms, PO Box 369, Richvale CA 95974

VEGETABLE GLYCERIN (coconut derived): Herb Craft, 11253 Trade Center Drive, Rancho Cordova, CA 95742

Major Manufacturers

Arrowhead Mills, PO Box 2059, Hereford, TX 79045

Cascadian Farms, 719 Metcalf Street, Rockport, WA 98283

Eden Food Inc., 701 Clinton-Tecumseh Highway, Clinton, MI 49236

Fantastic Foods Inc., 1250 North McDowell Boulevard, Petaluma, CA 94954

Hain Pure Food Co., 16100 Foothill Boulevard, Los Angeles, CA 90061

Health Valley Foods Inc., 16100 Foothill Boulevard, Los Angeles, CA 90061

Westbrae Natural Foods Co., PO Box 48006, Gardenia, CA 90040

Products For Health

CANNING: Vitantonio Manufacturing Co., 34355 Vokes Drive, Eastlake, OH 44095 (800) 732-4444

DEHYDRATORS: Emergency Essentials, 165 South Mountain Way Drive, Orem, UT 84058-5119

Nutriflex Magic Air II, 1515 South 400 West, South Salt Lake City, UT, 84115

Perfect Health, Products Division, 5423 Driftwood Street, Oxnard, CA 93035

Ronco Food Dehydrator, PO Box 4120, Carlsbad, CA 92018

Richard Yolles Distribution, 1834 South Bertley Avenue, Suite 307, Los Angeles, CA 90025-4361

FRUIT AND VEGETABLE JUICERS: Krup's, 7 Pearl Court, Allendale, NJ 07401

Perfect Health, Products Division, 5423 Driftwood Street, Oxnard, CA 93035

Vita Mix Corp., 8615 Usher Road, Department YJO792, Cleveland, OH 44138

GRAIN MILLS: K-Tec, 370 East 1300 Street, Orem, UT 84058
Nutriflex Magic Mill, 1515 South 400 West, South Salt Lake City,
UT, 84115
Perfect Health, Products Division, 5423 Driftwood Street, Oxnard,
CA 93035
Richard Yolles Distribution, 1834 South Bertley Avenue, Suite 307,
Los Angeles, CA 90025-4361
SPROUT EQUIPMENT: The Sprout House, 40 Railroad Street, Great
Barrington, MA 01230
STEAM JUICER: Back to Basics Products, Inc., 11660 South State,
Draper, UT 84020

Ecological Helps

AIR CONDITIONERS: Berner Air Products Inc., PO Box 5410, New
Castle, PA 16105
CARPET: Naturlich, Old Mill Station R, Sebastopol, CA 95472
FURNACE AND AIR CONDITIONING UNITS: Thurmond Air
Quality Systems, PO Box 23037, Little Rock, AK 72221
MAGNETIC WATER SYSTEMS AND BEDS: E.T.M., PO Box 761,
Healdsburg, CA 95448
VACUUM CLEANERS: Rainbow Vacuum Distributors, Aqua-Tex
Enterprises, PO Box 395, Addison, TX 75001
WATER PURIFIER SYSTEMS: Multi-Pure Corporation, 21339
Nordhoff Street, Chatsworth, CA 91311
Pure Health Concepts, 2430 Herodian Way, Smyrna, GA 30080

General Information

Accu-Chem Laboratories, J. Laseter, Ph.D., 990 North Bowser Suite
800, Richardson, TX 75081, (214) 234-5577
Allergy Product Directory, PO Box 640, Menlo Park, CA 94026, (415)
322-1663
Allergy Specialists Referrals, Immuno Laboratories Patient Service,
1620 West Oakland Park Boulevard, Fort Lauderdale, FL 33311,
(800) 231-9197
California Certified Organic Farmers, 303 Potrero Street, Suite 51,
Santa Cruz, CA 95060, (408) 423-2263

Citizens Commission on Human Rights, 5265 Fountain Avenue, Suite 2, Los Angeles, CA 90029, (800) 522-0247

Dentists, Physicians, and Chiropractors for Environmental Illnesses, Hal Huggins, 5080 List Drive, Colorado Springs, CO 80919 (800) 331-2303

Earth Options, PO Box 1542, Sebastopol, CA 95473, (707) 829-4554

Environmental Health Network, Linda King, PO Box 1628, Harvy, LA 70058, (504) 340-2321

Environmental Protection Agency, 75 Hawthorne Street, San Francisco, CA 94501, (415) 744-1500

Health Food Business Annual Purchasing Guide, Howmark Publishing Corporation, 567 Morris Avenue, Elizabeth, NJ 07208, (908) 353-7461

Living Source, 3500 MacArthur Drive, Waco, TX 76708, (817) 756-6341

Mountain Ark Trading Co., 120 Southeast Avenue, Fayetteville, AZ 72701, (800) 643-8909

National Pesticide Telecommunication Network, Agricultural Chemistry Extension, Oregon State University, Weniger Hall 333, Corvallis, OR 97331-6502, (800) 858-7378

Natural Building Materials Network, Susan Hendrixson, 71020 Keating Avenue, Sebastapol, CA 95473, (707) 829-3959

Practical Allergy Research Foundation, Dorris J. Rapp, M.D., Assistant Professor of Pediatrics, State University of New York, Buffalo, NY 14214, (716) 645-2000

Sierra Group for Environmental Products, 433 Rivers Edge Court, Mishawaka, IN 46544, (800) 234-9517

Diagnostic Testing Laboratories

Great Smokies Diagnostic Laboratory, 18 Regent Park Boulevard, Asheville, NC 28896, (800) 522-4762

Spectra Cell Laboratories, Inc., 515 Post Oak Boulevard, Suite 830, Houston, TX 77027, (800) 227-5227

Allergy Testing Labs

Immuno Laboratories, Inc., 620 West Oakland Park Boulevard, Suite 301, Fort Lauderdale, FL 33311, (800) 231-9197

🦋 References

Part I: Food Addictions and Changing Your Ways

Badley, Lawrence E. *Healing AIDS Naturally.* Foster City, CA: Human Energy Press, 1987.

Balch, James F. and Phyllis A. Balch. *Prescription For Nutritional Healing.* Garden City, NY: Avery Publishing Group, 1990.

Braly, James. *Dr. Braly's Food Allergy and Nutrition Revolution.* New Canaan, CT: Keats Publishing, 1992.

Buist, Robert A. *Food Chemical Sensitivity.* Garden City, NY: Avery Publishing Group, 1988.

Buist, Robert A. *Food Intolerance: What Is It and How To Cope With It.* Sidney, Australia: Harper & Row, 1984.

Chaitow, Leon. *Candida Albicans.* Northhamptonshire, England: Thorsons Publishers, 1987.

Covey, Stephen R. *How to Succeed With People.* Salt Lake City, UT: Dessert Book Company, 1971.

Covey, Stephen R. *The 7 Habits of Highly Effective People.* New York, Simon & Schuster, 1989.

Covey, Stephen R. *Spiritual Roots of Human Relations.* Salt Lake City, UT: Dessert Book Company, 1970.

Crook, William G. *The Yeast Connection.* Jackson, TN: Professional Books, 1985.

Crook, William G. *Are You Allergic?* Jackson, TN: Professional Books, 1978.

Crook, William G. *Tracking Down Hidden Food Allergies.* Jackson, TN: Professional Books, 1978.

Dadd, Debra Lynn. *The Non-Toxic Home.* Los Angeles: Jeremy P. Tarcher, 1985.

David, Marc. *Nourishing Wisdom.* New York: Harmony Books, 1991.

Feingold, B. F. *Why Your Child Is Hyperactive.* New York:Random House, 1975.

Friends in Recovery. *The Twelve Steps–A Spiritual Journey.* San Diego, CA: Recovery Publications, 1988.

Gregory, Scott, *A Holistic Protocol for the Immune System: HIV/ARC/AIDS, Candidiasis, Epstein Barr, Herpes, and Other Opportunistic Infections.* Joshua Tree, CA: Tree of Life, 1992.

Griffin, La Dean. *Is Any Sick Among You?* Provo, UT: Bi-World Publishers, 1976.

Hunt, Douglas. *No More Cravings.* New York: Warner Books, 1988.

Hunter, Linda M. *The Healthy Home.* New York: Pocket Books, 1990.

Katherine, Anne. *Anatomy of a Food Addiction.* New York: Prentice Hall, 1991.

Kidd, Parris M. and Wolfgang Huber. *Living With the AIDS Virus: A Strategy for Long Term Survival.* Berkeley, CA: HK-Biomedical, 1991.

Levine, Stephen and Parris Kidd. *Antioxidant Adaptation and Its Role in Free Radical Pathology.* San Leandro, CA: Bio Currents Division, Allergy Research Group, l985.

Mandell, Marshall and Lynne Walker Scanlon. *Dr. Mandell's 5-Day Allergy Relief System.* New York: Pocket Books, 1980.

Milam, James R. and Katherine Ketcham. *Under the Influence.* Seattle, WA: Madrona Publishers, 1981.

Orenstein, Neil S. and Sarah Bingham. *Food Allergies: How to Tell If You Have Them, What To Do About Them If You Do.* New York: Putnam Books, 1987.

Oski, Frank A. *Don't Drink the Milk.* Brushton, NY: TEACH Services, 1983.

Peck, M. Scott. *The Road Less Traveled.* New York: Simon & Schuster, 1978.

Randolph, Theron and Ralph W. Moss. *An Alternative Approach to Allergies.* New York: Bantam Books, 1980.

Randolph, Theron. *Human Ecology and Susceptibility to the Chemical Environment.* Springfield, IL: Charles C. Thomas Publishers, 1972.

Randolph, Theron, H. J. Rinkel and M. Zeller. *Food Allergy.* Norwork, CT: New England Foundation of Allergic and Environmental Diseases, 1951.

Rapp, Doris. *Allergies and the Hyperactive Child.* New York: Simon and Schuster, 1979.

Reno (Gunner), Elizabeth. "The Hidden Epidemic–Candida Albicans." *The Nutrition and Dietary Consultant,* September 1989.

———"Correlation Between Alcoholism and Eating Disorders." *The Nutrition and Dietary Consultant,* July 1991.

———"Eating Disorders and Food Addictions." *The Nutrition and Dietary Consultant,* February 1992.

———"Nutrition and Alcoholism." *The Nutrition and Dietary Consultant,* February 1988.

———"Alcoholism and Nutrition." *The Nutrition and Dietary Consultant,* March 1988.

Rousseau, Daniel and W. J. Rea et al. *Your Home, Your Health and Well-Being.* Berkeley, CA: Ten Speed Press, 1989.

Smith, Lendon H. *Improving Your Child's Behavior Chemistry.* New York: Simon and Schuster, 1977.

Staff, J. and C. R. Pellergrine. *Chronic Fatigue Syndrome–The Hidden Epidemic.* New York: HarperCollins, 1988.

Weissman, Joseph D. *Choose to Live.* New York: Penguin Books, 1988.

Williams, Roger J. *The Prevention of Alcoholism Through Nutrition.* New York: Bantam Books, 1981.

Part II: The Healthy Diet and Tools for Change

Alletess Medical Laboratories. *A Guide to Processed Foods.* Rockland, MA: Alletess Medical Laboratories, 1990.

Berger, Stuart M. *Dr. Berger's Immune Power Diet.* New York: New American Living Library, 1985.

Berthold-Bond, Annie. *Clean and Green.* Woodstock, NY: Ceres Press, 1990.

Braly, James. *Dr. Braly's Food Allergy and Nutrition Revolution.* New Canaan, CT: Keats Publishing, 1992.

Brody, Jane E. *Jane Brody's Nutrition Book.* New York: W. W. Norton, 1990.

Cousens, Gabriel. *Conscious Eating.* Santa Rosa, CA: Vision Books International, 1992.

Dunne, Lavon J. *Nutrition Almanac, Third Edition.* New York: McGraw-Hill Publishing, 1990.

Elkington, John et al. *The Green Consumer.* New York: Penguin Books, 1990.

Goodman, Robert. *A Quick Guide to Food Additives.* San Diego, CA: Silvercat Publications, 1989.

Haas, Elson M. *Staying Healthy With Nutrition.* Berkeley, CA: Celestial Arts, 1992.

Jacobson, Michael F. *Safe Food.* Venice, CA: Living Planet Press, 1991.

Lappe, Frances Moore. *Diet for A Small Planet.* New York: Ballantine Books, 1975.

Nelson, Dennis. *Food Combining Simplified.* Santa Cruz, CA: Nelson Books, 1983.

Oski, Frank A. *Don't Drink the Milk.* Brushton, NY: TEACH Services, 1983.

Ornish, Dean. *Dr. Dean Ornish's Program for Reversing Heart Disease.* New York: Random House, 1990.

Schwartz, George R. *In Bad Taste–The MSG Syndrome.* Santa Fe, NM: Health Press, 1988.

Shelton, Herbert M. *Food Combining Made Easy.* San Antonio, TX: Willow Publishing, 1982.

Part III: Food and Recipes

Allen, Francine. *Eating Well in A Busy World.* Berkeley, CA: Ten Speed Press, 1986.

Ball Corporation. *Ball Canning Information.* (Obtain from PO Box 2729, Muncie, IN, 47307)

Birnker, Katherine. *Breaking the Sugar Habit Cookbook.* San Antonio, TX: Panic Stress Therapy Center, 1989.

Balch, James F. and Phyllis A. Balch. *Prescription for Cooking and Dietary Wellness.* Greenfield, IN: PAB Books, 1992.

Brody, Jane. *Jane Brody's Good Food Gourmet.* New York: Bantam Books, 1987.

Bumganer, Marlene A. *The Book of Whole Grains.* New York: St. Martin's Press, 1976.

Burton, Gail. *The Candida Control Cookbook.* New York: Penguin Books, 1989.

Cosper, Nancy. *You Can Can With Honey.* Eugene, OR: Sahalie Publishing, 1986.

Diamond, Marilyn. *American Vegetarian Cookbook from Fit For Life Kitchen.* New York: Warner Books, 1990.

Ferre, Julia. *Basic Macrobiotic Cooking.* Oreville, CA: George Oksawa Macrobiotic Foundation, 1987.

Greenberg, Ron and Angela Nori. *Freedom From Allergy Cookbook.* Vancover, Canada: Blue Poppy Press, 1990.

Gewanter, Vera and Dorothy Parker. *Home Preserving Made Easy.* New York: Viking Press, 1975.

Gourmet Distributing. *The Gourmet Cookbook Vol. I & II.* New York, Gourmet Distributing Corporation, 1965.

Haas, Elson M. *A Diet for All Seasons.* Berkeley, CA: Celestial Arts, 1995.

Hooker, Allan. *The Vegetarian Gourmet.* San Francisco, CA: 101 Productions, 1970

Katzen, Mollie. *The Enchanted Broccoli Forest.* Berkeley, CA: Ten Speed Press, 1982.

Kerr Canning. *Kerr Canning Book.* Sands Springs,OK: Kerr Canning Corporation, 1983.

Kulvinskas, Viktoras P. *Sprout for the Love of Everybody.* Wethersfield, CT: Omango D' Press, 1978.

MacRae, Norma M. *Canning and Preserving Without Sugar.* Seattle, WA: Pacific Search Press, 1982.

Madison, Deborah. *The Greens Cookbook.* New York: Bantam Books, 1987.

Madison, Deborah. *The Savory Way.* New York: Bantam Books, 1990.

Montagne, Prosper and editor Charlotte Turgeon. *Laurousse Gastronomique.* New York: Crown Publishers, 1961.

Newman, Laura. *Make Your Juicer Your Drugstore.* New York: Benedict Lust Publications, 1970.

Ortho Book Series. *12 Months Harvest.* San Francisco, CA: Ortho Books, 1975.

Pickarski, Brother Ron. *Friendly Foods.* Berkeley, CA: Ten Speed Press, 1991.

Pickarski, Ron. *Eco Cuisine.* Berkeley, CA: Ten Speed Press, 1995.

Robertson, Laurel. *New Laurel's Kitchen.* Berkeley, CA:Ten Speed Press, 1986.

Saltzman, Joanne. *Amazing Grains.* Tiburon, CA: H. J. Kramer, 1990.

Shattuck, Ruth R. *The Allergy Cookbook.* New York: New American Library, 1984.

Stoner, Carol H. *Stocking Up by the staff of Organic Gardening and Farming.* Emmaus, PA: Rodale Press, 1977.

Turner, Kristine. *Self-Healing Cookbook.* Vashon Island, WA: Earthtones Press, 1989.

Walker, N. W. *Raw Vegetable Juices.* New York: Pyramid Books, 1970.

❦ Bibliography

Allen, Francine. *Eating Well In A Busy World.* Berkeley, CA: Ten Speed Press, 1986.

Angier, Natalia. "Vitamins Win Support as Potent Agents of Health." *The New York Times,* 10 March 1992.

Bagley, Robert T. "Alcoholism, A Reflection of Adaptive Failure." *Journal of Orthomolecular Medicine,* Volume 2, Number 2, 1987.

Balch, James F. and Phyllis A. Balch. *Prescription for Nutritional Healing.* Garden City, NY: Avery Publishing Group, 1990.

Beard, James. *The James Beard Cookbook.* New York: Dell Publishing, 1959.

Berger, Stuart. "How I Lost 20 Pounds." *Parade Magazine,* 31 March 1985.

Bland, Jeffrey. *Medical Applications of Clinical Nutrition.* New Caanan, CT: Keats Publishing, 1983.

_____. *Your Health Under Siege: Using Nutrition to Fight Back.* Brattleboro, VT: Stephen Green Press, 1982.

Braly, James. *Dr. Braly's Food Allergy and Nutrition Revolution.* New Canaan, CT: Keats Publishing, 1992.

Bowerman, W. Maurice. "Milk and Thought Disorder." *Journal of Orthomolecular Psychiatry,* Volume 9, Number 4, 1990.

Bralley, J. Alexander and Richard S. Lord. *Treatment of CFS with Specific Amino Acid Supplementation.* Atlanta, GA: The Center for Continuing Education, The University of Georgia and North American Nutrition and Preventive Medicine Association, 1991.

Brighthope, Ian. "AIDS–Remissions by Using Nutrient Therapies and Megadose Intravenous Ascorbate." *International Clinical Nutrition Review,* Volume 7, Number 2, April 1987.

Bryce-Smith, D. and R.D. Simpson. "Zinc Supplementation in Anorexia Nervosa." *International Clinical Nutrition Review,* Volume 5, Number 2, April 1985.

Buist, Robert A. "Nutritional Supplementation for AIDS Victims and Those With High Risk." *International Clinical Nutrition Review,* Volume 5, Number 4, October 1985.

_____. "Food Intolerance—A Growing Phenomenon: Current Concepts in Development, Manifestation and Treatment." *International Clinical Nutrition Review,* Volume 6, Number 1, January, 1986.

_____. *Food Chemical Sensitivity.* Garden City, NY: Avery Publishing Group, 1988.

_____. "Anxiety Neurosis—The Lactate Connection." *International Clinical Nutrition Review,* Volume 5, Number l, January 1985.

_____ and C.H. Campbell. "Alcoholic Lacticacidosis Resulting from Thiamine Deficiency." *International Clinical Nutrition Review,* Volume 5, Number 2, April 1985.

_____ and Orian C. Truss. "Production of Acetaldehyde by Candida Albicans and Its Toxic Effects." *International Clinical Nutrition Review,* Volume 5, Number 2, April 1985.

Burton, Gail. *The Candida Control Cookbook.* Markham, Ontario: New American Library, 1989.

Chaltin, Luc. "Is AIDS an Autoimmune Disease?" *Similia Newsletter,* Volume 1, Number 2, January-February 1992.

Chandra, Robert K. and V. K. Jain. "Does Nutritional Deficiency Predispose to Acquired Immune Deficiency Syndrome?" *Nutrition Research,* June 4, 1984.

Cordray, Priscilla. "Focus on the Immune System." *Nutrition and Dietary Consultant,* November 1988.

Crook, William G. *The Yeast Connection: A Medical Breakthrough, Revised Edition.* New York: Vintage Books, 1986.

Dadd, Debra Lynn. *Nontoxic, Natural and Earthwise.* Los Angeles, CA: Jeremy Tarcher, 1990.

Diamond, Marilyn. *The American Vegetarian Cookbook—From The Fit For Life Kitchen.* New York: Warner Books, 1990.

Dinsmore, W. W., J. T. Alderdice, and D. McMaster, et al. "Zinc Absorption in Anorexia Nervosa." *The Lancet,* 1041-1042, 1985.

Doctor's Update. "Important Nutritional Factors for Improving Gastrointestinal Health." *Doctor's Update,* Second Quarter, 1991.

Dowling, Lynne. *Food Addiction as Crippling as Alcohol, Drugs: Father Joseph Martin's Story.* Boston, MA: 1985.

Durko, Irene, et al. "Antioxidant Enzyme Levels in Red Blood Cells of Chronic Alcoholic Men Patients During Oral Niacin Therapy." *Journal of Orthomolecular Medicine,* Volume 5, Number 4, 1990.

Frater, Marijke. "What is the Immune System?" *Doctor's Report,* Winter 91/92.

Gerrard, J. "Food Intolerance and Chronic Disorders." *International Clinical Nutrition Review,* Volume 5, Number 2, April 1985.

Goodman, Robert. *A Quick Guide to Additives.* San Diego, CA: Silvercat Publications, 1989.

Gottlieb, Bob. "Food Addiction: Hooked on Unhappiness." *Prevention Magazine,* June 1979.

Goulart, Frances Sheridan. "How Toxic Is Your Home?" *Nutrition and Dietary Consultant,* April 1987.

_____. "Radon: Protection Against It." *Nutrition and Dietary Consultant,* December 1986.

Greenberg, Ron and Angela Nori. *Freedom From Allergy Cookbook.* Vancouver, BC: Blue Poppy Press, 1985.

Gunner, Elizabeth. "Candida Albicans—The Hidden Epidemic." *Nutrition and Dietary Consultant,* September 1989.

_____. "Alcoholism and Nutrition—Biochemistry of Alcohol." *Nutrition and Dietary Consultant,* February 1988.

_____. "Alcoholism and Nutrition—Physiology of Alcohol." *Nutrition and Dietary Consultant,* March 1988.

Guyton, Arthur C. *Textbook of Medical Physiology.* Philadelphia, PA: W. B. Saunders Co., 1971.

Harvey, Daniel. "Cow's Milk, Diabetes Linked." *Santa Rosa Press Democrat,* July 30, 1992.

Hills, Sandra. "The Immune System." *Nutrition and Dietary Consultant,* April 1987.

Hooker, Alan. *Vegetarian Gourmet Cookery.* San Francisco, CA: 101 Productions, 1970.

Jaffe, Russell. "Clinical and Laboratory Suggestions for CFS." *International Clinical Nutrition Review.* Volume 11, Number 2, April 1991.

Jaroff, Leon. "Allergies–Nothing To Sneeze At." *Time Magazine,* 22 June 1992.

Kaslow, J.E., L. Rucker, and R. Onishi. "CFS: More Recognition But Still No Cure." International Clinical Nutrition Review, Volume 10, Number 3, July 1990.

Kidd, Parris. *Nutrition as Medicine: Containment of HIV-1 and Other Chronic Viruses.* Atlanta, GA: The Center for Continuing Education, The University of Georgia and North American Nutrition and Preventive Medicine Association, 1991.

_____ and Wolfgang Huber. "Egg Lipids (Phospholipids) as Therapies in AIDS Senescence and Other Membrane-Related Syndromes." *International Clinical Nutrition Review,* Volume 10, Number 1, January 1990.

Krohn, Jacqueline. *The Whole Way to Allergy Relief and Prevention.* Vancouver, BC: Hartley and Marks, 1991.

Levine, Stephen A. and Michael Hefferman. "Allergy Update." *Nutrition News,* 1992.

_____ and Parris Kidd. "Biochemical Pathologies Initiated by Free Radical Oxidant Compounds in the Aetiology of Food Hypersensitivity Disease." *International Clinical Nutrition Review,* Volume 5, Number 1, January, 1985.

_____ and Jay Parker. "Selenium and Human Chemical Hypersensitivity: Preliminary Findings." *International Journal of Biosocial Research,* Volume 3, Number 1, 1982.

_____ and Jeffrey H. Reinhardt. "Biochemical Pathology Initiated by Free Radicals, Oxidant Chemicals, and Therapeutic Drugs in the Etiology of Chemical Hypersensitivity Disease." *Journal of Orthomolecular Psychiatry,* Volume 12, Number 3, 1983.

_____. "Oxidants/Anti-oxidants and Chemical Hypersensitivities (Part One)." *International Journal of Biosocial Research,* Volume 4, Number 1, 1983.

_____. "Oxidants/Anti-oxidants and Chemical Hypersensitivities (Part Two)." *International Journal of Biosocial Research,* Volume 4, Number 2, 1983.

_____. *Food Addiction, Food Allergy and Overweight.* San Leandro, CA: Allergy Research Group, 1982.

_____. *More About Allergy and Addiction.* San Leandro, CA: Allergy Research Group, 1984.

MacPhail, David. "New Insights into Chemical Hypersensitivity." *Environmental Allergy Society Newsletter,* 1992.

Madison, Deborah. *The Greens Cookbook.* New York: Bantam Books, 1987.

_____. *The Savory Way.* New York: Bantam Books, 1990.

Mandell, Marshall and Lynne Waller Scanlon. *5-Day Allergy Relief System.* New York: Pocket Books, 1980.

McCabeb, Rob. "Enchinacea for the Immune System." *Doctor's Update,* September 1991.

Milam, James R. and Katherine Ketcham. *Under the Influence.* Seattle, WA: Madrona Publishers, 1981.

Naples Research and Counseling Center. *Mini-Guide to Food Addiction.* Naples, FL: Naples Research and Counseling Center, 1984.

Norwood, Robin. *Women Who Love Too Much.* New York: Pocket Books, 1986.

Nusbaum, Margaret. "Food for Thought: The Problem Anorexia Nervosa and Bulimia." *Journal of Orthomolecular Medicine,* Volume 1, Number 4, August, 1986.

Orbach, Susie. *Hunger Strike: The Anorexic's Struggle as a Metaphor for Our Age.* New York: W. W. Norton, 1986.

Oski, Frank A. *Don't Drink the Milk.* Brushton, NY: TEACH Services, 1983.

Pfeiffer, Carl C. *Mental and Elemental Nutrients.* New Canaan, CN: Keats Publishing, 1975.

Poulos, C. Jean. "Anorexia Nervosa." *Nutrition and Dietary Consultant,* November 1986.

_____. "Bulimia." *Nutrition and Dietary Consultant,* February 1987.

Raeburn, Paul. "Pistachio Ice Cream Neurotransmitter." *American Health,* December 1987.

Randolph, Theron. *An Alternative Approach to Allergies.* New York: Bantam Books, 1981.

_____. *Human Ecology and Susceptibility to the Chemical Environment.* Springfield, IL: Charles C. Thomas Publisher, 1981.

Rogers, Sherry A. "Zinc Deficiency as Model for Developing Chemical Sensitivity." *International Clinical Nutrition Review,* Volume 10, Number 1, January 1990.

_____. *The Environmental Illness Syndrome.* Syracuse, NY: Prestige Publishers, 1986.

Sampson, H.A. and P.L. Jolie. "Plasma Histamine and Food Allergy Detection." *International Clinical Nutrition Review,* Volume 5, Number 2, April, 1985.

Schnert, Keith. "That Amazing Immune System." *Nutrition and Dietary Consultant,* September 1990.

Schwartz, George R. *In Bad Taste–The MSG Syndrome.* Santa Fe, NM: Health Press, 1988.

Simon, Balkan and Akar N. Derlet Hastares. "Evidence for Zinc Deficiency in Anorexia Nervosa." *International Clinical Nutrition Review,* Volume 5, Number 3, July 1985.

Smith, Lendon H. *Improving Your Child's Behavior Chemistry.* New York: Simon and Schuster, 1977.

Task Force of Nutrition Support in AIDS. "An Overview of Nutrition Support in AIDS." *Nutrition and Dietary Consultant,* August 1989.

Tortora, Gerard J. *Principles of Human Anatomy, Second Edition.* New York: Harper and Row, 1980.

Toth, Jennifer N. "Crack Cocaine Lures Overweight Women to Drugs." *Press Democrat,* August 6, 1990.

Truss, Orian. "Production of Acetaldehyde by Candida Albicans and Its Toxic Effects." *International Clinical Nutrition Review,* Volume 5, Number 2, April 1985.

Updike, Earl F. *The Mormon Diet.* Orem, UT: CFI, 1991.

_____. *A Word of Wisdom.* Orem, UT: CFI, 1991.

_____. *14 Days to New Vigor and Health.* Orem, UT: CFI, 1991.

_____. *Best Possible Health.* Orem, UT: CFI, 1991.

Wellness Staff. "Can A Building Really Make You Sick?" *University of California at Berkeley Wellness Letter.* Volume 7, Issue 10, July 1991.

Whitney, Hamilton. *Understanding Nutrition.* New York: West Publishers, 1981.

Williams, Roger J. and Dwight K. Kalita. *A Physician's Handbook on Orthomolecular Medicine.* New Caanan, CT: Keats Publishing, 1979.

_____. *Prevention of Alcoholism Through Nutrition.* New York: Bantam, 1986.

Wright, Jonathan V. *Dr. Wright's Guide to Healing with Nutrition.* Eramus, PA: Rodale Press, 1984.

🦋 Index to Recipes

✖ Index